Antibiotic Resistance: A One-Health Approach

Antibiotic Resistance: A One-Health Approach

Editor

Piera Anna Martino

MDPI • Basel • Beijing • Wuhan • Barcelona • Belgrade • Manchester • Tokyo • Cluj • Tianjin

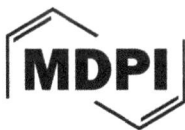

Editor
Piera Anna Martino
Biomedical, Surgical and
Dental Sciences
Università degli Studi
di Milano
Milan
Italy

Editorial Office
MDPI
St. Alban-Anlage 66
4052 Basel, Switzerland

This is a reprint of articles from the Special Issue published online in the open access journal *Antibiotics* (ISSN 2079-6382) (available at: www.mdpi.com/journal/antibiotics/special_issues/ Antibiotic_Health).

For citation purposes, cite each article independently as indicated on the article page online and as indicated below:

LastName, A.A.; LastName, B.B.; LastName, C.C. Article Title. *Journal Name* **Year**, *Volume Number*, Page Range.

ISBN 978-3-0365-6032-8 (Hbk)
ISBN 978-3-0365-6031-1 (PDF)

© 2023 by the authors. Articles in this book are Open Access and distributed under the Creative Commons Attribution (CC BY) license, which allows users to download, copy and build upon published articles, as long as the author and publisher are properly credited, which ensures maximum dissemination and a wider impact of our publications.

The book as a whole is distributed by MDPI under the terms and conditions of the Creative Commons license CC BY-NC-ND.

Contents

About the Editor vii

Preface to "Antibiotic Resistance: A One-Health Approach" ix

Lauren L. Wind, Jonathan S. Briganti, Anne M. Brown, Timothy P. Neher, Meghan F. Davis and Lisa M. Durso et al.
Finding What Is Inaccessible: Antimicrobial Resistance Language Use among the One Health Domains
Reprinted from: *Antibiotics* **2021**, *10*, 385, doi:10.3390/antibiotics10040385 1

Smitha Gudipati, Marcus Zervos and Erica Herc
Can the One Health Approach Save Us from the Emergence and Reemergence of Infectious Pathogens in the Era of Climate Change: Implications for Antimicrobial Resistance?
Reprinted from: *Antibiotics* **2020**, *9*, 599, doi:10.3390/antibiotics9090599 19

Mohamed Rhouma, Michelle Tessier, Cécile Aenishaenslin, Pascal Sanders and Hélène Carabin
Should the Increased Awareness of the One Health Approach Brought by the COVID-19 Pandemic Be Used to Further Tackle the Challenge of Antimicrobial Resistance?
Reprinted from: *Antibiotics* **2021**, *10*, 464, doi:10.3390/antibiotics10040464 27

Ingeborg Björkman, Marta Röing, Jaran Eriksen and Cecilia Stålsby Lundborg
Swedish Efforts to Contain Antibiotic Resistance in the Environment—A Qualitative Study among Selected Stakeholders
Reprinted from: *Antibiotics* **2022**, *11*, 646, doi:10.3390/antibiotics11050646 35

Steward Mudenda, Sydney Malama, Musso Munyeme, Bernard Mudenda Hang'ombe, Geoffrey Mainda and Otridah Kapona et al.
Awareness of Antimicrobial Resistance and Associated Factors among Layer Poultry Farmers in Zambia: Implications for Surveillance and Antimicrobial Stewardship Programs
Reprinted from: *Antibiotics* **2022**, *11*, 383, doi:10.3390/antibiotics11030383 51

Said Abukhattab, Haneen Taweel, Arein Awad, Lisa Crump, Pascale Vonaesch and Jakob Zinsstag et al.
Systematic Review and Meta-Analysis of Integrated Studies on Salmonella and Campylobacter Prevalence, Serovar, and Phenotyping and Genetic of Antimicrobial Resistance in the Middle East—A One Health Perspective
Reprinted from: *Antibiotics* **2022**, *11*, 536, doi:10.3390/antibiotics11050536 63

Patrick Butaye, Iona Halliday-Simmonds and Astrid Van Sauers
Salmonella in Pig Farms and on Pig Meat in Suriname
Reprinted from: *Antibiotics* **2021**, *10*, 1495, doi:10.3390/antibiotics10121495 81

Joanna Pławińska-Czarnak, Karolina Wódz, Magdalena Kizerwetter-Świda, Janusz Bogdan, Piotr Kwieciński and Tomasz Nowak et al.
Multi-Drug Resistance to *Salmonella* spp. When Isolated from Raw Meat Products
Reprinted from: *Antibiotics* **2022**, *11*, 876, doi:10.3390/antibiotics11070876 89

Julio A. Benavides, Marília Salgado-Caxito, Andrés Opazo-Capurro, Paulina González Muñoz, Ana Piñeiro and Macarena Otto Medina et al.
ESBL-Producing *Escherichia coli* Carrying CTX-M Genes Circulating among Livestock, Dogs, and Wild Mammals in Small-Scale Farms of Central Chile
Reprinted from: *Antibiotics* **2021**, *10*, 510, doi:10.3390/antibiotics10050510 103

Zoi Athanasakopoulou, Katerina Tsilipounidaki, Marina Sofia, Dimitris C. Chatzopoulos, Alexios Giannakopoulos and Ioannis Karakousis et al.
Poultry and Wild Birds as a Reservoir of CMY-2 Producing *Escherichia coli*: The First Large-Scale Study in Greece
Reprinted from: *Antibiotics* **2021**, *10*, 235, doi:10.3390/antibiotics10030235 117

Yusuf Wada, Azian Binti Harun, Chan Yean Yean and Abdul Rahman Zaidah
Vancomycin-Resistant Enterococci (VRE) in Nigeria: The First Systematic Review and Meta-Analysis
Reprinted from: *Antibiotics* **2020**, *9*, 565, doi:10.3390/antibiotics9090565 129

Anna-Rita Attili, Alessandro Bellato, Patrizia Robino, Livio Galosi, Cristiano Papeschi and Giacomo Rossi et al.
Analysis of the Antibiotic Resistance Profiles in Methicillin-Sensitive *S. aureus* Pathotypes Isolated on a Commercial Rabbit Farm in Italy
Reprinted from: *Antibiotics* **2020**, *9*, 673, doi:10.3390/antibiotics9100673 145

About the Editor

Piera Anna Martino

Piera Anna Martino is Associate Professor at One Health Unit, Dept. of Biomedical, Surgical and Dental Sciences, Università degli Studi di MIlano.

From 1991 Doctor in Biological Sciences, Università degli Studi di Milano, Italy.

From 1992 Licence to practice (Biological Sciences).

From 1999 PhD in "Zootechnical Sciences", Università degli Studi di Milano, Italy.

From 2002 Specialist in "Laboratory Animals Sciences", Università degli Studi di Milano, Italy.

Research interests: Bacteriology and mycology, in all aspects (theoretical, pratical-applicatory and comparative), in pets, domestic and exotic animals; Research and teaching interests lie in the fields of clinical and diagnostic microbiology, particularly new diagnostic technologies, emerging veterinary pathogens, and antimicrobial resistance; Antimicrobial resistence evaluation and discovery of antimicrobial activities of novel molecules; Transmissible spongiform encephalopathies (TSE) in their pathogenetic, diagnostic, prophylactic and therapeutic aspects.

Preface to "Antibiotic Resistance: A One-Health Approach"

Antimicrobial resistance and emergent multi-drug resistance consitute a multifaceted and critical global problem, considered one of the most urgent challenges that needs to be solved. The use of antibiotics forces selective pressure on pathogens and also on commensal microorganisms, favoring the emergence of resistant strains. For years, farms and intensive breeding systems, together with the increasing spread of food-borne diseases, were seen as the unique sources of this global problem. The One Health concept focuses on issues at the human, animal (both domestic and wildlife), and environmental levels. This concept is not old and highlights the connection between human, animal, and environmental health in a rapidly changing world. Human and Veterinary medicine must work together to control antimicrobial resistance. The One Health approach offers a crucial part of the solution. The development of new antibiotics is known to be time-consuming, but new alternative therapies are ongoing among the scientific community and can be though as the new promising protagonists in this panorama. The "full-length genome sequencing" and the molecular revolution based on high-throughput platforms will describe new molecular targets as candidates for more precise pharmacological therapies, providing in-depth knowledge about pivotal bacterial molecular pathways.

This Special Issue promotes our understanding of antimicrobial resistance in both Human and Veterinary medicine, in a harmonized One Health approach; the description of antimicrobial resistance profile and the development of novel therapies have an high impact on the scientific world.

Piera Anna Martino
Editor

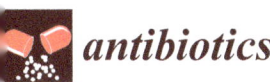

Article

Finding What Is Inaccessible: Antimicrobial Resistance Language Use among the One Health Domains

Lauren L. Wind [1,*], Jonathan S. Briganti [2], Anne M. Brown [2], Timothy P. Neher [3], Meghan F. Davis [4], Lisa M. Durso [5], Tanner Spicer [2] and Stephanie Lansing [6]

1. Department of Biological Systems Engineering, Virginia Tech, Blacksburg, VA 24060, USA
2. University Libraries, Virginia Tech, Blacksburg, VA 24060, USA; jonbrig@vt.edu (J.S.B.); ambrown7@vt.edu (A.M.B.); tanner9@vt.edu (T.S.)
3. Department of Agricultural and Biosystems Engineering, Iowa State University, Ames, IA 50011, USA; tpneher@iastate.edu
4. Johns Hopkins Bloomberg School of Public Health, Baltimore, MD 21205, USA; mdavis65@jhu.edu
5. USDA-ARS, Lincoln, NE 68583, USA; lisa.durso@usda.gov
6. Department of Environmental Science and Technology, University of Maryland, College Park, MD 20742, USA; slansing@umd.edu
* Correspondence: wlauren@vt.edu

Abstract: The success of a One Health approach to combating antimicrobial resistance (AMR) requires effective data sharing across the three One Health domains (human, animal, and environment). To investigate if there are differences in language use across the One Health domains, we examined the peer-reviewed literature using a combination of text data mining and natural language processing techniques on 20,000 open-access articles related to AMR and One Health. Evaluating AMR key term frequency from the European PubMed Collection published between 1990 and 2019 showed distinct AMR language usage within each domain and incongruent language usage across domains, with significant differences in key term usage frequencies when articles were grouped by the One Health sub-specialties (2-way ANOVA; $p < 0.001$). Over the 29-year period, "antibiotic resistance" and "AR" were used 18 times more than "antimicrobial resistance" and "AMR". The discord of language use across One Health potentially weakens the effectiveness of interdisciplinary research by creating accessibility issues for researchers using search engines. This research was the first to quantify this disparate language use within One Health, which inhibits collaboration and crosstalk between domains. We suggest the following for authors publishing AMR-related research within the One Health context: (1) increase title/abstract searchability by including both antimicrobial and antibiotic resistance related search terms; (2) include "One Health" in the title/abstract; and (3) prioritize open-access publication.

Keywords: one health; antimicrobial resistance; antibiotic resistance; human; animal; environment; text data mining; natural language processing; common language; AMR; AR

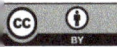

1. Introduction

Recently, global interdisciplinary efforts to treat infectious diseases and prolong the efficacy of antimicrobial drugs are starting to be conceptualized using the One Health model [1,2]; the collaborative and transdisciplinary approach to connect human, animal, and plant health to their environmental health [3]. Success of these efforts is often dependent on effective communication across the One Health disciplines at local, regional, national, and global scales; and among scientists, policy makers, and the public. Historically, human and animal health have been viewed and treated as two distinct disciplines [4], typically segregated among practitioners, policy makers, and academics despite acknowledgment of their linkages through 'One Medicine' [4]. However, the need to address emerging zoonotic diseases with an interdisciplinary approach has become increasingly evident. An interdisciplinary approach is especially needed and called for with the emergence and reemergence of pathogens and drug-resistant pathogens, such as Escherichia coli O157:H7, avian flu H5N1, swine flu H1N1 [5], and more recently with SARS–CoV–2 (COVID–19) [6]. Now called One Health, the concept integrates human, animal, and environmental health, including both natural sciences and human dimensions, in a single holistic approach to address public health concerns, including antimicrobial resistance (AMR) [2].

A One Health approach is key to addressing the complex, overlapping, and embedded subsets of problems associated with AMR [7]. The overwhelming success of antimicrobial drugs in treating infectious diseases during the last century contributed to their wide adoption in both human and veterinary medicine [8], and plant agriculture [9]. The same trend has been observed for anti-viral treatments, such as those used to treat AIDS, as well as antifungal and antiparasitic drugs [10–12]. The biological phenomenon of resistance was noted almost immediately following the discovery of antibiotics [13], and it is well established that the use of antimicrobial drugs, even prudent use, selects for microbial resistance to the drugs [14–16]. Complicating efforts to control drug resistant pathogenic microorganisms is the fact that the resistance mechanisms can also be found in non-pathogenic bacteria and pristine environments [7,17], and the genes coding for AMR often reside on mobile genetic elements with the potential to be shared [18]. The environment then becomes a source and a sink of antibiotic resistant bacteria (ARB) and antibiotic resistance genes (ARGs) that can have serious consequences for human and animal health.

As with any multi-disciplinary approach, the individual disciplines use similar vocabularies, but each may have different preferred terms or ascribe the same words with different meanings or connotations [19], leading to potential miscommunication and barriers to collaborative success [20]. For example, using the word "environment" in human medicine may be directly related to the operating room to which a patient is exposed [21]. Within environmental health disciplines, the word "environment" corresponds to the physical, chemical, and biological external factors that may impact behavior and overall health [22], while in environmental science disciplines, "environment" refers to components of nature that support life, including soil, water, and air [22]. Specific to AMR research, some disciplines within the One Health approach use "antimicrobial resistance," whereas others use "antibiotic resistance." Researchers may or may not state the distinctions between these two terms, which challenges interdisciplinary communication and collaboration.

One Health bridges a widespread cohort of disciplines, which include but are not limited to environmental health, ecology, veterinary medicine, public health, human medicine, microbiology, and health economics [23]. There is a general consensus that the key terms and practices used in each of the One Health disciplines will inherently be different [24]. A One Health evaluation was conducted at the University of Copenhagen Research Centre for Control of Antibiotic Resistance (UC–CARE) to analyze how researchers from fourteen departments over four years could come together to produce new knowledge to reduce AMR [25]. Léger et al. [25] found that most interviewees had increased awareness and general understanding of AMR from a One Health lens. However, the challenges of information sharing, collaboration, and methods hindered the productivity of producing novel AMR findings. Additionally, the problems that arose from communication, and/or lack thereof, were linked to the overarching issue that there was no common scientific language across disciplines [25]. This evaluation highlights that language disparity among One Health domains needs to be quantified to identify language gaps. Understanding these disparities will aid in creating consistency and a common language within the One Health framework to increase AMR communication, support productive discussions, and enhance knowledge transfer across disciplines. As stated by Mendelson et al. [24], "Antibiotic Resistance has a language problem."

The aim of the current study was to evaluate the variations in language usage among One Health researchers and their relevant disciplines (i.e., human, animal, environment).

Specifically, the following questions were addressed: (1) Are there dissimilarities in key term frequency usage within the AMR published literature across the One health domains; (2) Does AMR associated language usage increase at similar rates across the One Health domains from 1990–2019, and (3) Are the AMR language usage frequency trends similar in open-access articles compared to non-open-access articles in the One Health domain? Quantifying the scale of language disparities among the One Health domains will improve future searchability and accessibility to create a more inclusive and collaborative understanding, while continuing to promote interdisciplinarity within AMR research. This quantification using neutral and replicable methods necessitated bringing together an interdisciplinary group of scholars across the One Health domains and experts in text data mining (TDM) and natural language processing (NLP). The team performed an open-access search of all One Health and AMR relevant available publications in European PubMed Central (Europe PMC), and analyzed the results across the three One Health domains (human, animal, environment). This study is novel in its application of natural text parsing and large data analytics to the One Health domains which, to our knowledge, has not been attempted before this effort. By including experts across the One Heath domain with data scientists from project conception through data analysis, this team was able to show the impact of language use dissimilarities on effective communication and publication access across the One Health disciplines.

2. Results and Discussion

The TDM analysis of open access AMR publications confirmed that language continues to be a significant barrier to communication across the One Health domains. We found that when writing about antibiotic resistance, each of the four term bins (Human, Animal, Environment, and the combined bin of One Health) had its own common language (i.e., theme) that did not overlap with the other bins. Additionally, the majority of articles recovered in our search used the term "antibiotic resistance" instead of "antimicrobial resistance," regardless of the domain. We also identified temporal trends in language and acronym use from our investigation. The next sections summarize key findings in each of these areas and describe factors that may be important to consider for future research and language harmonization efforts within the One Health domains.

2.1. Language Use across the One Health Domains

There is broad support among national and international groups to adopt an interdisciplinary and One Health approach in efforts to address AMR [26], with calls for a review of AMR terminology across disciplines to facilitate a productive and coordinated global response [24]. Using TDM, we analyzed key term frequency within 20,000 representative AMR articles to determine consistent, and at times inconsistent, language use within articles categorized into four independent term bins (Human, Animal, Environmental, and One Health bins). As language use is key to interdisciplinary group dynamics, terminological imprecision can result in dissimilar vocabulary that presents a barrier to moving to the shared cognition required for strategic interdisciplinary problem solving [19,25,27–30], particularly as it relates to AMR [24]. We identified that when using a consistent search term string, the key term usage deviated amongst the individual domains, with search term clusters shown within each bin (Figure 1). Term frequency and usage becomes increasingly less consistent with articles containing terms from multiple domains. Articles that used human and animal terms in the title and abstract used the term 'human' 2x more and 'ecosystem' 11x less on average within the article body than articles with human and environment title and abstract terms. ContentMine identified search terms that were specific to each of the four bins. However, there was no distinct overlap in the language used across the One health domains. The limited overlap observed in the title and abstract key terms highlights the lack of shared language, and potentially shared cognition, among AMR researchers in different One Health domains (Figure 1).

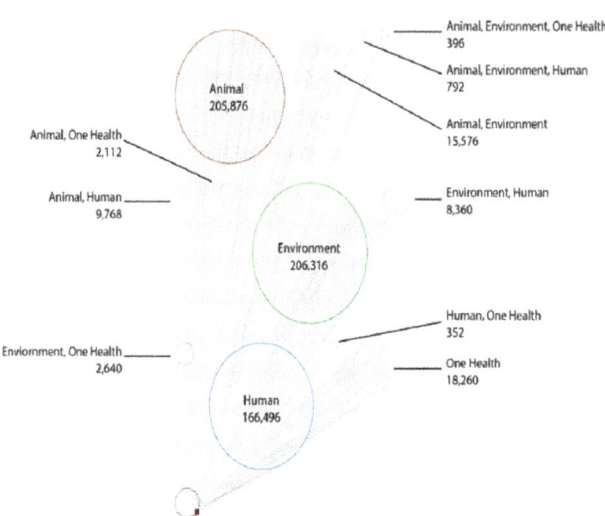

Figure 1. Network of the similar and/or dissimilar language usage among One Health groups. The Group Attributes Network Layout groups articles into bins and places each bin on the graph in relation to how similar the bins are to one another. Each bin represents different combinations of search terms found in the articles' titles and abstracts. For instance, the Human group are articles that exclusively used human-binned terms in their title or abstract. Larger groups (and group counts) indicate the number of articles within that group. Bins plotted closer together share similar patterns of term frequency and usage within the articles' body. The number within each circle indicate how many occurrences of those terms occurred in the articles (i.e., the terms in the human term bin occurred 166,496 times in the articles that exclusively used human terms in their title and abstracts).

These results highlight the information gap among fields. Open-access, peer-reviewed AMR research content largely focuses on a singular domain concept, with primarily superficial links between the disciplines, which others have noted [20,31]. The new findings from this current study on language use frequency also support this claim. It should be noted that this method of text processing is not encompassing of the totality of how NLP can be applied. This foundational work determined language trends and the methods of how new analyses types, such as NLP, can be applied to the One Health field. In order to overcome the language use barriers, we recommend the following: (1) researchers from specialized disciplines be trained to search for multiple search terms encompassing each One Health domain in title/abstract literature searches, and (2) researchers be trained to include multiple search terms encompassing all of the One Health domains in their title/abstracts when writing AMR focused papers.

2.2. Trends in "Antimicrobial Resistance" Language Use over Time

The raw number of peer-reviewed One Health-related AMR articles indexed in Europe PMC increased almost five-fold from 1990 (n = 33,362 articles) to 2019 (n = 165,516). Each One Health discipline or sub-discipline had different underlying assumptions and understandings of the terms "antibiotic resistance" and "antimicrobial resistance." In the representative 20,000 articles used for TDM analysis, the search term group for antibiotic resistance, consisting of "antibiotic resistance" and the known associated acronym ("AR") was used on average 18 times more often than the antimicrobial resistance term group consisting of "antimicrobial resistance" and its known acronym ("AMR") (Figure 2). However, since 2009, there has been a marginal, yet discernable, increase in other resistance related terms being used (i.e., multidrug resistance, one health, antimicrobial resistance) and a substantial decrease (26%) in the frequency of the antibiotic resistance term group

(Figure 2). This was unexpected, but the decrease in frequency use of "antibiotic resistance" and "AR" key terms suggests that authors may be narrowing their scope of AMR research to identify more closely with specific research objectives (e.g., limited to a single gene) rather than a broader scope discussing "antibiotic resistance" in general. Additionally, Krockow [32] argued that a new name is needed for AMR due to the inconsistent use of AMR in the literature, difficulty in pronunciation, and unclear meaning to lay audiences, but a new name was not suggested. Our analysis shows that the literature is already starting to move away from the more general AMR term to more specific terms within sub-fields in the One Health context.

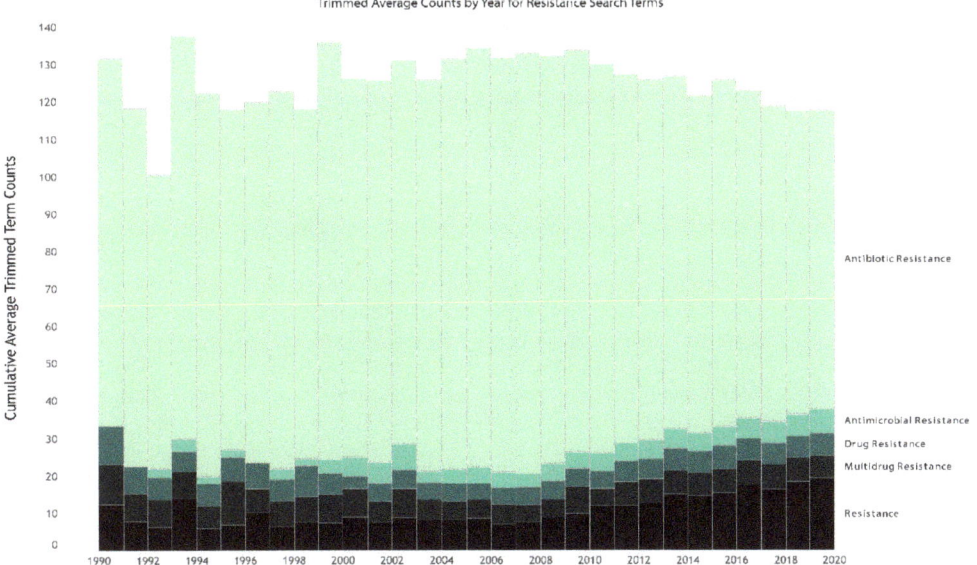

Figure 2. The average trimmed term counts of resistance-related search terms each year used per article. Trimmed search term counts, top and bottom 10%, were removed as assumed outliers.

2.3. Trends in Acronym Use over Time

We identified that acronyms (e.g., AMR) are used commonly in text rather than in the title/abstract title/abstract among the included articles. Researchers within the AMR One Health field have worked towards creating a common glossary of terms and acronyms related to "antibiotic resistance" [33–35]; however, the study results show there is still a lack of consensus on the meaning of many terms and disagreement, or inconsistency, in which term or acronym should be used when publishing in a One Health context. In addition to "AMR" and "AR", "MDR" is widely used for "multidrug resistance." We found fluctuations in the popularity of "AMR" vs. "MDR" vs. "AR" over time (Figure 2). The median frequency of "AR," "AMR," and "MDR" after TDM averaged 230.0, 9.5, and 13.5 average term counts for each article, respectively (Table S1). This supports the concept that the acronym usage remains consistent overtime (i.e., researchers are using "antibiotic resistance" and "AR"), but that subfields within each domain have seen increased popularity over time for other related resistance terms. Creating a common language will aid to bridge communication gaps between the domains. Potential solutions to language barriers include harmonization to a single term/abbreviation and/or training researchers to include both "AR" and "AMR" in title/abstract to increase searchability across domains.

2.4. Trends in Language Use among the One Health Domains

Over the twenty–nine year span studied in this work, there was an upward trend in the usage frequency of the term "One Health," indicating that more articles include the One Health concept in their studies or are using "One Health" within their AMR related research articles. Consistent with prior work [36], our analysis further indicates that Human-associated key terms were two times more likely to be used than environmental and animal associated key terms in articles addressing AMR (Figure 3A–D). In 2013, the Animal and Environmental-associated search terms began to increase, while the human-associated search term frequency began to decrease in all articles. It is unsurprising that the human associated search terms were more frequently being used at the beginning of this study period due to the larger focus on AMR research in human and clinical studies in the 1990s. Using TDM, we identified that the Animal, Environment, and One Health binned associated search terms began developing in the late 2000s and continued to increase in frequency over time. This trend correlates with broader adoption of the One Health concept and an increase in funding for animal and environmental AMR research, which began in the late 2000s and is ongoing with the creation of national and international One Health funding programs and initiatives, such as the Joint Programming Initiative on Antimicrobial Resistance, the US Center for Disease Control (CDC) AMR Fund, and the US Department of Agriculture's National Institute of Food and Agriculture (USDA-NIFA) AMR funding initiative [37–39]. Although Human-associated key terms were used more frequently in human grouped articles over the 29-year analysis period, there was no significant difference between the average usage frequency of key terms between Human, Animal, Environmental, and One Health binned articles (2-way ANOVA; $p = 0.482$; Table S2). However, when all overlapping domain (i.e., animal-human, human-environment, environment-animal, animal-environment, etc.) articles were considered, there were significant differences between key term usage frequency and binned domain (2-way ANOVA; $p < 0.001$; Table S2). This suggests that once articles are grouped by sub-specialties within each One Health domain, differences in common language use throughout the entire article can be identified.

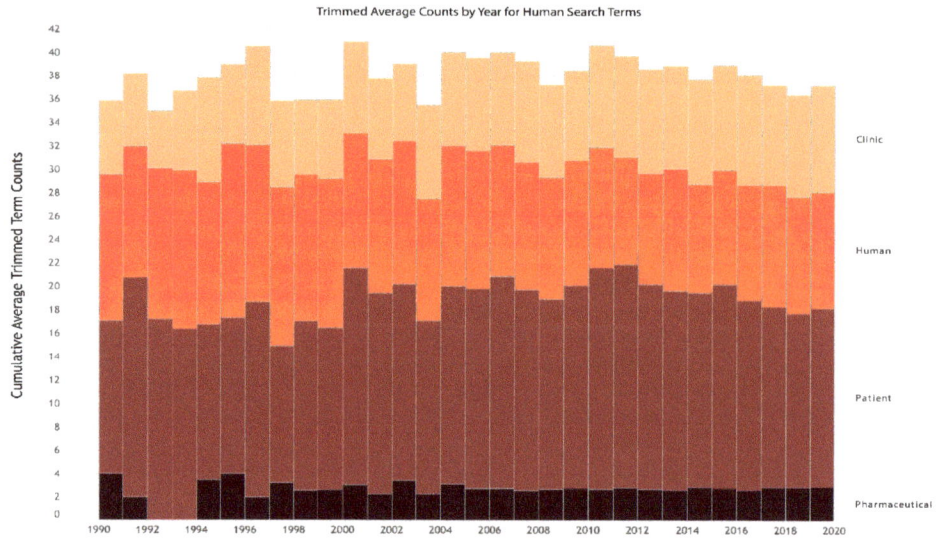

A.

Figure 3. *Cont.*

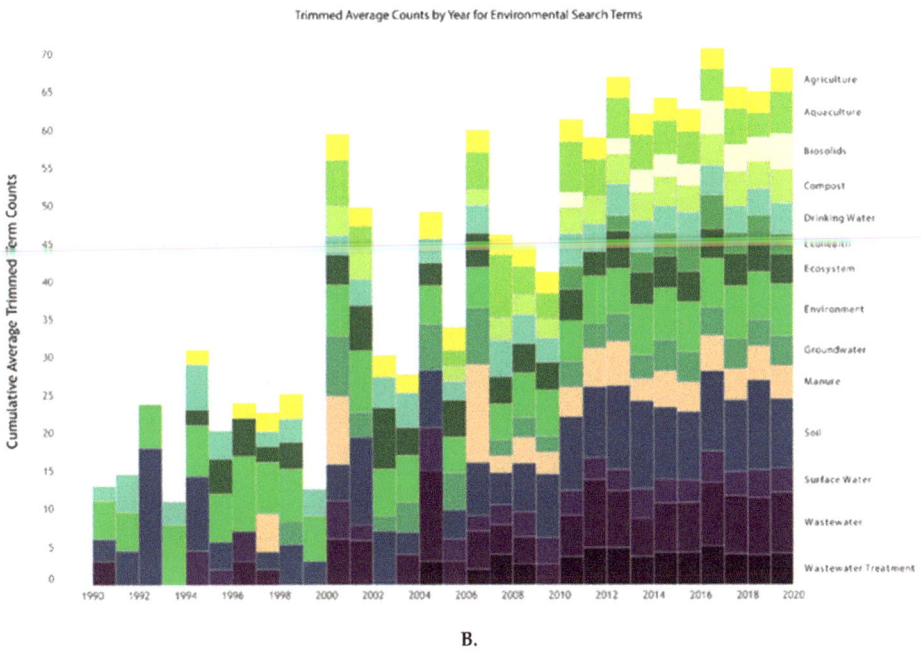

B.

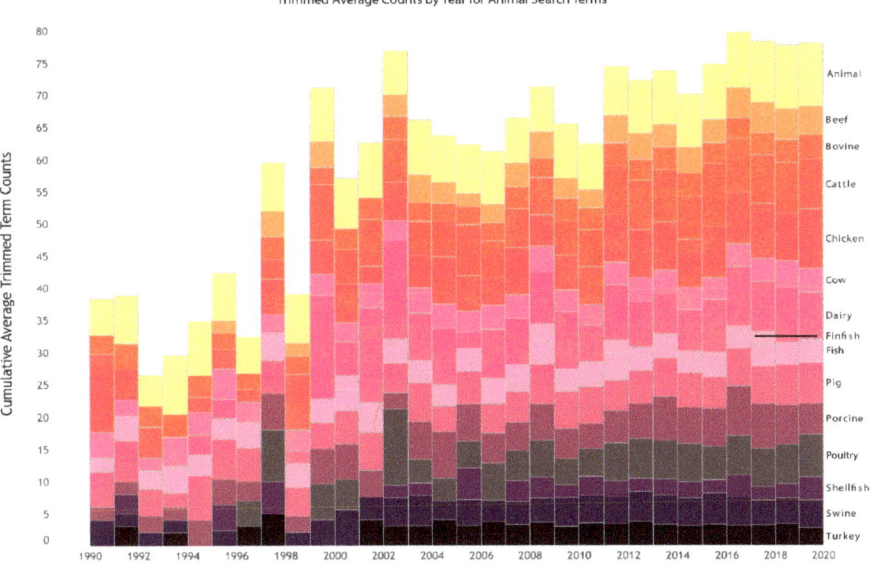

C.

Figure 3. *Cont.*

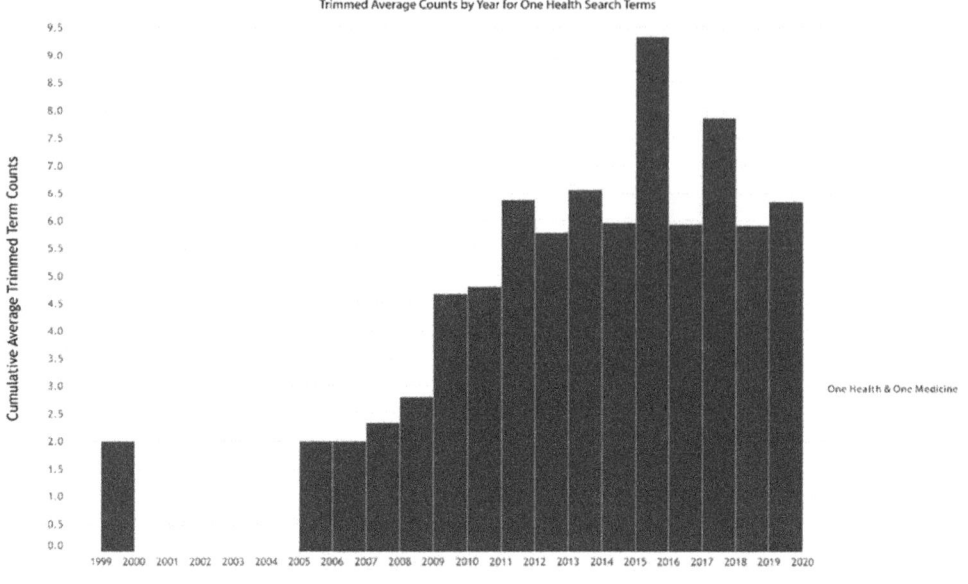

D.

Figure 3. The cumulative average trimmed (top and bottom 10 percentile omitted) term ounts from 1990 to 2019, binned by the One Health domains. Returned articles that contained search terms related to antimicrobial resistance in title and/or abstract are shown based on bins: (**A**) Human-associated, (**B**) Environmental-associated, (**C**) Animal-associated, and (**D**) One Health associated.

For each One Health domain, the most and least frequently used search terms from 1990–2019 ranged from 6.9–3.9 average trimmed counts within AMR related articles (Figure 4, Table S1). For Human binned articles, "patient" was the most frequently used (16.7 trimmed counts) and "pharmaceutical" was the least frequently used (2.8 trimmed counts) search terms. For Animal binned articles, "dairy" was the most frequently used (7.7 trimmed counts) and "finfish" was the least frequently used (2.3 trimmed counts) search terms. Interestingly, within the Animal binned articles, "dairy," "cattle," and "chicken" were the top three search terms and had similar frequencies (7.7, 7.6, 7.3 trimmed counts, respectively). For Environmental binned articles, "soil" was the most frequently used (9.4 trimmed counts) and "agriculture" was the least frequently used (2.8 trimmed counts) search terms. A notable similarity among the three bins is that the most frequently used search term was associated with the physical environment that each bin influences, suggesting the journal articles on AMR research continue to direct their discussions only on the physical environments in their associated domain and fail to widen the discussion to the One Health context. The term environment is a known rich point that has different meanings among domains [20], which is supported by our word frequency analysis results. Future NLP analyses contextualizing how the word environment is used in One Health domains could elucidate these distinctions and patterns.

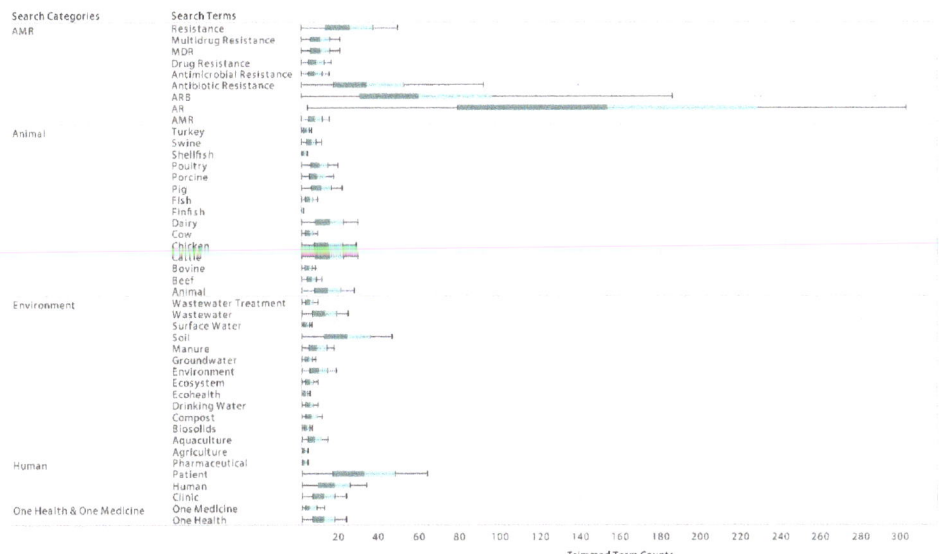

Figure 4. Box and whiskers of the top and bottom term counts in each of the term bins.

2.5. Accessibility of AMR Articles, Publication Preferences, and Potential Biases among the One Health Domains

2.5.1. Non-Open/Restricted Access vs. Open Access Journals

A TDM analysis relies on unrestricted access to literature. To explore potential biases among the used methods that only include open access literature, we performed a case study of a non-open access journal in the Animal domain, as the Animal domain had a higher proportion of non-open access journals related to AMR. The Journal of Dairy Science (JDS), a non-open access journal, was selected for the case study, with language usage in articles from JDS compared to the studied set of open-access articles. As non-open access journals are available only to subscribers, the audience has a more focused expertise, likely to convey a more niche perspective than open-access audiences. The comparison between resistance (i.e., "AMR," "AR," and "MDR") search terms in open-access journals and JDS showed that the language usage patterns were similar overall. The term "antibiotic resistance" was used more frequently over time in open-access journals compared in JDS, however, the term "antibiotic resistance" was the most frequently used AMR term in the analyzed JDS articles. Interestingly, the search term "resistance" increased in usage in both datasets, but was proportionately used more frequently in JDS, suggesting that other terms relating to resistance (i.e., viral, pesticide, etc.) are populating the field recently (Figure S1). "One Health" or "multidrug resistant" were not used in any of the JDS subset articles, in contrast to the open-access articles. This result may be indicative of JDS authors obtaining funding from sources that do not require open access publications, and/or the more subject-specific focus of researchers publishing in JDS compared to open-access sources. Furthermore, while "antimicrobial resistance" usage was rising in the open-access journals, it was steady over time (1990–2019) in JDS. The range of One Health associated search terms used in JDS was expected to be smaller compared to the large dataset of open-access journals due to the niche JDS audience. However, the result that the term "One Health" was not found in journal articles from JDS may suggest that One Health articles are more likely to be published in journals specifically geared towards the One Health concept rather than in animal-specific journals. While not all search terms were present within the JDS sample, the represented search terms maintained a similar average term count throughout the time span studied, suggesting that the omission of non-open/restricted access journals in this study potentially biases towards the overuse of One-health related terms, but not resistance search terms.

2.5.2. Publication Preferences

The 1.2 million articles returned on Europe PMC were retrieved from 4239 unique journals (Tables S3–S7). The inherent diversity and potential bias in choosing where to publish highlights the importance of using appropriate search terms and key words to find relevant articles. For example, a scientist studying the effects of antibiotic usage in dairy cows may never find a useful, relevant article if they only searched within animal science and not One Health or environment-associated journals. PLOS ONE, Frontiers in Microbiology, and One Health were the open-access journals that returned the most One Health binned articles in our TDM analysis (Table S3). In another example, there were not any One Health binned articles (i.e., one-health, one-medicine) from the British Journal of Cancer, which highlights that articles that specifically use "One Health" or "One Medicine" in their title/abstract are not publishing in the same journals as the Human, Animal, and Environmental subdisciplines. This finding mirrors what was identified with the JDS case study. As the One Health domains gradually become more communicative and use common language, the focus on where to publish to reach the most researchers in Human, Animal, and Environmental disciplines will become more judicious. To increase communication and common language usage within One Health a preference should be given to publishing open access.

2.5.3. Potential Biases among the One Health Domains

Providing data lake application programming interfaces (APIs) and NLP processing tools with a specific set of search terms inherently introduces bias into the results. These terms were iteratively collated by the domain experts and referenced against ontologies to provide potential synonyms. Without providing these tools with an initial direction, these results would culminate in discovering the most commonly used word, overall, in the EuroPMC repositories. This search term bias is unavoidable at project conception, but can be mitigated by future programmatically driven analysis to identify alternative principal agents that may be responsible for the trends seen. While we cannot state that all findings are concisely linked to the terms we have identified, there is confidence that these results do indicate that term usage discrepancies exist, and that the dissimilarities must first be identified consistently before domain-level changes can be made.

Additional biases can be shown by authors or search term users through both Journal choice for publication, and more importantly, when searching for relevant AMR literature using search terms in title/abstract. The search strings used for the four binned groups in this study came from multiple brainstorming sessions with the authors, librarians, and a group of AMR-focused researchers, veterinarians, economists, and extension specialists from a USDA-NIFA funded workshop (detailed at https://osf.io/g7amj/, accessed on 1 April 2021). After using TDM to gather the count frequency of the search terms from the queries, the top 100 words from each domain were analyzed. The NLP analysis identified several terms that were not part of our search queries (Table S8). Among these, the word "cell" occurred most frequently in all three domains (Human, Animal, and Environment), with "study," "gene," and "protein" also found in all three domains. The human and animal group shared four additional terms ("patient," "cancer," "human," and "expression"), possibly due to the conceptual links and overall health goals of both human and veterinary medicine. In contrast, the human and environment group only shared one additional term ("treatment"). We suspect that the term refers to caring for a patient in the Human domain and processing wastewater in the Environmental domain, another example of how the same word conveys different meanings across One Health teams. The Human and Animal groups each had one word in the top ten list that was unique to their group ("disease" and "level,", respectively). The Environment group had four terms that were unique, highlighting fundamentally different perspectives and subject matter of the environmental pillar compared to the other two groups. Interestingly, the search term "resistance" was within the top ten search terms found only in the Animal and Environmental groups. The top ten words returned among all the binned articles included words specific to molecular research levels (i.e., cell, gene, protein, expression, and cancer) (Table S8).

Within the last decade, AMR articles have shifted to focus on specific microbial, genetic, ecological, public health, and disease mechanisms as critical research questions. The TDM analysis illuminated this shift and can be used to help researchers and policy makers within the One Health domains better understand which AMR related research areas are growing and which areas of growth are needed within each domain and across domains. One hypothesis for the unique and rather clumped molecular and medically related terms being more frequently used in all the analyzed articles may be related to funding sources within each domain. For example, the National Institute of Health (NIH) established Public Access Policy in 2008 that required all research funded by NIH to be published in an open-access format [40]. However, most Animal and Environmental AMR funding sources (i.e., US USDA, and US CDC) do not require research to be published open access. Promotion of open-access publishing among the animal and environmental domains could partially address this gap.

2.5.4. Implications for Accessing the Literature

Given the differences in language use among the domains and over time, barriers likely exist for researchers to access publications from different disciplines. Differences exist in how major search engines identify publications based on keywords and/or controlled language [41]. For example, in PubMed, a search for antibiotic resistance returns the following search: "drug resistance, microbial" [MeSH Terms] OR antibiotic resistance [Text Word]. In contrast, a search for antimicrobial resistance returns a different search string: "anti-infective agents" [All Fields] OR "anti-infective agents" [MeSH Terms] OR antimicrobial [Text Word] AND resistance [All Fields]. This work identifies a need for researchers to consider using keywords and controlled language that may be outside their discipline, with the understanding that different assumptions and search algorithms of the various databases (Europe PMC, PubMed, Agricola, Scopus, Web of Science, etc.) will not capture all relevant publications across the One Health domains when language use is domain specific. This lack of a common language used in AMR-related articles limits results being produced from search that span across disciplines, which limits engaging in interdisciplinary team science due to the lack of common language usage across the One Health domain.

2.6. Using Text Data Mining to Predict Patterns of Historical and Future Events

TDM was valuable in detecting a decreasing trend in use of "antibiotic resistance" following 2009, which highlights the importance of understanding potential associated historical events that may have substantial effects on language usage in the One Health arena. In 2009, the Pandemic A(H1N1) outbreak occurred, claiming the lives of 123,000–395,600 people worldwide [42]. While this could be coincidental, it is also possible that the resources being used to study AMR within the One Health domains shifted to focus on the influenza outbreak, decreasing antibiotic-resistance related research and ultimately publications in 2009 and beyond [43,44]. The TDM analysis provided critical insight into a potential shift in research within the One Health domains after the 2009 H1N1 pandemic, which resulted in a 26% decrease in resistance related terms in 2010. At the time of publication of this work, the outbreak of the novel COVID-19 coronavirus is ongoing. It will be interesting to consider whether this trend may be seen again in coming years as research shifts focus to antiviral associations, despite concerns with breakdowns in antimicrobial stewardship given new reliance on telemedicine [45,46].

The relationships between AMR common terms and common misconceptions may be another communication issue for One Health moving forward. For example, antimicrobial soaps and sanitizers have been marketed for COVID-19 protection [47], and AMR is now being linked to COVID-19 [48,49]. This COVID-19 era highlights the importance of communication and having a common language to inform all stakeholders (i.e., essential workers, health care workers, school teachers etc.) of the current situation. Although AMR research is 20-30 years ahead of the COVID-19 pandemic, there is not a consensus surrounding AMR language within the One Health domains. Similar to the AMR research conducted here, TDM and NLP techniques can be used in the future to understand the beginning trends of COVID-19 research and how common language, or inconsistent language, was used during the COVID-19 pandemic. Currently, there is not enough academic literature to conduct this analysis, but in time, this type of study can be used to identify and coalesce a common language for COVID-19 related research without having to wait a quarter of a century to do so.

3. Materials and Methods

3.1. Open Access Data Collection

ContentMine's GetPapers [50] was utilized to create a text data lake (centralized repository) of relevant academic articles based on our search terms (Table 1) for each One Health domain. GetPapers is an open-source text mining tool, ran on NodeJS, designed to identify and retrieve open-access, peer-reviewed, full-text articles from Europe PMC [51]. GetPapers can pull the full text and metadata from Europe PMC, IEEE, ArXic, and Crossref via their respective APIs (application programming interface). These APIs allow for large scale recursive search and retrieval of articles without the need to manually do so via the website. This enabled automated replicable data collection to mine the large numbers of articles necessary. By using GetPapers, our search queries had the same functionality and parameters as searching those repositories directly with the added benefit of automating the large-scale collection. An example of the GetPapers Europe PMC query syntax can be found in the Supporting Information (Figure S2). Multiple terms related to the same topic, such as "multi-drug resistance" and "antibiotic resistance" were pulled/retrieved if the domain experts felt that the terms are used interchangeably or in different frequencies within the term bins. The intention of this data pull was to pull as many related articles to these search terms, and redundant terms increased the potential search sample. Each search domain category (Human, Animal, Environment, One Health) is classified as a term bin. The search was restricted to articles written in English. Full-text articles were returned as both PDF and JavaScript Object Notation (JSON)-formatted files that were binned into groups (i.e., bins), initially, based on the One Health search domains. NodeJS was used to run the ContentMine library. Workflow of the data collection, processing, and visualization is detailed in Figure S3.

Table 1. Specific search key terms binned by One Health domains used to query and return articles from ContentMine containing the key terms in the title or abstract, with at least one word from the 'AND' row in the article's title or abstract and not articles returned with words from the 'NOT' row.

Term Bin	Human	Animal	Environment	One Health
Search Terms	Human, patient, pharmaceutical, clinic [1]	Animal, dairy, cow, beef, cattle, poultry, swine, chicken, pig, turkey, fish, porcine, bovine, finfish, shellfish	Ecosystem, ecohealth, environment, soil, agriculture, wastewater, drinking water, groundwater, surface water, compost, manure, biosolids, aquaculture, wastewater treatment	One health, one medicine
AND	antimicrobial resistance, antibiotic resistance, drug resistance, multi-drug resistance, resistance, AMR, ARB, AR, MDR			
NOT	Herbicide, pesticide, disease resistance			

[1] all possible endings to the root of "clinic" were included.

Initially, One Health specific key terms (i.e., one health, one medicine) were included in each binned search query. However, that resulted in the binned queries occasionally returning articles that only contained One Health terms in the title or abstract, and not being related to AMR. These hits artificially raised the total counts per bin without providing data that informed the experimental questions related to AMR language use across the One Health domains. To enhance relevant sample size and text representation in all domains, One Health as a search term was added as a fourth term bin (i.e., domain), and articles were further processed downstream to confirm utilization of One Health terms and utilization with respect to AMR as an additional group (Table 1).

In total, 1.2 million articles were returned from the Europe PMC search queries for all articles by search term bins (Human, Animal, Environment, and One Health; n = 4) by title/abstract. To create a workable and representative sample size, up to 2000 articles were pulled from Europe PMC for each search term bin for every year from 2000–2019. Additionally, a data pull was done for each search term bin for the years 1990–1999, again with a 2000 article cap. As there were less articles in Europe PMC during that duration, one pull was sufficient to gather the majority of the articles. All pulled articles were used to create a data lake of up to 168,000 total articles with full text and metadata. It was not possible to search the terms for each bin without yearly constraints, as the EuroPMC API defaults to providing the most recent articles first. By specifying and running multiple queries per term bin, we were able to ensure that every year was represented, and no year was overly represented in the sample, as long as papers with those terms existed during that year. From this article data lake, 5000 randomly selected articles were pulled for each term bin to create a dataset of 20,000 articles for downstream TDM analysis. This created fixed, uniform sample sizes for each term bin that could then be analyzed.

3.2. Non-Open Access Data Collection

The Journal of Dairy Science (JDS) was used to descriptively compare the TDM results from open-access vs. non-open/restricted access articles within the animal domain using the same search queries as the ContentMine data mining process presented above (Table 1). As stated in Buyalskaya et al. [52], the silos that exist within journals that cater to the readership of a specific discipline may limit access to information for interdisciplinary researchers within the One Health context. JDS was chosen as an example discipline-specific journal, because the manual review of an initial search revealed that the animal domain more frequently had relevant AMR articles in non-open/restricted access journals compared to the other domains surveyed. In addition to its clear categorization within the animal domain of the One Health triad, the JDS data structure allowed for an automated search via EBSCOhost database using the same queries that were used to search Europe PMC via ContentMine. Unlike the millions of open-access articles returned from Europe PMC that were subset into 5,000 articles per topic bin from 1990–2019, the JDS search queries returned 689 Human, 1,853 Animal, 340 Environment, and 14 One Health binned articles. A sample (40%) of each topic bin was randomly downloaded for returned articles (saved as PDF) using EndNote, and the saved PDFs were used to compare the language and key term frequency use between open vs. non-open/restricted access articles.

3.3. Text Data Mining Processing

A total of 20,000 open-access articles from Europe PMC and 972 non-open/restricted access articles from Journal of Dairy Science were collected as PDFs in the four topic bins and further analyzed. All search queries, keyword binning, manuscript retrieval and processing methods, script files, and raw data can be found on our Open Science Framework (OSF) site (https://osf.io/g7amj/, accessed on 1 April 2021). While our search queries specified open access articles, which primarily have a CC BY license attached, we have not provided the individual text articles, as the exact copyright requirements for each document cannot be assumed. These search queries are specific and will pull a near identical set to the data we collected.

Natural Language Processing (NLP) trained libraries were used to extract data from published peer-reviewed articles. NLP, among other functions, creates structure out of unstructured text through analyzing, understanding, and deriving meaning from human written language [53]. Using NLP can give researchers insight into the meaning, purpose, sentiment, and more of natural (i.e., human-written) text information that was previously locked primarily behind individual or group manual interpretation. Downloaded PDFs were first converted to plain text files using the python package pdf2text. The NLP package NLTK (www.nltk.org) was then used to create consistency with letter case style, remove punctuation, tokenize, remove stop words, and lemmatize the text. Lemmatization, in NLP context, means to reduce alternate forms of a word, for example "am", "are", and "is" are all grouped together under the verb "be", and "cars", "car", and "car's" are all grouped together under the noun "car."

The clean data were then merged with metadata (i.e., DOI, article title, year published, journal, PMC ID) from the paired JSON files for each article, and a combination of Pandas, a popular python library with integrated data processing functions, data frames and NLTK processing were used to calculate the term counts per article. Terms that were comprised of two or more words (i.e., antibiotic resistance) were counted with text processed in bi-grams. The total number of words per article was used to provide a percentage of term counts related to each unique article. Percentages based on the total word count were used to standardize against differing article lengths. Data were trimmed to remove articles that comprised the bottom and top 10% of search term frequencies. This was done to further normalize the data and omit outliers (i.e., a 48-page review on antibiotic usage in agriculture and related public health implications that used the word "resistance" 409 times (PMC6017557, [54]) compared to the average and standard deviation term count (16 ± 28) across all articles analyzed.

3.4. Data and Statistical Analysis

Tableau Desktop (Tableau Software, Seattle, WA) was used to process and analyze the merged data after cleaning [55]. Two-Way Analysis of Variance (ANOVA) was used to determine the variance between the top 25 search key terms frequencies counted (Text S1), as well as the key term frequency usage among their associated topic bins. The correlation coefficient was used to determine similarity of total key term frequencies between the topic bins. Additionally, correlation coefficients between the top 25 key terms (Text S1) were used to determine the potential of terms co-existing within an article, regardless of the articles' original topic bin. Interactive Tableau visualizations to explore all avenues of the dataset can be found at the publicly available collection within the OSF site (https://osf.io/g7amj/, accessed on 1 April 2021). Cytoscape software (www.cytoscape.org) was used to create a network graph [56]. This network graph plotted the frequency in which each article used any of the search key terms (Table 1) in their title or abstract and allowed visualization of potential overlap in key term use between the four One Health domains.

4. Conclusions

Using TDM methods, our study highlights what many researchers in the One Health domains already perceive with respect to AMR: we do not communicate well outside of our trained disciplines, and this is reflected in the peer-reviewed literature. This is in part due to the differences in our use of key search terms, where we publish, and how we identify interdisciplinary and transdisciplinary research articles. Moving forward, we suggest the following for authors publishing AMR-related research within the One Health context: (1) increase title/abstract searchability by including both antimicrobial and antibiotic related search terms; (2) include "One Health" in the title/abstract and keywords; and (3) prioritize publishing open-access. Additionally, we suggest that in order to bridge the gap between the One Health domains, researchers need to incorporate specific, and multiple, search terms when looking for relevant AMR research (i.e., include both antibiotic and antimicrobial resistance term groups). Table 1 from this study can be used as a guide for choosing relevant terms. Throughout this article, we specifically chose to use antimicrobial resistance as our key term to include bacterial, fungal, parasitic, and viral resistance representation, following the common language used by the World Health Organization (WHO) for AMR global action plan and the World Organization for Animal Health (OIE). While we chose to use AMR here, our study found that antibiotic resistance was the more frequently used key term, suggesting that the use of different derivatives of this term (i.e., antimicrobial, multidrug, etc.) may not be accessed by One Health researchers actively searching for antibiotic and not antimicrobial. The keywords used to collect the articles, and in turn the data used, were intentionally terms that are broadly used throughout the One Health domain. This study acts as a first milestone on this research, reaffirming the notion that disparate language use within One Health is prohibitory towards collaboration and crosstalk between domains. With that milestone, a crucial next step will be to replicate this research and data collection with a new list of terms specific to one domain or research area to isolate examples of this happening, and begin qualifying and quantifying the language discrepancies.

Using the data produced from the TDM analysis in this study, we propose future research analyzes that address connotations of the language found in these articles using NLP techniques, such as sentiment analysis, topic modeling, and summarization. Further, these methods, both search term frequency and context, can be incorporated when analyzing writing intended for a greater audience (i.e., not solely peer-reviewed articles). This study can be scaled to include consumer and extension databases, web pages, blogs, and trade magazines to understand how AMR is communicated to those outside academia. Our python scripts have been made open source and are readily adaptable to new search terms, articles, or domains, enabling future language studies by researchers seeking to understand how topics and terms differ across disciplinary lines. Additionally, the links to our interactive Tableau dashboards can be found on our OSF site (https://osf.io/g7amj/, accessed on 1 April 2021). The strength of NLP lies in the fact that it can be used to predict the direction of the field based on past research. We hope that once a common language is established within One Health for AMR research, NLP can be used to predict the gaps and next steps to holistically address AMR globally through team science that is truly interdisciplinary; this starts with understanding differences in language use and language context.

Supplementary Materials: The following are available online at https://www.mdpi.com/article/10.3390/antibiotics10040385/s1, Figure S1: JDS resistance search term frequency over time, Figure S2: Example of search query used within bin terms in ContentMine, Figure S3: Workflow, Text S1: The reduced list of the top 25 search terms, Table S1: Summary statistics of all searched terms, Table S2: ANOVA results, Table S3: Top "One Health" domain journals, Table S4: Top 10 "Animal" domain journals, Table S5: Top 10 "Environment" domain journals, Table S6: Top "Human" domain journal, Table S7: Top 10 combined journals for domain groups, Table S8: Top 10 words not searched for in the four binned queries.

Author Contributions: Conceptualization, L.L.W., T.P.N., M.F.D., L.M.D., and S.L.; methodology, L.L.W., J.S.B., and A.M.B.; software, J.S.B., A.M.B., and T.S.; validation, J.S.B. and A.M.B.; formal analysis, J.S.B., A.M.B., and T.S.; resources, L.L.W., J.S.B., and A.M.B.; data curation, J.S.B., A.M.B., and T.S.; writing—original draft preparation, L.L.W., J.S.B., A.M.B., T.P.N., M.F.D., L.M.D., and S.L.; writing—review and editing, L.L.W., J.S.B., A.M.B., T.P.N., M.F.D., L.M.D., and S.L.; visualization, J.S.B. and A.M.B.; supervision, S.L.; project administration, L.L.W.; funding acquisition, S.L. All authors have read and agreed to the published version of the manuscript.

Funding: This research was funded by USDA-NIFA grant number 2019-67017-29114 and 2018-68003-27467. The authors thank the Virginia Tech University Libraries Open Access Subvention Fund for supporting us to publish open access.

Institutional Review Board Statement: Not applicable.

Informed Consent Statement: Not applicable.

Data Availability Statement: Data is contained within the article.

Acknowledgments: The authors acknowledge Allison Woods, Erin Smith, and Nathaniel Porter of Virginia Tech University Libraries for their early assistance in project ideation, search query generation, and data organization. Additionally, Amy Pruden was central in the conceptualization of this project. This manuscript is the result of collaborations formed during the Human Dimensions of Antimicrobial Resistance in Agriculture Workshop in Nebraska City, NE, USA in May 2019. This Workshop was funded by the USDA-NIFA grant entitled 'Surveys and Communication of AMR: Human Dimensions Conference' (NIFA Award # 2019-67017-29114).

Conflicts of Interest: The authors declare no conflict of interest. The funders had no role in the design of the study; in the collection, analyses, or interpretation of data; in the writing of the manuscript, or in the decision to publish the results.

References

1. Van Puyvelde, S.; Deborggraeve, S.; Jacobs, J. Why the antibiotic resistance crisis requires a One Health approach. *Lancet Infect. Dis.* **2018**, *18*, 132–134. [CrossRef]
2. Robinson, T.P.; Bu, D.P.; Carrique-Mas, J.; Fèvre, E.M.; Gilbert, M.; Grace, D.; Hay, S.I.; Jiwakanon, J.; Kakkar, M.; Kariuki, S.; et al. Antibiotic resistance is the quintessential One Health issue. *Trans. R. Soc. Trop. Med. Hyg.* **2016**, *110*, 377. [CrossRef]
3. American Veterinary Medical Association. *One Health: A New Professional Imperative*; American Veterinary Medical Association: Schaumburg, IL, USA, 2008.
4. Schwabe, C.W. *Veterinary Medicine and Human Health*; Williams & Wilkins: Philadelphia, PA, USA, 1967.
5. Gibbs, E.P.J. Emerging zoonotic epidemics in the interconnected global community. *Vet. Rec.* **2005**, *157*, 673–679. [CrossRef] [PubMed]
6. Mackenzie, J.S.; Smith, D.W. COVID-19: A novel zoonotic disease caused by a coronavirus from China: What we know and what we don't. *Microbiol. Aust.* **2020**, *41*, 45. [CrossRef] [PubMed]
7. Collignon, P.J.; McEwen, S.A. One Health—Its Importance in Helping to Better Control Antimicrobial Resistance. *Trop. Med. Infect. Dis.* **2019**, *4*, 22. [CrossRef]
8. Aminov, R.I. A Brief History of the Antibiotic Era: Lessons Learned and Challenges for the Future. *Front. Microbiol.* **2010**, *1*, 134. [CrossRef]
9. McManus, P.S.; Stockwell, V.O.; Sundin, G.W.; Jones, A.L. Antibiotic use in plant agriculture. *Annu. Rev. Phytopathol.* **2002**, *40*, 443–465. [CrossRef] [PubMed]
10. Bauer, D.J. A History of the Discovery and Clinical Application of Antiviral Drugs. *Br. Med. Bull.* **1985**, *41*, 309–314. [CrossRef]
11. Odds, F.C. Antifungal agents: Their diversity and increasing sophistication. *Mycologist* **2003**, *17*, 51–55. [CrossRef]
12. Campbell, W.C. Lessons from the History of Ivermectin and Other Antiparasitic Agents. *Annu. Rev. Anim. Biosci.* **2016**, *4*, 1–14. [CrossRef]
13. Mohr, K.I. History of Antibiotics Research. *Curr. Top. Microbiol. Immunol.* **2016**, *398*, 237–272.
14. Witte, W. Selective pressure by antibiotic use in livestock. *Int. J. Antimicrob. Agents* **2000**, *16* (Suppl. 1), S19–S24. [CrossRef]
15. Kolár, M.; Urbánek, K.; Látal, T. Antibiotic selective pressure and development of bacterial resistance. *Int. J. Antimicrob. Agents* **2001**, *17*, 357–363. [CrossRef]
16. Mainardi, J.-L.; Villet, R.; Bugg, T.D.; Mayer, C.; Arthur, M. Evolution of peptidoglycan biosynthesis under the selective pressure of antibiotics in Gram-positive bacteria. *FEMS Microbiol. Rev.* **2008**, *32*, 386–408. [CrossRef] [PubMed]
17. Van Goethem, M.W.; Pierneef, R.; Bezuidt, O.K.I.; Van De Peer, Y.; Cowan, D.A.; Makhalanyane, T.P. A reservoir of "historical" antibiotic resistance genes in remote pristine Antarctic soils. *Microbiome* **2018**, *6*, 40. [CrossRef]
18. Partridge, S.R.; Kwong, S.M.; Firth, N.; Jensen, S.O. Mobile Genetic Elements Associated with Antimicrobial Resistance. *Clin. Microbiol. Rev.* **2018**, *31*, e00088-17. [CrossRef] [PubMed]
19. Sheehan, D.; Robertson, L.; Ormond, T. Comparison of language used and patterns of communication in interprofessional and multidisciplinary teams. *J. Interprof. Care* **2007**, *21*, 17–30. [CrossRef]
20. Durso, L.M.; Cook, K.L. One Health and Antibiotic Resistance in Agroecosystems. *Ecohealth* **2018**, *16*, 414–419. [CrossRef]
21. Ritter, M.A. Operating Room Environment. *Clin. Orthop. Relat. Res.* **1999**, *369*, 103. [CrossRef]
22. Yassi, A.; Kjellström, T.; de Kok, T.; Guidotti, T.L. *Basic Environmental Health*; Oxford University Press: Oxford, UK, 2001.
23. One Health Initiative. Available online: https://onehealthinitiative.com/about/ (accessed on 9 April 2020).
24. Mendelson, M.; Balasegaram, M.; Jinks, T.; Pulcini, C.; Sharland, M. Antibiotic resistance has a language problem. *Nature* **2017**, *545*, 23–25. [CrossRef]
25. Léger, A.; Stärk, K.D.C.; Rushton, J.; Nielsen, L.R. A One Health Evaluation of the University of Copenhagen Research Centre for Control of Antibiotic Resistance. *Front. Vet. Sci* **2018**, *5*, 194. [CrossRef] [PubMed]
26. UN Announces Interagency Group to Coordinate Global Fight against Antimicrobial Resistance. Available online: https://news.un.org/en/story/2017/03/553412-un-announces-interagency-group-coordinate-global-fight-against-antimicrobial (accessed on 26 October 2020).

27. Cheruvelil, K.S.; Soranno, P.A. Data-intensive ecological research is catalyzed by open science and team science. *BioScience* **2018**, *68*, 813–822. [CrossRef]
28. Jakobsen, C.H.; McLaughlin, W.J. Communication in ecosystem management: A case study of cross-disciplinary integration in the assessment phase of the interior Columbia Basin Ecosystem Management Project. *Environ. Manag.* **2004**, *33*, 591–605. [CrossRef] [PubMed]
29. Van Swol, L.M.; Kane, A.A. Language and group processes: An integrative, interdisciplinary review. *Small Group Res.* **2019**, *50*, 3–38. [CrossRef]
30. Wray, A. The language of dementia science and the science of dementia language. *J. Lang. Soc. Psychol.* **2017**, *36*, 80–95. [CrossRef]
31. Destoumieux-Garzón, D.; Mavingui, P.; Boetsch, G.; Boissier, J.; Darriet, F.; Duboz, P.; Fritsch, C.; Giraudoux, P.; Le Roux, F.; Morand, S.; et al. The One Health Concept: 10 Years Old and a Long Road Ahead. *Front. Vet. Sci.* **2018**, *5*, 14. [CrossRef]
32. Krockow, E.M. Nomen est omen: Why we need to rename 'antimicrobial resistance'. *JAC Antimicrob. Resist.* **2020**, *2*. [CrossRef]
33. Glossary of Terms Related to Antibiotic Resistance |NARMS| CDC. Available online: https://www.cdc.gov/narms/resources/glossary.html (accessed on 13 July 2020).
34. Katrime Integrated Health Glossary of Terms: Antimicrobial Resistance. Available online: https://nccid.ca/publications/glossary-terms-antimicrobial-resistance/ (accessed on 13 July 2020).
35. Encyclopaedia. Available online: https://revive.gardp.org/resources/encyclopaedia/ (accessed on 26 October 2020).
36. Davis, M.F.; Rankin, S.C.; Schurer, J.M.; Cole, S.; Conti, L.; Rabinowitz, P. COHERE Expert Review Group Checklist for One Health Epidemiological Reporting of Evidence (COHERE). *One Health* **2017**, *4*, 14–21. [CrossRef]
37. Kelly, R.; Zoubiane, G.; Walsh, D.; Ward, R.; Goossens, H. Public funding for research on antibacterial resistance in the JPIAMR countries, the European Commission, and related European Union agencies: A systematic observational analysis. *Lancet Infect. Dis.* **2016**, *16*, 431. [CrossRef]
38. The AMR Fund. Available online: https://www.cdcfoundation.org/what/programs/amr-fund (accessed on 26 February 2021).
39. Manure & Nutrient Management Programs. Available online: https://nifa.usda.gov/program/manure-nutrient-management-programs (accessed on 9 September 2020).
40. When and How to Comply. Available online: https://publicaccess.nih.gov/ (accessed on 9 September 2020).
41. MeSH. Available online: https://www.ncbi.nlm.nih.gov/mesh/?term=antibiotic+resistance (accessed on 26 October 2020).
42. Fineberg, H.V. Pandemic preparedness and response—Lessons from the H1N1 influenza of 2009. *N. Engl. J. Med.* **2014**, *370*, 1335–1342. [CrossRef]
43. CDC. Ten Years of Gains: A Look Back at Progress Since the 2009 H1N1 Pandemic. Available online: https://www.cdc.gov/flu/spotlights/2018-2019/decade-since-h1n1-pandemic.html (accessed on 9 September 2020).
44. Congress Approves $7.65 Billion for Pandemic Flu Response. Available online: https://www.cidrap.umn.edu/news-perspective/2009/06/congress-approves-765-billion-pandemic-flu-response (accessed on 9 September 2020).
45. Rawson, T.M.; Moore, L.S.P.; Castro-Sanchez, E.; Charani, E.; Davies, F.; Satta, G.; Ellington, M.J.; Holmes, A.H. COVID-19 and the potential long-term impact on antimicrobial resistance. *J. Antimicrob. Chemother.* **2020**, *75*, 1681–1684. [CrossRef]
46. Khor, W.P.; Olaoye, O.; D'Arcy, N.; Krockow, E.M.; Elshenawy, R.A.; Rutter, V.; Ashiru-Oredope, D. The Need for Ongoing Antimicrobial Stewardship during the COVID-19 Pandemic and Actionable Recommendations. *Antibiotics* **2020**, *9*, 904. [CrossRef]
47. Studies: Hand Sanitizers Kill COVID-19 Virus, E-Consults Appropriate. Available online: https://www.cidrap.umn.edu/news-perspective/2020/04/studies-hand-sanitizers-kill-covid-19-virus-e-consults-appropriate (accessed on 9 September 2020).
48. Getahun, H.; Smith, I.; Trivedi, K.; Paulin, S.; Balkhy, H.H. Tackling antimicrobial resistance in the COVID-19 pandemic. *Bull. World Health Organ.* **2020**, *98*, 442. [CrossRef] [PubMed]
49. Nieuwlaat, R.; Mbuagbaw, L.; Mertz, D.; Burrows, L.; Bowdish, D.M.E.; Moja, L.; Wright, G.D.; Schünemann, H.J. COVID-19 and Antimicrobial Resistance: Parallel and Interacting Health Emergencies. *Clin. Infect. Dis.* **2020**. [CrossRef]
50. Richard Smith-Unna, P.M.-R. The ContentMine Scraping Stack: Literature-scale Content Mining with Community-maintained Collections of Declarative Scrapers. *D-Lib Mag.* **2014**, *20*. [CrossRef]
51. The Europe PMC Consortium. Europe PMC: A full-text literature database for the life sciences and platform for innovation. *Nucleic Acids Res.* **2015**, *43*, D1042. [CrossRef] [PubMed]
52. Buyalskaya, A.; Gallo, M.; Camerer, C.F. The golden age of social science. *Proc. Natl. Acad. Sci. USA* **2021**, *118*. [CrossRef]
53. Collobert, R.; Weston, J.; Bottou, L.; Karlen, M.; Kavukcuoglu, K.; Kuksa, P. Natural Language Processing (Almost) from Scratch. *J. Mach. Learn. Res.* **2011**, *12*, 2493–2537.
54. Manyi-Loh, C.; Mamphweli, S.; Meyer, E.; Okoh, A. Antibiotic Use in Agriculture and Its Consequential Resistance in Environmental Sources: Potential Public Health Implications. *Mol. A J. Synth. Chem. Nat. Prod. Chem.* **2018**, *23*, 795. [CrossRef]
55. Tableau (version. 9.1). *J. Med. Libr. Assoc.* **2016**, *104*, 182–183. [CrossRef]
56. Shannon, P.; Markiel, A.; Ozier, O.; Baliga, N.S.; Wang, J.T.; Ramage, D.; Amin, N.; Schwikowski, B.; Ideker, T. Cytoscape: A software environment for integrated models of biomolecular interaction networks. *Genome Res.* **2003**, *13*, 2498–2504. [CrossRef] [PubMed]

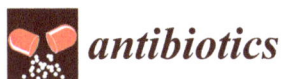

Perspective

Can the One Health Approach Save Us from the Emergence and Reemergence of Infectious Pathogens in the Era of Climate Change: Implications for Antimicrobial Resistance?

Smitha Gudipati *, Marcus Zervos and Erica Herc

Department of Infectious Disease, Henry Ford Hospital, Detroit, MI 48202, USA; mzervos1@hfhs.org (M.Z.); Eherc1@hfhs.org (E.H.)
* Correspondence: sgudipa2@hfhs.org; Tel.: +1-313-932-5065

Received: 29 July 2020; Accepted: 11 September 2020; Published: 14 September 2020

Abstract: Climate change has become a controversial topic in today's media despite decades of warnings from climate scientists and has influenced human health significantly with the increasing prevalence of infectious pathogens and contribution to antimicrobial resistance. Elevated temperatures lead to rising sea and carbon dioxide levels, changing environments and interactions between humans and other species. These changes have led to the emergence and reemergence of infectious pathogens that have already developed significant antimicrobial resistance. Although these new infectious pathogens are alarming, we can still reduce the burden of infectious diseases in the era of climate change if we focus on One Health strategies. This approach aims at the simultaneous protection of humans, animals and environment from climate change and antimicrobial impacts. Once these relationships are better understood, these models can be created, but the support of our legislative and health system partnerships are critical to helping with strengthening education and awareness.

Keywords: climate change; One Health; *Candida auris*; COVID 19; emerging pathogens; antimicrobial resistance

---

Climate change has become a controversial topic in today's media despite decades of warnings from climate scientists [1,2]. Reports of "The Hottest Month Ever Recorded," "Glaciers Melting" and "Earth's Food Supply Under Threat" are news headlines with which people have become familiar [3]. Most recently, the Australian wildfires are another example of the urgency to address climate change. Additionally, several studies suggest climate change is contributing to infectious disease emergence [4]. The Centers for Disease Control and Prevention stated that the impact of climate change on human health is significant [5]. Increasing temperatures have led to extreme weather resulting in rising sea and carbon dioxide levels, which contributes to increased prevalence of infectious agents. These changes affect adaptations in vector ecology, water quality and decreased nutritional supply that are associated with infectious diseases such as tickborne encephalitis, cryptosporidiosis and leptospirosis [2,6]. It also contributes to increased antimicrobial resistance [7]. We analyze the One Health approach, which focuses on the simultaneous protection of humans, animals and the environment from climate change and antimicrobial impact [8].

The relationship between global warming and infectious pathogens dates back many years. For example, Roman aristocrats used to vacation in the summer at hill resorts to avoid malaria [9]. Although humans thought they could "outsmart" these infections, many viruses, bacteria, protozoa and multicellular parasites have evolved to the human species as their natural reservoir through vector-borne transmission [10]. These infectious agents adapt to their optimal climate that includes temperature, precipitation, elevation and daylight duration. According to the Centers for Disease

Control and Prevention, about 75% of emerging diseases and 60% of known human infectious diseases originate in animals. It is imperative that we learn to diagnose and control zoonotic infections, while evaluating the impact of human activity and environmental change on nonhuman reservoirs of disease [11].

Even though climate change impact and its effect on infectious diseases are well reported, it is occurring at an accelerated rate. Legionnaires' disease, a waterborne illness, is rising with a rate of reported cases increasing 5.5 times from 2000 to 2017 [12]. Vector-borne infections such as Zika, Chagas disease, dengue and chikungunya that are usually localized to tropical climates as they require higher temperatures to complete their life cycle, are slowly migrating towards temperate climates, such as the United States, as global temperatures are increasing even in winter months [13]. Malaria is the most prevalent vector-borne disease globally [14,15]. Temperature and humidity are among the most important factors for disease transmission and extrinsic incubation period, and are facilitating the spread of malaria into areas that are currently malaria-free large urban highland populations [9]. Similarly, dengue viruses are traditionally transmitted in the tropics because frost and sustained cold weather kills adult mosquitoes and overwintering eggs and larvae [16,17]. Warming trends are shifting the vector and disease distribution to higher latitudes and altitudes. Warmer temperatures reduce the larval size of the *Aeagypti* mosquito as well, requiring the adult to feed more frequently, increasing bite rates and spread of infection [18,19]. Additionally, mosquito-borne diseases, such as West Nile virus, that typically occur during the rainy season are now occurring during the drought season. This shift is occurring because mosquitoes are brought into proximity with birds at scarce water sources, enhancing the transmission of the virus in the enzootic cycle [13,20,21].

Tickborne infections that were once thought to be confined to the Northeast United States are now expanding throughout the Midwest and further West. This is in part due to increased temperatures, which are increasing the survival and activity period of ticks, allowing extension of the range of both the reservoir and tick hosts. Additionally, this prolongs the duration of the season when people are exposed to the ticks [22]. Bacterial and protozoan tickborne diseases doubled in the United States between 2004 and 2016 as reports of both *Ixodes scapularis* and *Amblyomma americanum* ticks are expanding to new areas [23,24]. These ticks are known to transmit infections such as Lyme disease, *Anaplasma phagocytophilum*, babesiosis, human monotrophic ehrlichiosis and tularemia.

Diarrheal diseases such as *Campylobacter*, *Salmonella* and cholera survive better in warmer temperatures and, with the increasing temperatures in our water systems, we have seen the reemergence of these diarrheal infections in recent years [20,25]. This is particularly alarming as we already have significant antimicrobial resistance to these Gram-negative pathogens, and as these bacteria evolve, treatment options may be limited [20,26–28]. For example, there have already been numerous outbreaks of *Salmonella typhi* with resistance to several key therapeutic antimicrobials such as ciprofloxacin; however, now nontyphoidal salmonellas, which are being frequently transmitted by means of contaminated water supply, have developed decreased susceptibility to fluoroquinolone antimicrobials in developing countries [29]. Additionally, Gonzalez et al. found that *Campylobacter jejuni* survives in well water for long periods of time and the effect of ciprofloxacin resistance was temperature-dependent as the resistance mechanisms in vitro increased as temperatures went from 4 to 25 °C [30].

A well-known infection that is hypothesized to have arisen from climate change is *Candida auris*, which previously existed as a plant saprophyte and gained thermotolerance and salinity tolerance from the effects of climate change on the wetland ecosystem [31,32]. *C. auris* was first isolated in 2009 from a human ear and since then has been associated with human disease in many countries and exhibited nonsusceptibility to antifungal agents [32]. This new thermotolerant *C. auris* was proposed to have been transplanted by birds across the globe to rural areas where humans and birds are in constant contact. Human migration likely led to the emergence of *C. auris* into urban healthcare environments in which antimicrobial resistance and infection control issues have arisen. *C. auris* is the only *Candida* species that has isolates shown to be resistant to all four classes of antifungal drugs, which has created higher risks for clinical infections and breakthrough infections during antifungal treatment and prophylaxis [33]. These infections have the potential to result in significant morbidity and mortality and could be on the rise as climate change continues [3].

SARS-COV-2, the virus responsible for COVID-19, originated from the interplay between humans and animals. The likely transmission of the virus came from bats and potentially used an intermediate source, the pangolin, to transmit the virus to humans [34]. Many of the initial cases had a common exposure to the Huanan wholesale seafood market that also traded live animals. On 7 January 2020, the virus was sequenced and was found to have >95% homology with the bat coronavirus [35]. Through travel and community spread, it has become a global pandemic. Bats are especially vulnerable to climate change due to low reproductive output, ecological specialization and high trophic positions [36]. Their large surface area of noninsulated wings create significant water loss that is higher than in other small animals [37]. Thus, with climate change, increased aridity and prolonged droughts in their endemic areas bats migrate to more populated areas in search of insect prey, thereby increasing their interaction with humans, and as a result, may transmit virulent infections [37,38]. Additionally, although the prevalence of confirmed community-onset bacterial coinfections are low in patients with COVID-19, 56.6% of hospitalized patients in 38 Michigan hospitals received empiric antibiotic therapy [38]. This study and many others bring to light the urgency of antimicrobial stewardship principles to prevent antimicrobial resistance during the COVID-19 era [39].

The implications of antimicrobial resistance due to the emergence and reemergence of infectious pathogens from climate change are complex as the decreasing effectiveness of antibiotics has accelerated in recent years [40]. In 2016, a U.K government-commissioned report estimated that if no action were taken, by 2050, antimicrobial resistance would cause up to 10 million annual deaths globally, reduce gross domestic product by 2% to 3.5% and cost 100 trillion US dollars [41]. A key feature of antimicrobial resistance and climate change is that antibiotic consumption and carbon use will bring about adverse future consequences [42]. Tackling this issue has led to the establishment of a global innovation fund for both antimicrobial resistance research and investing in new drugs; however, both developments are financially competing against each other [43].

Recent evidence shows that higher temperatures are associated with higher resistance levels in common pathogens such as *Escherichia coli*, *Klebsiella pneumoniae* and *Staphylococcus aureus* [44]. In an unadjusted analysis, MacFadden et al. demonstrated an increase of 10°C across all regions in the United States was associated with increased resistance of 5.1%, 3.4% and 3.1% for *E. coli*, *K. pneumoniae* and *S. aureus* respectively [45]. This association postulates that due to horizontal gene transfer, warmer temperatures could affect the way bacteria respond to certain drug mechanisms [45]. Another recent study suggested an association between temporal climate developments and carbapenem-resistance in *Pseudomonas aeruginosa* in Europe [7]. Climate change and antimicrobial resistance are also driven by the consumption of carbon and antibiotics that can provide people with valuable short term benefits but impose long term costs [44,46]. Although both antimicrobial resistance and climate change are not wholly comparable, both issues require participation from the local, national and international organizations to help solve their challenges [47].

Additionally, animal and environmental compartments play a significant role in antimicrobial resistance [48]. There are multiple links between humans, animals and environmental compartments allowing for movement and alteration of genetic elements of bacteria and creating resistance to antimicrobials [45,49]. Industrial agriculture relies heavily on the widespread use of antimicrobials for livestock farms for therapeutics, prophylactics and controversially growth promotion [48]. Agricultural usage of antimicrobials exceeds and rivals medical usage in the United States and Europe respectively, and observational studies and surveillance reports have described antimicrobial resistance in farm animals resulting from misuse [40,48]. Small doses of antibiotics from urine, feces, manure and pharmaceutical waste are also being released into the environment through rivers, lakes and soil [50]. These sublethal doses allow for antimicrobial resistance to occur as they do not reach "cidal" concentrations [51].

With the emergence and the reemergence of these infectious pathogens, our hospital systems need to be equipped with the proper resources and education. Infection control and antimicrobial stewardship efforts will need to adapt and be prepared for these pathogens as they become more resistant to antimicrobials and cause "outbreaks" in hospital settings. Sentinel, vector, syndromic and real-time surveillance will be necessary to monitor changes related to climate change to help hospitals prepare for the emergence of new pathogens [25]. Evidence-based epidemic intelligence with early identification of infectious disease threats related to climate change is crucial to help with adaptation and preparedness for these outbreaks [25]. Microbiology laboratories will need to develop advanced capacity to identify these new organisms. As more infections are transmitted from animal reservoirs, communication between veterinarians and clinicians will be necessary in order to prevent animal transmission to humans that could lead to significant morbidity and mortality [8].

Although these new infectious pathogens and potential for increased antimicrobial resistance are alarming, we can still reduce the burden of infectious disease in the era of climate change if we focus on One Health strategies. We must acknowledge both the fragility of our healthcare systems and the healthcare's own large carbon footprint [52]. One Health is an approach that recognizes that the health of people is closely connected to the health of animals and our shared environment. This is not a new concept, but one that is becoming important in recent years as human populations are growing and expanding into new geographic areas [8,53]. More people are now living in close contact with wild and domestic animals, both livestock and pets. Close contact with animals and their environments provides more opportunities for diseases to pass between animals and people. Additionally, our planet has experienced changes such as deforestation and intensive farming practices because of climate change. Disruptions in environmental conditions and habitats can provide new opportunities for diseases to pass to animals. Finally, the movement of people, animals and animal products has increased from international travel and trade leading to global transmission of pathogens as we are now seeing with COVID-19 [53–55].

The One Health concept is gaining recognition in the United States and globally as an effective way to fight health issues at the human–animal–environment interface. Preventative One Health strategies, such as mass vaccinations of animal populations can help reduce livestock-mediated zoonoses, and is both feasible and cost-effective [56]. Livestock vaccination against brucellosis and leptospirosis has been effective in reducing the burden of disease in many parts of the world where diagnosis and treatment of these diseases are limited [56–58]. International implementation by the World Health Organization has already utilized the One Health approach for Influenza A H1N1 in 2009, Polio in 2014, Ebola in 2014 and the Zika virus in 2016 by declaring them potential public health emergencies of international concern. This approach has had relative success by incorporating aspects of human, animal and environmental health to help with mitigation of these diseases [59]. However, there is controversy if One Health will be enough to fight climate change [8]. To implement this protection, we need to learn more about the underlying complex relationships of these pathogens and vectors and develop well-designed mitigation measures. Successful public health interventions require the cooperation of human, animal, and environmental health partners. Professionals within these sectors need to communicate, collaborate and coordinate activities [53,54]. Once these relationships are better understood, these models can be created, but the support of our legislative and health system partnerships are critical to helping with strengthening education and awareness.

Author Contributions: S.G. contributed as the primary author of writing and researching the topics of interest. E.H. and M.Z. made intellectual contributions to the design and analysis of the article. All authors have read and agreed to the published version of the manuscript.

Funding: This research received no external funding.

Conflicts of Interest: The authors declare no conflict of interest.

References

1. Salas, R.N. The climate crisis and clinical practice. *N. Engl. J. Med.* **2020**, *382*, 589–591. [CrossRef]
2. Altizer, S.; Ostfeld, R.S.; Johnson, P.T.; Kutz, S.; Harvell, C.D. Climate change and infectious diseases: From evidence to a predictive framework. *Science* **2013**, *341*, 514–519. [CrossRef]
3. Casadevall, A.; Pirofski, L.A. Benefits and costs of animal virulence for microbes. *mBio* **2019**, *10*, e00863-19. [CrossRef]
4. Baylis, M. Potential impact of climate change on emerging vector-borne and other infections in the UK. *Environ. Health* **2017**, *16*, 112. [CrossRef]
5. Centers for Disease Control and Prevention. Ecology and Epidemiology of Tickborne Pathogens, Washington, USA, 2011–2016. Available online: https://wwwnc.cdc.gov/eid/article/26/4/19-1382_article (accessed on 2 March 2020).
6. Eisen, L. Stemming the rising tide of human-biting ticks and tickborne diseases, United States. *Emerg. Infect. Dis.* **2020**, *26*, 641–647. [CrossRef]
7. Kaba, H.E.J.; Kuhlmann, E.; Scheithauer, S. Thinking outside the box: Association of antimicrobial resistance with climate warming in Europe—A 30 country observational study. *Int. J. Hyg. Environ. Health* **2020**, *223*, 151–158. [CrossRef]
8. Zinsstag, J.; Crump, L.; Schelling, E.; Hattendorf, J.; Maidane, Y.O.; Ali, K.O.; Muhummed, A.; Umer, A.A.; Aliyi, F.; Nooh, F.; et al. Climate change and One Health. *FEMS Microbiol. Lett.* **2018**, *365*, fny085. [CrossRef]
9. Patz, J.A.; Epstein, P.R.; Burke, T.A.; Balbus, J.M. Global climate change and emerging infectious diseases. *JAMA* **1996**, *275*, 217–223. [CrossRef]
10. Almeida, A.P.; Goncalves, Y.M.; Novo, M.T.; Sousa, C.A.; Melim, M.; Gracio, A.J. Vector monitoring of Aedes aegypti in the Autonomous Region of Madeira, Portugal. *Euro Surveill.* **2007**, *12*, E071115.6. [CrossRef]
11. Sarkar, A. Climate change: Adverse health impacts and roles of health professionals. *Int. J. Occup. Environ. Med.* **2011**, *2*, 4–7.
12. Centers for Disease Control and Prevention. National Notifiable Diseases Surveillance System. Available online: https://wwwn.cdc.gov/nndss/ (accessed on 2 March 2020).
13. Shuman, E.K. Global climate change and infectious diseases. *N. Engl. J. Med.* **2010**, *362*, 1061–1063. [CrossRef] [PubMed]
14. Institute of Medicine; Committee for the Study on Malaria Prevention and Control; Division of International Health; Oaks, S.C., Jr.; Mtichell, V.S.; Pearson, G.W.; Carpenter, C.C. (Eds.) *Malaria: Obstacles and Opportunities*; National Academies Press: Washington, DC, USA, 1991.
15. Alonso, P.L.; Smith, T.; Schellenberg, J.R.; Masanja, H.; Mwankusye, S.; Urassa, H.; Bastos de Azevedo, I.; Chongela, J.; Kobero, S.; Menendez, C.; et al. Randomised trial of efficacy of SPf66 vaccine against Plasmodium falciparum malaria in children in southern Tanzania. *Lancet* **1994**, *344*, 1175–1181. [CrossRef]
16. Macdonald, W.W.; Rajapaksa, N. A survey of the distribution and relative prevalence of Aedes aegypti in Sabah, Brunei, and Sarawak. *Bull. World Health Organ.* **1972**, *46*, 203–209. [PubMed]
17. Scott, T.W.; Chow, E.; Strickman, D.; Kittayapong, P.; Wirtz, R.A.; Lorenz, L.H.; Edman, J.D. Blood-feeding patterns of Aedes aegypti (Diptera: Culicidae) collected in a rural Thai village. *J. Med. Entomol.* **1993**, *30*, 922–927. [CrossRef]
18. Rueda, L.M.; Patel, K.J.; Axtell, R.C.; Stinner, R.E. Temperature-dependent development and survival rates of Culex quinquefasciatus and Aedes aegypti (Diptera: Culicidae). *J. Med. Entomol.* **1990**, *27*, 892–898. [CrossRef] [PubMed]
19. Shope, R. Global climate change and infectious diseases. *Environ. Health Perspect.* **1991**, *96*, 171–174. [CrossRef]
20. Omazic, A.; Bylund, H.; Boqvist, S.; Hogberg, A.; Bjorkman, C.; Tryland, M.; Evengard, B.; Koch, A.; Berggren, C.; Malogolovkin, A.; et al. Identifying climate-sensitive infectious diseases in animals and humans in Northern regions. *Acta Vet. Scand.* **2019**, *61*, 53. [CrossRef]
21. Zeman, P. Prolongation of tick-borne encephalitis cycles in warmer climatic conditions. *Int. J. Environ. Res. Public Health* **2019**, *16*, 4532. [CrossRef]
22. Bouchard, C.; Dibernardo, A.; Koffi, J.; Wood, H.; Leighton, P.A.; Lindsay, L.R. N Increased risk of tick-borne diseases with climate and environmental changes. *Can. Commun. Dis. Rep.* **2019**, *45*, 83–89. [CrossRef]

23. Molaei, G.; Little, E.A.H.; Williams, S.C.; Stafford, K.C. Bracing for the worst—Range expansion of the lone star tick in the northeastern United States. *N. Engl. J. Med.* **2019**, *381*, 2189–2192. [CrossRef]
24. Ogden, N.H.; Radojevic, M.; Wu, X.; Duvvuri, V.R.; Leighton, P.A.; Wu, J. Estimated effects of projected climate change on the basic reproductive number of the Lyme disease vector Ixodes scapularis. *Environ. Health Perspect.* **2014**, *122*, 631–638. [CrossRef] [PubMed]
25. Semenza, J.C.; Menne, B. Climate change and infectious diseases in Europe. *Lancet Infect. Dis.* **2009**, *9*, 365–375. [CrossRef]
26. Jobling, M.G. Trust but verify: Uncorroborated assemblies of plasmid genomes from next-generation sequencing data are likely spurious comment on "Diverse Plasmids Harboring blaCTX-M-15 in Klebsiella pneumoniae ST11 Isolates from Several Asian Countries," by So Yeon Kim and Kwan Soo Ko. *Microb. Drug. Resist.* **2019**, *25*, 1521–1524. [CrossRef] [PubMed]
27. Lipp, E.K.; Huq, A.; Colwell, R.R. Effects of global climate on infectious disease: The cholera model. *Clin. Microbiol. Rev.* **2002**, *15*, 757–770. [CrossRef] [PubMed]
28. Constantin de Magny, G.; Colwell, R.R. Cholera and climate: A demonstrated relationship. *Trans. Am. Clin. Climatol. Assoc.* **2009**, *120*, 119–128.
29. Threlfall, E.J. Antimicrobial drug resistance in Salmonella: Problems and perspectives in food- and water-borne infections. *FEMS Microbiol. Rev.* **2002**, *26*, 141–148. [CrossRef]
30. González, M.; Hänninen, M.-L. Effect of temperature and antimicrobial resistance on survival of Campylobacter jejuni in well water: Application of the Weibull model. *J. Appl. Microbiol.* **2012**, *113*, 284–293. [CrossRef]
31. Lockhart, S.R.; Etienne, K.A.; Vallabhaneni, S.; Farooqi, J.; Chowdhary, A.; Govender, N.P.; Colombo, A.L.; Calvo, B.; Cuomo, C.A.; Desjardins, C.A.; et al. Simultaneous Emergence of Multidrug-Resistant Candida auris on 3 Continents Confirmed by Whole-Genome Sequencing and Epidemiological Analyses. *Clin. Infect. Dis.* **2017**, *64*, 134–140. [CrossRef]
32. Casadevall, A.; Kontoyiannis, D.P.; Robert, V. On the emergence of Candida auris: Climate change, azoles, swamps, and birds. *mBio* **2019**, *10*, e01397-19. [CrossRef]
33. Pristov, K.E.; Ghannoum, M.A. Resistance of Candida to azoles and echinocandins worldwide. *Clin. Microbiol. Infect.* **2019**, *25*, 792–798. [CrossRef]
34. World Health Organization. Coronavirus disease 2019 (Covid-19) Situation Report—57. Available online: https://www.who.int/docs/default-source/coronaviruse/situation-reports/20200317-sitrep-57-covid-19.pdf?sfvrsn=a26922f2_4 (accessed on 18 March 2020).
35. Sun, P.; Lu, X.; Xu, C.; Sun, W.; Pan, B. Understanding of COVID-19 based on current evidence. *J. Med. Virol.* **2020**, *92*, 548–551. [CrossRef] [PubMed]
36. Jones, G.; Rebelo, H. *Responses of bats to climate change: Learning from the past and predicting the future In Bat Evolution, Ecology, and Conservation*; Adams, R.A., Pedersen, S.C., Eds.; Springer: New York, NY, USA, 2013; p. 549.
37. Van der Meij, T.; Strein, A.J.V.; Haysom, K.A.; Dekker, J.; Russ, J.; Biala, K.; Bihari, Z.; Jansen, E.; Langton, S.; Kurali, A.; et al. Return of the bats? A prototype indicator of trends in European bat populations in underground hibernacula. *Mamm. Biol.* **2015**, *80*, 170–177. [CrossRef]
38. Vaughn, V.M.; Gandhi, T.; Petty, L.A.; Patel, P.K.; Prescott, H.C.; Malani, A.N.; Ratz, D.; McLaughlin, E.; Chopra, V.; Flanders, S.A. Empiric Antibacterial Therapy and Community-onset Bacterial Co-infection in Patients Hospitalized with COVID-19: A Multi-Hospital Cohort Study. *Clin. Infect. Dis.* **2020**, ciaa1239. [CrossRef]
39. Beović, B.; Doušak, M.; Ferreira-Coimbra, J.; Nadrah, K.; Rubulotta, F.; Belliato, M.; Berger-Estilita, J.; Ayoade, F.; Rello, J.; Erdem, H. Antibiotic use in patients with COVID-19: A 'snapshot' Infectious Diseases International Research Initiative (ID-IRI) survey. *J. Antimicrob. Chemother.* **2020**, dkaa326. [CrossRef] [PubMed]
40. Laxminarayan, R.; Duse, A.; Wattal, C.; Zaidi, A.K.; Wertheim, H.F.; Sumpradit, N.; Vlieghe, E.; Hara, G.L.; Gould, I.M.; Goossens, H.; et al. Antibiotic resistance-the need for global solutions. *Lancet Infect. Dis.* **2013**, *13*, 1057–1098. [CrossRef]
41. de Kraker, M.E.; Stewardson, A.J.; Harbarth, S. Will 10 Million People Die a Year due to Antimicrobial Resistance by 2050? *PLoS Med.* **2016**, *13*, e1002184. [CrossRef] [PubMed]

42. Roope, L.S.J.; Smith, R.D.; Pouwels, K.B.; Buchanan, J.; Abel, L.; Eibich, P.; Butler, C.C.; Tan, P.S.; Walker, A.S.; Robotham, J.V.; et al. The challenge of antimicrobial resistance: What economics can contribute. *Science* **2019**, *364*, eaau4679. [CrossRef] [PubMed]
43. Turner, B. Tackling antimicrobial resistance and climate change. *Lancet* **2018**, *392*, 2435–2436. [CrossRef]
44. Pearce, W.; Mahony, M.; Raman, S. Science advice for global challenges: Learning from trade-offs in the IPCC. *Environ. Sci. Policy* **2018**, *80*, 125–131. [CrossRef]
45. MacFadden, D.R.; McGough, S.F.; Fisman, D.; Santillana, M.; Brownstein, J.S. Antibiotic Resistance Increases with Local Temperature. *Nat. Clim. Chang.* **2018**, *8*, 510–514. [CrossRef]
46. Frederick, S.; Loewenstein, G.; O'donoghue, T. Time discounting and time preference: A critical review. *J. Econ. Lit.* **2002**, *40*, 351–401. [CrossRef]
47. The Lancet Respiratory, M. Antimicrobial resistance-what can we learn from climate change? *Lancet Respir. Med.* **2016**, *4*, 845. [CrossRef]
48. Woolhouse, M.; Ward, M.; van Bunnik, B.; Farrar, J. Antimicrobial resistance in humans, livestock and the wider environment. *Philos. Trans. R. Soc. Lond. Ser. B Biol. Sci.* **2015**, *370*, 20140083. [CrossRef] [PubMed]
49. Woolhouse, M.E.; Ward, M.J. Microbiology. Sources of antimicrobial resistance. *Science* **2013**, *341*, 1460–1461. [CrossRef] [PubMed]
50. Rodríguez-Verdugo, A.; Lozano-Huntelman, N.; Cruz-Loya, M.; Savage, V.; Yeh, P. Compounding Effects of Climate Warming and Antibiotic Resistance. *iScience* **2020**, *23*, 101024. [CrossRef]
51. Andersson, D.I.; Hughes, D. Microbiological effects of sublethal levels of antibiotics. *Nat. Rev. Microbiol.* **2014**, *12*, 465–478. [CrossRef]
52. Costello, A.; Abbas, M.; Allen, A.; Ball, S.; Bell, S.; Bellamy, R.; Friel, S.; Groce, N.; Johnson, A.; Kett, M.; et al. Managing the health effects of climate change: Lancet and University College London Institute for Global Health Commission. *Lancet* **2009**, *373*, 1693–1733. [CrossRef]
53. One Health Initiative. About the One Health Intiative. Available online: http://www.onehealthinitiative.com/about.php (accessed on 2 March 2020).
54. Centers for Disease Control and Prevention. One Health Basics. Available online: https://www.cdc.gov/onehealth/basics/index.html?CDC_AA_refVal=https%3A%2F%2Fwww.cdc.gov%2Fonehealth%2Fabout.html (accessed on 2 March 2020).
55. Chen, Z.L.; Zhang, Q.; Lu, Y.; Guo, Z.M.; Zhang, X.; Zhang, W.J.; Guo, C.; Liao, C.H.; Li, Q.L.; Han, X.H.; et al. Distribution of the COVID-19 epidemic and correlation with population emigration from Wuhan, China. *Chin. Med. J.* **2020**, *133*, 1044–1050. [CrossRef]
56. Cleaveland, S.; Sharp, J.; Abela-Ridder, B.; Allan, K.J.; Buza, J.; Crump, J.A.; Davis, A.; Del Rio Vilas, V.J.; de Glanville, W.A.; Kazwala, R.R.; et al. One Health contributions towards more effective and equitable approaches to health in low- and middle-income countries. *Philos. Trans. R. Soc. Lond. B Biol. Sci.* **2017**, *372*, 20160168. [CrossRef]
57. Dean, A.S.; Crump, L.; Greter, H.; Schelling, E.; Zinsstag, J. Global burden of human brucellosis: A systematic review of disease frequency. *PLoS Negl. Trop. Dis.* **2012**, *6*, e1865. [CrossRef]
58. Allan, K.J.; Biggs, H.M.; Halliday, J.E.; Kazwala, R.R.; Maro, V.P.; Cleaveland, S.; Crump, J.A. Epidemiology of Leptospirosis in Africa: A Systematic Review of a Neglected Zoonosis and a Paradigm for 'One Health' in Africa. *PLoS Negl. Trop. Dis.* **2015**, *9*, e0003899. [CrossRef] [PubMed]
59. Phelan, A.L.; Gostin, L.O. Law as a fixture between the One Health interfaces of emerging diseases. *Trans. R. Soc. Trop. Med. Hyg.* **2017**, *111*, 241–243. [CrossRef] [PubMed]

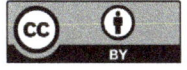

© 2020 by the authors. Licensee MDPI, Basel, Switzerland. This article is an open access article distributed under the terms and conditions of the Creative Commons Attribution (CC BY) license (http://creativecommons.org/licenses/by/4.0/).

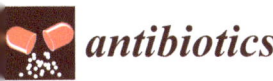

Perspective

Should the Increased Awareness of the One Health Approach Brought by the COVID-19 Pandemic Be Used to Further Tackle the Challenge of Antimicrobial Resistance?

Mohamed Rhouma [1,2,*], Michelle Tessier [2,3], Cécile Aenishaenslin [1,2,4], Pascal Sanders [5] and Hélène Carabin [1,2,4]

1. Department of Pathology and Microbiology, Faculty of Veterinary Medicine, Université de Montréal, 3200 Sicotte, Saint-Hyacinthe, QC J2S 2M2, Canada; cecile.aenishaenslin@umontreal.ca (C.A.); helene.carabin@umontreal.ca (H.C.)
2. Groupe de Recherche en Épidémiologie des Zoonoses et Santé Publique, Université de Montréal, 3200 Sicotte, Saint-Hyacinthe, QC J2S 2M2, Canada; michelle.tessier@canada.ca
3. Public Health Agency of Canada, 3200 Sicotte, Saint-Hyacinthe, QC J2S 2M2, Canada
4. Centre de Recherche en Santé Publique de l'Université de Montréal et du CIUSSS du Centre-Sud-de-l'Île-de-Montréal, Montréal, Québec, QC H3N 1X9, Canada
5. Laboratory of Fougères, French Agency for Food, Environmental and Occupational Health & Safety, ANSES, 35306 Fougères, France; pascal.sanders@anses.fr
* Correspondence: mohamed.rhouma@umontreal.ca; Tel.: +1-(450)-7738521 (ext. 52416)

Abstract: Several experts have expressed their concerns regarding the potential increase in antimicrobial resistance (AMR) during the COVID-19 pandemic as a consequence of the increase in antimicrobial and biocide use in humans globally. However, the impact of the pandemic on antimicrobial use (AMU) and AMR in animals has yet to be discussed and evaluated. Indeed, veterinary practices have been hugely impacted by the pandemic and its restrictive measures around the world. In this perspective, we call for more research to estimate the impact of COVID-19 on AMU and AMR in both humans and animals, as well as on the environment, in coherence with the One Health approach. In addition, we argue that the current pandemic is an opportunity to accelerate the implementation of a One Health approach to tackle the AMR crisis at the global scale. Indeed, the momentum created by the increased general awareness of both the public and decision-makers for the development and maintenance of effective drugs to treat human infections, as well as for the importance of a One Health approach to prevent the emergence of infectious diseases, should be used as a lever to implement global collaborative and sustainable solutions to the complex challenges of AMR.

Keywords: antimicrobial use; antimicrobial resistance; COVID-19; SARS-CoV-2; farm animals; one health

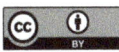

1. Introduction

When first identified in December 2019, in Wuhan (Hubei, China), coronavirus disease 2019 (COVID-19), caused by the severe acute respiratory syndrome coronavirus 2 (SARS-CoV-2), was described as a mystery viral pneumonia outbreak [1]. A few months after, the World Health Organization (WHO) declared a global pandemic on 11 March 2020. The uncertainties surrounding the severity, mortality, treatment, transmission dynamics, risk factors, individual and herd immunity of this new global threat led some to qualify it as one of "unknown unknowns" [2]. As of March 2021, there is still no solid evidence about the effectiveness of existing antivirals or other drugs for the treatment of COVID-19, nor is there any long term study about the duration of protective immunity after infection with SARS-CoV-2 or following vaccination against the disease [3]. Moreover, the recent emergence of SARS-CoV-2 variants, which could escape naturally in induced or vaccine-induced immunity, is a current global concern [4].

Multiple countries experienced multiple waves of cases and hospitalizations, pushing authorities to implement strict public health measures. This unprecedented global health issue is exerting a colossal pressure on scientists and physicians to develop and use therapeutic and prophylactic strategies to counter the severe consequences of this infection, so that societies can return to some form of normality and the economy can be restarted. Increasing evidence suggests that this context has resulted in an increase in both AMU and AMR in humans, followed by an increase in AMR bacteria shed into the environment [5–7]. It is noteworthy that AMR is a complex issue affecting the health of humans, animals and the environment on a global scale. Thereby, addressing this problem requires a coordinated multisectoral and multidisciplinary approach, such as the One Health approach [8,9]. This approach recognizes that human health and animal health are interconnected and linked to their shared environment [8]. According to the WHO, the areas of interest in which a One Health approach is particularly relevant include food safety and the control of both zoonoses and AMR [10].

In this perspective we: (i) give an overview of the trends in AMU during this pandemic and its consequences on humans and the environment; (ii) explore the potential consequences of the pandemic on AMU/AMR in veterinary medicine; and (iii) explain how the pandemic is an opportunity to strengthen the One Health approach for AMR prevention and control.

2. Impact of the COVID-19 Pandemic on Antimicrobial Use and Antimicrobial Resistance in Humans and in the Environment

In May 2016, an independent review on AMR reported that AMR infections in humans were estimated to cause at least 700,000 deaths per year and this number is projected to increase up to 10 million deaths per year by 2050 globally, overtaking the number of people dying from cancer (8.2 million each year) [11]. In the United States, it is estimated that each year at least 2.8 million people get an antibiotic-resistant infection, and that more than 35,000 people die as a consequence of these resistant infections [12]. The Council of Canadian Academies estimated that AMR had caused 5400 human deaths (almost 15 human death per day) in Canada and cost the Canadian healthcare system nearly CAD 1.4 billion in 2018 [13]. On the other hand, many publications reported that the majority of hospitalized patients with COVID-19 were treated with antimicrobials, mostly to prevent or to treat secondary bacterial and fungal infections, despite a low proportion of these coinfections [14–16]. Indeed, Chen et al. have reported that around 71% of the hospitalized COVID-19 patients, admitted at Jinyintan Hospital in Wuhan (China) from 1 January to 20 January 2020, had received antimicrobial drugs (cephalosporins, quinolones, carbapenems, tigecycline, linezolid, and antifungal drugs), while only 1% and 4% demonstrated secondary bacterial or fungal coinfections, respectively [14]. Moreover, in a large multicenter Chinese study, 58% of patients admitted to hospitals as of 29 January 2020, received intravenous antimicrobials (without specification regarding the molecules used) [16]. Moreover, Wu et al. reported that, in three hospitals of Jiangsu Province, China (from 22 January to 14 February 2020), all patients were treated empirically with a single antibiotic, mainly moxifloxacin, for a period of 3 to 12 days (median 7 days) [15]. In addition, an international survey, performed in April 2020 amongst 166 participants from 23 countries and 82 different hospitals, suggested that broad-spectrum antimicrobials were commonly used in patients with COVID-19 [7]. Rawson et al. performed a review of the medical literature published between 1 January 2020, and 18 April 2020, to explore commonly reported bacterial/fungal coinfections in patients admitted to hospitals with lower respiratory tract infections associated with coronavirus [6]. The results of this review showed that the use of broad-spectrum antimicrobial therapy was widely reported, with 72% of COVID-19 cases receiving antibacterial therapy, while only 8% of the patients were reported as experiencing bacterial/fungal coinfections [6]. As such, prescribing of antimicrobials is significantly higher than the prevalence of bacterial/fungal coinfections, suggesting an empirical use of antimicrobials in patients with COVID-19, and such practice could increase the emergence of multidrug-resistant microorganisms as well as the development of other microbial infections (e.g., *Clostridioides difficile* infection) [17,18]. Consequently, in July 2020, the WHO warned of the risk of AMR spread as well as an impairment to antimicrobial stewardship as a result of the misuse of antimicrobials during this pandemic [19]. While some studies, mostly from Asia and the United States, have shown evidence about the negative impact of COVID-19 on AMR, other studies from France and Spain did not show an increase in infections with multidrug-resistant bacteria during the COVID-19 pandemic [20]. This conflicting evidence highlights that the impact of the pandemic on AMR in humans remains largely unknown, thereby more research is needed to better estimate the consequences of the unnecessary use, in just a few months, of high levels of antimicrobials on AMR development and spread worldwide.

In addition, considerable amounts of these antimicrobials could reach the environment in their active forms and might exert selection for resistant bacteria [21,22]. Moreover, the use of sanitizers and other biocidal agents (e.g., quaternary ammonium compounds (QACs), hydrogen peroxide, sodium hypochlorite, peroxyacetic acid, chlorine dioxide) has dramatically increased during the COVID-19 pandemic [23], hand hygiene and surface disinfection being among the most important preventative measures used globally to reduce SARS-CoV-2 transmission. Antimicrobial soaps and disinfectant cleaners could contaminate the environment, mostly through wastewater, in high concentrations and could select for AMR microorganisms [23–25]. Indeed, cross-resistance to clinically used antimicrobials has occurred following bacterial exposure and adaptation to some biocides [26]. It should be noted that quaternary ammonium compounds (QACs) constitute the highest percentage of biocidal agents in EPA approved disinfectant products for COVID-19 disinfection [27]. Many studies reported a cross-resistance to QACs and antimicrobials in *E. coli*, *Salmonella* and *Pseudomonas* strains [28,29]. In fact, a subinhibitory concentrations of some QACs (e.g., benzalkonium chloride (BAC), didecyl dimethyl ammonium chloride (DDAC)) can select for bacteria resistant to medically important antibiotics such as ampicillin, cefotaxime, ceftazidime, ciprofloxacin and colistin [28,29]. Moreover, it was reported that the exposure of *Pseudomonas aeruginosa* isolates to increasing concentrations of BAC selected for mutations in the polymyxin resistance (*pmrB*) gene, as well as for some physiological adaptations (including an overexpression of *mexCD-oprJ* multidrug efflux pump genes), contributing to a higher tolerance to polymyxin B and to other antimicrobials (e.g., ciprofloxacin, chloramphenicol, and rifampin) [30]. Common mechanisms such as bacterial membrane alterations and upregulation of efflux pumps are the most documented mechanisms responsible for bacterial cross-resistance to biocides and antimicrobials [26,31]. In addition, the use of these household cleaners, disinfectants, and sanitizers may be implemented globally for a prolonged time even beyond the COVID-19 pandemic, due to the change in world population's behavior regarding hygiene, and such use could exert further selection for resistant bacteria to both antimicrobials and biocides.

3. Potential Impact of the COVID-19 Pandemic on Antimicrobial Use and Antimicrobial Resistance in Food-Producing Animals

In farm animals, antimicrobials are used therapeutically (to treat clinically sick animals) for prophylaxis (to healthy animals at risk of infection), for metaphylaxis (to prevent infection among healthy animals in contact with infected animals), and some are still used for growth promoting purposes [9,32]. In 2010, the global antibiotic consumption in the livestock sector was estimated at 63,151 tons, with some models suggesting that it could increase by 67% to reach 105,596 tons by 2030 [33]. In the United States, antimicrobial use in farm animals was estimated to account for 80% of the nation's annual antimicrobial consumption in 2010 [33]. The Public Health Agency of Canada estimated in 2018 that the livestock sector accounts for 79% of the total antimicrobial use in Canada [34]. It is noteworthy that of the 41 antimicrobials (including ionophores) that are approved for used in food-producing animals by the Food and Drug Administration (FDA), 31 are categorized as being medically important for human use [11]. While there is mounting evidence of a link between the preventative/growth promotion use of antimicrobials in animal production and the occurrence of AMR bacteria in humans and in animals [32,35,36], the relative contribution, in this issue, of AMU in farm animals remains unknown [37]. Despite this uncertainty, considerable efforts have been made in veterinary medicine to limit the spread of AMR bacteria and to preserve the effectiveness of antimicrobials [38–40]. Research on alternatives to the use of preventative antimicrobials in farm animals has increased in the recent years [41], especially following the ban of several classes of antimicrobials as growth promoters in several countries [38].

The impact of the COVID-19 pandemic on the global efforts to control AMU and AMR in animals is unknown. The following factors could have contributed to an increase in AMU and ultimately an increase in AMR. First, veterinary services were not considered essential in several countries implementing lockdowns, at least during the first wave of the pandemic, and consequently veterinarians were not able to offer preventative care, including vaccination, to their clients (farmers, pet owners, etc.). This could have resulted in animals developing infections which would normally be prevented and hence an increase in AMU in animal production. Second, the unavailability of veterinary services, particularly during the first lockdown, could increase self-medication as well as off-label use of antimicrobials on farms. Furthermore, the pandemic has also resulted in instances where animals were kept on farms for longer than usual due to large outbreaks in slaughterhouses and the disruption of inter-regional and international transportation. This situation might lead to an increase in AMU in animal production as a consequence of the increase in animal density on farms, which could facilitate the spread of infectious diseases. In addition, all research and development activities of alternatives to antimicrobials and vaccines in animals could be disrupted worldwide during this pandemic, which could create more pressure on the AMU in animals in the long term.

On the other hand, the pandemic may have also resulted in a decrease in AMU in farm animals. Indeed, access to antimicrobials (or their molecules or ingredients) could have been disrupted by commerce and transport limitations. Moreover, the pandemic may have caused a breach in surveillance for AMU and AMR in food systems globally. For example, in several countries (Canada and France, for example), the majority of animal health laboratories were redirected towards COVID-19 diagnoses in support of the public health laboratories. Food safety regulatory agencies also faced a huge challenge related to staff shortages, resulting in a reorientation of the inspection and the sampling activities towards certain sectors (e.g., meat processing plants), rather than sampling for AMR monitoring, to avoid further overloading of the human health systems with foodborne infections. Sampling along the food chain (on farms, at slaughterhouses, and from retail meats) and the analysis for the surveillance of AMR for some foodborne pathogenic bacteria (e.g., *Salmonella*, *Campylobacter*, *E. coli*) were greatly altered by the pandemic and particularly during the first lockdown. The extent to which the pandemic led to an increase or a decrease in AMU and ultimately its impact on AMR in animal populations should be urgently assessed in future studies.

4. Lessons Learned from the COVID-19 Pandemic to Strengthen the One Health Approach for the Control of Antimicrobial Resistance

By the end of February 2021, more than 100 million people had been diagnosed with SARS-CoV-2 and 2.5 million people had died of the disease it causes globally [42]. The ongoing pandemic constantly reminds the public of the importance of hand-washing and there has been a growing interest in vaccination against influenza and pneumococcal disease, which, in combination with the current efforts to social distance and wear masks, will likely decrease the spread of other airborne infections [43]. Moreover, to prevent COVID-19 contamination, several interesting communication tools (e.g., brochures, flyers, advertising spot) have been developed by health authorities around the world in order to educate, while simplifying the information, all citizens, even those in the most remote regions of the planet, so they adhere to some precautionary COVID-19 measures (e.g., wearing a face mask, social distancing). This has been accompanied by important media coverage, investigations and interviews with experts regarding emerging infections, zoonoses, public health and the One Health approach. Such communication tools are also very relevant to raise awareness regarding AMU and AMR at the human–animal–environment interface. In fact, awareness campaigns on AMR through effective education and communication constitute the first goal of the WHO Global Action Plan on Antimicrobial Resistance [44]. In the current context, all humanity is very aware of the importance of having effective drugs to treat microbial infections and also the necessity to protect their effectiveness through time. This aspect is much more important in the current context of AMR, where multidrug-resistant bacteria have spread widely and the number of brand new drugs placed on the market is drastically decreasing. Indeed, the last new class of antimicrobial discovered is daptomycin (1986), which was only approved in 2003 by the US Food and Drug Administration (FDA), showing that antimicrobial agents found on the market in the last 30 years are associations or redevelopments of classic antimicrobials [45]. Thereby, it is the responsibility of all stakeholders involved in AMU (e.g., physicians, pharmacists, patients, veterinarians, agronomists, farmers and regulatory agencies) to develop various strategies ensuring the responsible use of antimicrobials in order to protect their effectiveness for as long as possible.

Environmental changes and ecosystem degradation across the planet (e.g., deforestation, intensified agriculture and livestock production, illegal and poorly regulated wildlife trade) increased the frequency of contacts between wild animals, domestic animals and humans, contributing to a zoonotic transfer of diseases [46]. Thereby, the COVID-19 pandemic is bringing to light the importance of protecting the environment and the ecosystem, which is of paramount importance in the context of AMR management. Indeed, there is growing evidence that the environment plays an important role in the transmission of AMR bacteria and/or AMR genes to humans and livestock in addition to serving as a reservoir of AMR microorganisms. For example, *Shewanella algae*, an environmental species from marine and fresh water, was identified as a reservoir of plasmid-mediated quinolone resistance (QnrA) in *Enterobacteriaceae* [47]. Cabello et al. suggested that mobile colistin resistance (*mcr*) genes may have originated in aquatic environments as a result of aquaculture activities, and these genes could have earned terrestrial bacteria by horizontal gene transfer to yield colistin-resistant bacteria in humans and animals [48]. It should be stressed here that the United Nations Environment Programme (UNEP) ranked environmental AMR first among the six emerging issues of concern (environmental dimensions of AMR, nanomaterials, protected marine areas, sand and dust storms, off-grid solar solutions, and environmental displacement) [49]. It is therefore essential to establish science-based standards regarding the acceptable antimicrobial concentrations (and AMR genes) in soil (manured or not), in aquaculture, in farm and hospital environments as well as in manufacturing effluents in order to better inform and involve policy-makers in the management of this issue [50].

Finally, by joining the few episodes of infectious diseases that have deeply shaped human history, the COVID-19 pandemic had succeeded, in an unprecedented way, in increasing awareness of both the public and decision-makers regarding the development and maintenance of effective drugs to treat human infections as well as for the importance of the One Health approach to prevent the emergence of infectious diseases. We believe that these prerequisites should be used as a lever to accelerate both the development of global collaborations and the implementation of sustainable solutions for the management of the current AMR crisis.

5. Conclusions

Antimicrobial resistance is a cross-sectoral complex problem affecting the health of humans, animals and the environment. We strongly believe that COVID-19 pandemic has generated a powerful incentive and momentum to address the AMR crisis by accelerating collaborations and interdisciplinary communication between concerned stakeholders (e.g., researchers, physicians, veterinarians, pharmacists, farmers, other health and environmental professionals, public and policy-makers), while taking into account the specificity of each sector during and beyond this pandemic. More research and retrospective analysis of surveillance data are needed in both humans and animals as well as in the environment to estimate the impact of COVID-19 on AMU and AMR in coherence with the One Health approach. One of the lessons of the COVID-19 pandemic is that acting too late carries serious costs to both health and the economy. Thereby, the colossal budgets allocated to human medicine worldwide for the control of this pandemic should not compromise efforts conducted to manage the current AMR crisis at the human–animal–environment interface. We stress here the paramount importance of the One Health approach to face the increasing threat of AMR, and we believe that this pandemic could be an excellent opportunity to accelerate its implementation for an effective surveillance, prevention and control of AMR at the global scale.

Author Contributions: M.R. conceived and designed the topic of interest and wrote the first draft of the manuscript. M.T. and H.C. designed the study and revised the paper. C.A. and P.S. critically revised the paper. All authors have read and agreed to the published version of the manuscript.

Funding: This research received no external funding.

Acknowledgments: The authors would like to thank the Groupe de recherche en épidémiologie des zoonoses et santé publique (Grezosp) for the financial support that allowed the publication of this perspective.

Conflicts of Interest: The authors declare no conflict of interest.

References

1. Dong, E.; Du, H.; Gardner, L. An interactive web-based dashboard to track COVID-19 in real time. *Lancet Infect. Dis.* **2020**, *20*, 533–534. [CrossRef]
2. Grech, V. Unknown unknowns—COVID-19 and potential global mortality. *Early Hum. Dev.* **2020**, *144*, 105026. [CrossRef] [PubMed]
3. Sette, A.; Crotty, S. Adaptive immunity to SARS-CoV-2 and COVID-19. *Cell* **2021**, *184*, 861–880. [CrossRef] [PubMed]
4. Garcia-Beltran, W.F.; Lam, E.C.; Denis, K.S.; Nitido, A.D.; Garcia, Z.H.; Hauser, B.M.; Feldman, J.; Pavlovic, M.N.; Gregory, D.J.; Poznansky, M.C. Multiple SARS-CoV-2 variants escape neutralization by vaccine-induced humoral immunity. *Cell* **2021**, *184*, 1–12.
5. Cox, M.J.; Loman, N.; Bogaert, D.; O'grady, J. Co-infections: Potentially lethal and unexplored in COVID-19. *Lancet Microbe* **2020**, *1*, e11. [CrossRef]
6. Rawson, T.M.; Moore, L.S.; Zhu, N.; Ranganathan, N.; Skolimowska, K.; Gilchrist, M.; Satta, G.; Cooke, G.; Holmes, A. Bacterial and fungal co-infection in individuals with coronavirus: A rapid review to support COVID-19 antimicrobial prescribing. *Clin. Infect. Dis.* **2020**, *71*, 2459–2468.
7. Beović, B.; Doušak, M.; Ferreira-Coimbra, J.; Nadrah, K.; Rubulotta, F.; Belliato, M.; Berger-Estilita, J.; Ayoade, F.; Rello, J.; Erdem, H. Antibiotic use in patients with COVID-19: A 'snapshot'Infectious Diseases International Research Initiative (ID-IRI) survey. *J. Antimicrob. Chemother.* **2020**, *75*, 3386–3390. [CrossRef]
8. Hernando-Amado, S.; Coque, T.M.; Baquero, F.; Martínez, J.L. Defining and combating antibiotic resistance from One Health and Global Health perspectives. *Nat. Microbiol.* **2019**, *4*, 1432–1442. [CrossRef] [PubMed]
9. Collignon, P.J.; McEwen, S.A. One health—Its importance in helping to better control antimicrobial resistance. *Trop. Med. Infect. Dis.* **2019**, *4*, 22. [CrossRef]
10. World Health Organization. One Health. Available online: https://www.who.int/news-room/q-a-detail/one-health (accessed on 14 April 2021).
11. O'Neill, J. Review on Antimicrobial Resistance. Tackling Drug-Resistant Infections Globally: Final Report and Recommendations. Available online: https://amr-review.org/ (accessed on 15 February 2021).
12. Centers for Disease Control and Prevention (CDC). Antibiotic/Antimicrobial Resistance (AR/AMR). Available online: https://www.cdc.gov/drugresistance/ (accessed on 18 January 2021).
13. Finlay, B.B.; Conly, J.; Coyte, P.C.; Dillon, J.-A.R.; Douglas, G.; Goddard, E.; Greco, L.; Nicolle, L.E.; Patrick, D.; Prescott, J.F. When Antibiotics Fail: The Expert Panel on the Potential Socio-Economic Impacts of Antimicrobial Resistance in Canada. Available online: https://cca-reports.ca/reports/the-potential-socio-economic-impacts-of-antimicrobial-resistance-in-canada/ (accessed on 15 February 2021).
14. Chen, N.; Zhou, M.; Dong, X.; Qu, J.; Gong, F.; Han, Y.; Qiu, Y.; Wang, J.; Liu, Y.; Wei, Y. Epidemiological and clinical characteristics of 99 cases of 2019 novel coronavirus pneumonia in Wuhan, China: A descriptive study. *Lancet* **2020**, *395*, 507–513. [CrossRef]
15. Wu, J.; Liu, J.; Zhao, X.; Liu, C.; Wang, W.; Wang, D.; Xu, W.; Zhang, C.; Yu, J.; Jiang, B.; et al. Clinical Characteristics of Imported Cases of Coronavirus Disease 2019 (COVID-19) in Jiangsu Province: A Multicenter Descriptive Study. *Clin. Infect. Dis.* **2020**, *71*, 706–712. [CrossRef] [PubMed]
16. Guan, W.-J.; Ni, Z.-Y.; Hu, Y.; Liang, W.-H.; Ou, C.-Q.; He, J.-X.; Liu, L.; Shan, H.; Lei, C.-L.; Hui, D.S. Clinical characteristics of coronavirus disease 2019 in China. *N. Engl. J. Med.* **2020**, *382*, 1708–1720. [CrossRef] [PubMed]

7. Sandhu, A.; Tillotson, G.; Polistico, J.; Salimnia, H.; Cranis, M.; Moshos, J.; Cullen, L.; Jabbo, L.; Diebel, L.; Chopra, T. Clostridioides difficile in COVID-19 patients, Detroit, Michigan, USA, March–April 2020. *Emerg. Infect. Dis.* **2020**, *26*, 2272. [CrossRef]
8. Langford, B.J.; So, M.; Raybardhan, S.; Leung, V.; Soucy, J.-P.R.; Westwood, D.; Daneman, N.; MacFadden, D.R. Antibiotic prescribing in patients with COVID-19: Rapid review and meta-analysis. *Clin. Microbiol. Infect.* **2021**, *27*, 520–531. [CrossRef] [PubMed]
9. Getahun, H.; Smith, I.; Trivedi, K.; Paulin, S.; Balkhy, H.H. Tackling antimicrobial resistance in the COVID-19 pandemic. *Bull. World Health Organ.* **2020**, *98*, 442. [CrossRef]
10. Monnet, D.L.; Harbarth, S. Will coronavirus disease (COVID-19) have an impact on antimicrobial resistance? *Eurosurveillance* **2020**, *25*, 2001886. [CrossRef] [PubMed]
11. Vidovic, N.; Vidovic, S. Antimicrobial resistance and food animals: Influence of livestock environment on the emergence and dissemination of antimicrobial resistance. *Antibiotics (Basel)* **2020**, *9*, 52. [CrossRef]
12. Larouche, E.; Généreux, M.; Tremblay, M.-È.; Rhouma, M.; Gasser, M.-O.; Quessy, S.; Côté, C. Impact of liquid hog manure applications on antibiotic resistance genes concentration in soil and drainage water in field crops. *Can. J. Microbiol.* **2020**, *66*, 549–561. [CrossRef]
13. Murray, A.K. The novel coronavirus covid-19 outbreak: Global implications for antimicrobial resistance. *Front Microbiol.* **2020**, *11*, 1020. [CrossRef]
14. Usman, M.; Farooq, M.; Hanna, K. Environmental side effects of the injudicious use of antimicrobials in the era of COVID-19. *Sci. Total Environ.* **2020**, *745*, 141053. [CrossRef]
15. Rezasoltani, S.; Yadegar, A.; Hatami, B.; Aghdaei, H.A.; Zali, M.R. Antimicrobial Resistance as a Hidden Menace Lurking Behind the COVID-19 Outbreak: The Global Impacts of Too Much Hygiene on AMR. *Front. Microbiol.* **2020**, *11*, 590683. [CrossRef] [PubMed]
16. Rhouma, M.; Romero-Barrios, P.; Gaucher, M.-L.; Bhachoo, S. Antimicrobial resistance associated with the use of antimicrobial processing aids during poultry processing operations: Cause for concern? *Crit. Rev. Food Sci. Nutr.* **2020**, *12*, 1–18. [CrossRef] [PubMed]
17. EPA. List N Advanced Search Page: Disinfectants for Coronavirus (COVID-19). Available online: https://www.epa.gov/coronavirus/list-n-advanced-search-page-disinfectants-coronavirus-covid-19 (accessed on 15 April 2021).
18. Soumet, C.; Méheust, D.; Pissavin, C.; Le Grandois, P.; Frémaux, B.; Feurer, C.; Le Roux, A.; Denis, M.; Maris, P. Reduced susceptibilities to biocides and resistance to antibiotics in food-associated bacteria following exposure to quaternary ammonium compounds. *J. Appl. Microbiol.* **2016**, *121*, 1275–1281. [CrossRef] [PubMed]
19. Nasr, A.M.; Mostafa, M.S.; Arnaout, H.H.; Elshimy, A.A.A. The effect of exposure to sub-inhibitory concentrations of hypochlorite and quaternary ammonium compounds on antimicrobial susceptibility of *Pseudomonas aeruginosa*. *Am. J. Infect. Control* **2018**, *46*, e57–e63. [CrossRef] [PubMed]
20. Kim, M.; Weigand, M.R.; Oh, S.; Hatt, J.K.; Krishnan, R.; Tezel, U.; Pavlostathis, S.G.; Konstantinidis, K.T. Widely used benzalkonium chloride disinfectants can promote antibiotic resistance. *Appl. Environ. Microbiol.* **2018**, *84*. [CrossRef] [PubMed]
21. Chen, B.; Han, J.; Dai, H.; Jia, P. Biocide-tolerance and antibiotic-resistance in community environments and risk of direct transfers to humans: Unintended consequences of community-wide surface disinfecting during COVID-19? *Environ. Pollut.* **2021**, *283*, 117074. [CrossRef]
22. Olaitan, A.O.; Dandachi, I.; Baron, S.A.; Daoud, Z.; Morand, S.; Rolain, J.-M. Banning colistin in feed additives: A small step in the right direction. *Lancet Infect. Dis.* **2021**, *21*, 29–30. [CrossRef]
23. Van Boeckel, T.P.; Brower, C.; Gilbert, M.; Grenfell, B.T.; Levin, S.A.; Robinson, T.P.; Teillant, A.; Laxminarayan, R. Global trends in antimicrobial use in food animals. *Proc. Natl. Acad. Sci. USA* **2015**, *112*, 5649–5654. [CrossRef]
24. Public Health Agency of Canada. Canadian Antimicrobial Resistance Surveillance System—Update 2020. Available online: https://www.canada.ca/content/dam/hc-sc/documents/services/drugs-health-products/canadian-antimicrobial-resistance-surveillance-system-2020-report/CARSS-2020-report-2020-eng.pdf (accessed on 30 January 2021).
25. Tang, K.L.; Caffrey, N.P.; Nóbrega, D.B.; Cork, S.C.; Ronksley, P.E.; Barkema, H.W.; Polachek, A.J.; Ganshorn, H.; Sharma, N.; Kellner, J.D. Restricting the use of antibiotics in food-producing animals and its associations with antibiotic resistance in food-producing animals and human beings: A systematic review and meta-analysis. *Lancet Planet Health.* **2017**, *1*, e316–e327. [CrossRef]
26. Dutil, L.; Irwin, R.; Finley, R.; Ng, L.K.; Avery, B.; Boerlin, P.; Bourgault, A.-M.; Cole, L.; Daignault, D.; Desruisseau, A. Ceftiofur resistance in *Salmonella enterica* serovar Heidelberg from chicken meat and humans, Canada. *Emerg. Infect. Dis.* **2010**, *16*, 48. [CrossRef] [PubMed]
27. Robinson, T.P.; Wertheim, H.F.; Kakkar, M.; Kariuki, S.; Bu, D.; Price, L.B. Animal production and antimicrobial resistance in the clinic. *Lancet* **2016**, *387*, e1–e3. [CrossRef]
28. Laxminarayan, R.; Van Boeckel, T.; Frost, I.; Kariuki, S.; Khan, E.A.; Limmathurotsakul, D.; Larsson, D.J.; Levy-Hara, G.; Mendelson, M.; Outterson, K. The Lancet Infectious Diseases Commission on antimicrobial resistance: 6 years later. *Lancet Infect. Dis.* **2020**, *20*, e51–e60. [CrossRef]
29. Rhouma, M.; Beaudry, F.; Theriault, W.; Letellier, A. Colistin in pig production: Chemistry, mechanism of antibacterial action, microbial resistance emergence, and One Health perspectives. *Front Microbiol.* **2016**, *7*, 1789. [CrossRef]

40. Rhouma, M.; Beaudry, F.; Letellier, A. Resistance to colistin: What is the fate for this antibiotic in pig production? *Int. J. Antimicrob. Agents.* **2016**, *48*, 119–126. [CrossRef]
41. Rhouma, M.; Fairbrother, J.M.; Beaudry, F.; Letellier, A. Post weaning diarrhea in pigs: Risk factors and non-colistin-based control strategies. *Acta Vet. Scand.* **2017**, *59*, 31. [CrossRef]
42. World Health Organization. Coronavirus Disease (COVID-19) Dashboard. Available online: https://covid19.who.int/ (accessed on 25 January 2021).
43. Grech, V.; Borg, M. Influenza vaccination in the COVID-19 era. *Early Hum. Dev.* **2020**, *148*, 105116. [CrossRef] [PubMed]
44. World Health Organization. Global Action Plan on Antimicrobial Resistance. Available online: https://www.who.int/antimicrobial-resistance/global-action-plan/en/ (accessed on 29 January 2021).
45. Durand, G.A.; Raoult, D.; Dubourg, G. Antibiotic discovery: History, methods and perspectives. *Int. J. Antimicrob. Agents.* **2019**, *53*, 371–382. [CrossRef] [PubMed]
46. Everard, M.; Johnston, P.; Santillo, D.; Staddon, C. The role of ecosystems in mitigation and management of Covid-19 and other zoonoses. *Environ. Sci. Policy.* **2020**, *111*, 7–17. [CrossRef] [PubMed]
47. Poirel, L.; Rodriguez-Martinez, J.M.; Mammeri, H.; Liard, A.; Nordmann, P. Origin of plasmid-mediated quinolone resistance determinant QnrA. *Antimicrob. Agents Chemother.* **2005**, *49*, 3523–3525. [CrossRef] [PubMed]
48. Cabello, F.C.; Tomova, A.; Ivanova, L.; Godfrey, H.P. Aquaculture and *mcr* colistin resistance determinants. *mBio.* **2017**, *8*. [CrossRef]
49. United Nations Environment Programme (UNEP). Antimicrobial Resistance from Environmental Pollution among Biggest Emerging Health Threats, Says UN Environment. 2017. Available online: https://www.unenvironment.org/news-and-stories/press-release/antimicrobial-resistance-environmental-pollution-among-biggest (accessed on 30 January 2021).
50. Topp, E.; Larsson, D.J.; Miller, D.N.; Van den Eede, C.; Virta, M.P. Antimicrobial resistance and the environment: Assessment of advances, gaps and recommendations for agriculture, aquaculture and pharmaceutical manufacturing. *FEMS Microbiol. Ecol.* **2018**, *94*, fix185. [CrossRef] [PubMed]

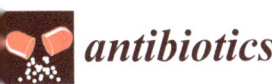

Article

Swedish Efforts to Contain Antibiotic Resistance in the Environment—A Qualitative Study among Selected Stakeholders

Ingeborg Björkman [1,*], Marta Röing [1], Jaran Eriksen [2,3] and Cecilia Stålsby Lundborg [4]

1. Department of Public Health and Caring Sciences, Health Services Research, Uppsala University, 751 22 Uppsala, Sweden; marta.roing@pubcare.uu.se
2. Department of Global Public Health, Karolinska Institutet, 171 77 Stockholm, Sweden; jaran.eriksen@ki.se
3. Department of Infectious Diseases/Venhalsan, Stockholm South General Hospital, 118 83 Stockholm, Sweden
4. Health Systems and Policy (HSP): Medicines, Focusing Antibiotics, Department of Global Public Health, Karolinska Institutet, Tomtebodavagen 18A, 171 77 Stockholm, Sweden; cecilia.stalsby.lundborg@ki.se
* Correspondence: ingeborg.bjorkman@nestorfou.se

Abstract: Antibiotic resistance is a serious global threat to human and animal health. In this study, we explored perceptions of work to contain antibiotic resistance with a focus on the environment. Nine stakeholders from six different areas were interviewed in 2018. A short information update was given by informants from four of the areas in 2021. Interview transcripts were analyzed by conventional content analysis. The stakeholders' perceptions were concluded in three categories: "examples of actions taken to combat antibiotic resistance", "factors influencing work", and "factors hindering work". All informants reported having a role to play. Some of them were very engaged in this issue, whereas among others, antibiotics and resistance were just one part of a general engagement. To be able to act, the policymaker stakeholders asked for more knowledge about antibiotics in the environment and possible actions to take. Actions from the government were requested by several informants. Coordination of the work to combat antibiotic resistance in the environment was not recognized and the One Health approach was known at policy level but not among practitioners. Still, actions seemed to be coordinated, but this was, according to the stakeholders, based on findings from research in their area rather than on strategies developed by national authorities.

Keywords: strategic action plan on antibiotic resistance; Swedish stakeholder perceptions; One Health; qualitative study

1. Introduction

Antibiotic resistance is a global threat to human and animal health [1,2]. The number of deaths at the global level associated with bacterial antimicrobial resistance in 2019 was estimated to 4.95 million [3]. The World Bank has described antibiotic resistance as a major threat to the world economy [4]. Antibiotic resistance can affect multiple sectors in society, as resistant bacteria can be transmitted between humans, animals, and the environment. Coordinated action has been suggested as a means of combating the threat of antibiotic resistance [5]. In 2015, the World Health Organization (WHO) published a Global Action Plan (GAP) based on a "One Health" approach [6]. The GAP set out five strategic objectives and stressed coordination between sectors and actors [6]. Member states were expected to develop and implement national action plans aligned with the GAP objectives [7]. The commitment of actors and stakeholders, for instance government authorities, policy makers, healthcare workers, university teachers, pharmaceutical companies and consumers, is essential [5], as well as multisectoral involvement, including human and animal health, together with the environment, trade, intellectual property, and innovation [8].

The Swedish government published its first action plan in 2016 [9]. When presented, it was based on a One Health approach, and had the overarching goal "To preserve the possibility of effective treatment of bacterial infections in people and animals". A quotation from the foreword reads, "It is a top priority for Sweden that the action plan is put into practice". This action plan was updated in 2020 [10]. Some years before the first action plan, in 2012, a national intersectoral coordinating platform was established to coordinate the work of national government agencies [9]. At that time, 21 government agencies were included in the platform [9], and some years later the number of government agencies involved was 25 [10].

This study is part of the ABRCARRO (A One Health Systems and Policy Approach to Antibiotic Resistance Containment: Coordination, Accountability, Resourcing, Regulation and Ownership)—an international project which aims to explore and describe how national action plans against antibiotic resistance were developed, implemented, monitored, and evaluated in Sweden, South Africa, and Swaziland. The project includes interviews with different categories of stakeholders, policymakers at government level, and professionals in human, animal, and environment/agriculture sectors, as well as policy document analyses. In this paper, we explore efforts to contain antibiotic resistance in the environment in Sweden.

Studying how actors and organizations work to contain the spread and development of antibiotic resistance in the environment is challenging. To begin with, it is known that the use of antibiotics has accelerated the development and spread of resistance in microbial populations [11]. However, the understanding of the role of the environment in the development and spread of antibiotic resistance is still limited [12]. At first, the role of the environment was recognized as a pathway for the spread of antibiotic resistance [5]. Later studies suggested that the environment is also involved in the development of antibiotic resistance [11,12]. Residual concentrations of antibiotics and resistant bacteria from human waste, animal waste, and manufacturing waste may end up in the environment [13]. Studies suggest that lakes can harbor antibiotic resistance genes, and also genes responsible for mobilization of genetic material [14].

Secondly, the problem of working to contain antibiotic resistance in the environment is multifaceted in such a way that multiple sectors must be involved to have some sort of impact. To reach effectiveness, organizations and actors generally not linked to each other most probably need to work together for the same goal. Research on how this can be experienced is sparse. Thus far, knowledge of actual Swedish efforts to contain antibiotic resistance in the environment, and how they are perceived, is limited. Further exploration is needed.

The aim of the present study was to explore and describe how informants working on environmental issues in a strategic selection of health and public sectors in Sweden perceive their own work, as well as other work in Sweden, to contain antibiotic resistance in the environment.

2. Method

2.1. Design

According to the explorative approach of the topic, a qualitative research design based on interviews was chosen [15,16]. By asking open-ended questions and letting the informant speak freely about the topic, data were collected as text, i.e., transcripts of the interviews. A content analysis approach was then chosen in the analysis and presentation of the findings of the transcribed interview texts. We used conventional content analysis with no predefined categories [17].

2.2. Informants

Our aim was to include informants involved in work to contain antibiotic resistance in the environment. We therefore approached individuals working at six strategically selected health and public service areas, see Table 1. Exploring their involvement and contributions can give insight into this work from their perspective, impart knowledge of the current situation in their area, and indicate directions for future efforts. Representatives from these selected areas were contacted by email and asked to participate. All approached persons accepted. In one case, the pharmaceutical company employee, the person first had to ask management for permission to take part in the interview. However, one informant withdrew the interview some years later. This was when the informant was asked to provide an update of the information (see below), explaining that they had no time to present an update and therefore chose not to participate at all.

Table 1. The informants and the rational for choosing the selected area of work.

Health and Public Service Area	Informants	Rational for Choice of Selected Area
Government authority	One analyst working at the Swedish Environmental Protection Agency	According to the agreement taken in the WHO, national governments should develop national action plans to combat antibiotic resistance. In Sweden, a national action plan was ready in 2016, and updated in 2020 [9,10]. Even so, written strategies must be put into practice, and authorities have an important role to stimulate action on behalf of the government.
Microbiology research	One researcher in medical microbiology and genetics	There is a need for new knowledge to understand the role of the environment in antibiotic resistance development and spread. Research in multiple fields is necessary, and one of the fields is medical microbiology and genetics. The focus of this researcher was basic research on how resistant genetic material is transmitted.
Pharmaceutical companies	One pharmaceutical company representative working in the company's medical department	The pharmaceutical industry plays an active role in research, discovery, and development of new drugs and medicines. It also has impact on production methods, and on the availability of drugs and medications on the market.
Pharmacies	Two pharmacy representatives responsible for quality management in their respective pharmacy chain	Consumers of antibiotics purchase their medications at a pharmacy. In addition to dispensing medications prescribed by physicians, pharmacists and pharmacy technicians can influence how consumers manage medications they purchase at the pharmacy. Another role for pharmacies is to collect consumer medical leftovers.
Hospitals	One environmental scientist working in a regional environmental department, responsible for environmental issues in hospitalsOne hospital environment department head.	Hospitals are major users of antibiotics and preventing pollution from hospitals seems to be essential. Patients in hospitals suffer from more complicated infections and are often treated with multiple and or broad-spectrum antibiotics. Many antibiotics used by hospital patients leave the body unmetabolized and end up in the wastewater.
Wastewater treatment	Two water treatment plant representatives responsible for municipal water quality control in two major Swedish cities	Wastewater plants are receivers of city wastewater, and their role is to remove undesirable chemicals and microorganisms, or reduce their concentration, so that water becomes clean enough to be released into the environment. They also treat sludge from wastewater, which after treatment is often used in agriculture.

2.3. Data Collection

A semi-structured interview guide was used, based on an interview guide previously used by the research group when studying perceptions of antibiotic resistance work in the human healthcare sector. Some questions were adapted to the purpose of the present study. The interview guide was first pilot tested on two informants working in the human and animal sectors, respectively. Results from these studies are presented elsewhere [18,19]. The main questions are presented in Table 2. The complete interview guide is available as Supplementary Material File S1.

Table 2. Interview guide, main questions.

1. What does antibiotic resistance mean to you?
2. How do you look upon your role in working to contain antibiotic resistance?
3. How do you look upon possibilities of limiting/preventing emergence and spread of antibiotic resistance?
4. What do you think are the main causes of antibiotic resistance?
5. How do you think antibiotic resistance spreads?
6. How do you look upon the use of antibiotics in humans, animals, or any other areas?
7. Have you heard of the concept of 'One Health'?
8. Do you have any comments to add?

During the interviews, informants spoke freely and shared their thoughts and understandings. The interviewer followed up with different probing questions, depending on what the informant was telling, for either more information or clarification. Author IB conducted the interviews during the period April to June 2018 at a place selected by the informant, usually at their workplace. The interviews lasted on average 47 min, with a range of 25 to 72 min. All interviews were tape recorded and transcribed verbatim by another person, and then the transcripts were checked and corrected, if necessary, by IB before the analysis process started.

2.4. Data Analysis

An inductive approach was used, with no predefined codes or categories. Author IB conducted the analysis, supported by author MR who acted as co-reader. The interviews were first read through to get an overview of the content. Next, interviews were read line by line and meaning units were picked out, given codes, and condensed. At this point each meaning unit and code was given an id-number to facilitate the analysis process. Meaning units were then sorted based on the codes, codes were merged and renamed in repeated steps, and codes that did not concern antibiotics or antibiotic resistance were taken away. Thereafter, all transcripts were sorted based on the new codes, and the content of each code was examined.

The codes were rearranged in subcategories and three main categories were chosen in a final step to organize and present the content of the interviews as follows: Informants' perceptions of actual efforts to contain antibiotic resistance in the environment, their perceptions of factors influencing their work, and factors hindering their work. All findings describe informants' perceptions.

2.5. Ethical Considerations

Ethical approval was sought from and granted by the Regional Ethics Board in Stockholm (Reg number: 2017/1999-31).

2.6. Contact with Informants in Autumn 2021 for Information Updating

Data collection took place in 2018 whereafter the interview material was analysed. However, the manuscript was not completed for a period of nearly four years. Thus, to be able to present current experiences, the authors felt that an update of the material would be of value. All informants were therefore contacted by email in the autumn of 2021. The aim was to obtain knowledge about the informants' experiences and engagement in efforts to contain antibiotic resistance, and if they differed or were similar as to the time of the first interview in 2018. To help recall what they had said at the first interview, each informant was shown the findings generated from their interview. The informants were asked three questions: (1) whether the informant or their organisation worked in the same way as they did in 2018, or if it had changed, and if so how; (2) whether the informant had noted any new function or organisation which coordinated work against antibiotic resistance development and spread in the environment; and (3) whether there were any changes in cooperation in the work to contain antibiotic resistance. The answers to the email questions are summarized at the end of the results section.

3. Findings

We present our findings in three main categories (Table 3). They are further described and illustrated by quotes from the interviews as follows.

Table 3. Main categories and subcategories describing the content of the interviews.

Categories	Subcategories	Area of Work Involved
Informants' examples of actions taken to combat antibiotic resistance	Monitoring and risk analysis	Government authorities
	Developing knowledge	Medical microbiological research Wastewater treatment
	Spreading knowledge	Medical microbiological research Pharmacies
	Reduce antibiotics and bacteria reaching the environment	Pharmacies Hospital environment department Wastewater treatment
	Activities for restrictive antibiotic use	Medical microbiological research Pharmaceutical companies Pharmacies Hospital environment department
Informants' perceptions of factors influencing work	Organisational and personal engagement Legislation, governance, and resources Cooperation and One Health	All areas of work contributed here.
Informants' perceptions of factors hindering work	Difficulties in setting environmental demands Lack of knowledge Lack of action Conflicting priorities	All areas of work contributed here.

3.1. Informants' Examples of Actions Taken to Combat Antibiotic Resistance

The informants talked about many different actions, which they thought could contribute to combat antibiotic resistance. These actions were identified as subcategories in our analysis. Due to the large differences in work areas involved, and for a better understanding of the contribution of each specific area, the following presentation of the content of this subcategory is sorted according to the informants' areas of work.

3.1.1. Actions Taken by Government Authority
Subcategories: Monitoring Environment Samples

The informant from the Environmental Protection Agency declared the agency had only recently become involved in this work and had so far found it difficult to find its role. The task of the agency was, according to the informant, to describe the state of the environment by sampling water, sediment, fish and wild animals, but antibiotics and antibiotic resistance were not a major issue.

> "This cooperation between agencies started a few years ago, it was around then that some people started to talk about it [...] and since then, it has grown [...] although just here it is really not a major question." (M2)

The informant gave examples of networks and platforms the agency was engaged in, both nationally, at EU level, and globally. According to this informant, antibiotics or antibiotic resistance were seldom the main focus in the environmental networks.

3.1.2. Actions Taken in Medical Microbiological Research
Subcategories: Developing Knowledge, Spreading Knowledge, Action for Restrictive Antibiotic Use

The medical research informant expressed explicit engagement in antibiotic resistance issues, and creating new knowledge in this field, for example, studying how genes are exchanged, and how resistance is spread through plasmids and viruses. We know that genes are spread by plasmids, the informant explained, and we do know that resistance can be transferred, but we do not know to what extent. The researcher informant furthermore described a role as a teacher at a medical school, teaching medical students to always think carefully before choosing infection treatment, and to always refrain from antibiotics when possible. To contain antibiotic resistance in the environment, as well in humans and animals, both safe use of antibiotics, and decreasing the use of antibiotics was required, stated the informant.

"I understand if you have, for example, a blood-poisoning and someone who is acutely ill, then I fully understand, it is clear then that antibiotics should be used I think, because then it is a matter of saving lives, it is the grey areas where I think you have to be more careful." (M9)

3.1.3. Actions Taken by Pharmaceutical Companies
Subcategory: Action for Restrictive Antibiotic Use

Safe antibiotic use, with narrow-spectrum antibiotics, and decreasing the use of antibiotics was brought up by the pharmaceutical company informant as ways to contain antibiotic resistance. It was therefore important to focus on keeping narrow-spectrum antibiotics commonly used in Sweden, as well as a wide assortment of dosage strengths and package sizes. According to this informant, individual adaption of antibiotics dispensed to patients, making sure the quantity of prescribed antibiotics does not exceed treatment duration, was fundamental for safe use and optimal antibiotic treatment.

"Our most important task is, right now, to maintain a large assortment and a wide range. Which is the basis for being able to eh, treat optimally and not drive resistance." (M10)

This informant noted that the company had been involved in starting up a multi-sectoral collaboration platform which gathered representatives from both healthcare and authorities, aiming to ensure access to antibiotics in Sweden. The company's interest here, the informant continued, was to enable discussions about which antibiotics the companies should fight to keep and develop, and which strengths and package sizes to focus on.

3.1.4. Actions Taken by Pharmacies
Subcategories: Action for Restrictive Antibiotic Use, Reduce Antibiotics and Bacteria Reaching the Environment, Spreading Knowledge

The pharmacy informants stated that decreasing the use of antibiotics, as well as safe use of antibiotics, were necessary to contain antibiotic resistance. Staff at pharmacies have a role here, informants said, and this was to provide patients packages of antibiotics adapted to their prescription, i.e., not give extra tablets that may be kept and used later for self-treatment, and by counselling patients on medication use and relief of adverse effects.

"You should be given an adapted amount to take home" [. . .] *"yes, we also sell lactic acid bacteria, and some can help during an antibiotic treatment, counteract diarrhoea and such that could be an obstacle to completing the cure, so it can actually help someone complete their treatment."* (M6)

Furthermore, the pharmacy informants brought up the fact that pharmacies have systems to collect medical waste, where all kinds of medicines are collected and sent for destruction, with no special focus on antibiotics. One informant worked in a pharmacy chain which had employed a specific person to work with environmental aspects of medicines, including antibiotic production. This chain was deeply involved in the issue of antibiotic waste at antibiotic production sites, and tried to reach the public, politicians and authorities through seminars, podcasts, YouTube films and newspaper articles, hoping to create debate. Another activity mentioned by the informant was a campaign driven in cooperation by pharmacy chains, directed to the public, to not take antibiotics for common colds.

3.1.5. Actions Taken in Hospital Environment Department

Subcategories: Reduce Antibiotics and Bacteria Reaching the Environment, Action for Restrictive Antibiotic Use

Hospitals have systems to manage medical waste, and the hospital wastewater is connected to the city wastewater treatment system, said informants working in this area. Medical waste, which included antibiotic waste, was collected in separate bins by the ward staff, and then sent for incineration. According to one hospital informant, the hospital environmental department focused on writing routines for collection, sorting and management of medical waste, and following-up whether they were adhered to by staff.

The hospital environment department was responsible for creating lists of approved products to be used in the hospital, one informant reported. One example of a product that the informant especially did not want in use at the hospital was detergents with silver, since, according to the informant, bacteria can develop resistance to silver, which can lead to increased antibiotic resistance. This hospital environmental department furthermore cooperated with the hospital's local Strama-group (Strama is the Swedish strategic programme against antibiotic resistance) in their efforts to reduce the use of fluoroquinolones. Another task of the environmental department, according to the informant, was to set environmental demands when ordering hospital food. The informant believed buying ecological meat was a way to support lower antibiotic usage in food-animal production.

> "There are certain substances, antibiotics that are extremely persistent in the environment, including fluoroquinolones that have long half-lives [. . .] because we see a connection to the external environment or that effect, we have seen that, yes it makes sense to raise it as an environmental goal as well, so we can pursue this together." (M8)

3.1.6. Actions Taken in Wastewater Treatment

Subcategories: Reduce Antibiotics and Bacteria Reaching the Environment, Developing Knowledge

Wastewater treatment plants did not have a special focus on antibiotic resistance, according to informants working at these plants. Both informants believed that the use of high-quality wastewater treatment methods can contribute to containing antibiotic resistance. Both said they worked at plants which had decided to study and install new technology to improve water treatment, methods that reduce the discharge of bacteria. One plant was installing effective membranes, and the other ozonation technology. The latter method will also reduce drug residues, according to the informant.

> "We had a project just a couple of years ago then, or yes, it ended well last year, [. . .] but then we had, among other things, sampling up there, where we looked at bacteria, how much bacteria comes out of the membranes and how much antibiotic-resistant bacteria comes out. And it was basically zero." (M1)

> "Ozone is a very powerful eh, oxidizing agent, it breaks down most drug residues eh, or drug molecules, eh, quite effectively. [. . .] It has a very strong effect on bacteria as well, they break down, so it is very effective." (M5)

Both informants described how sludge was managed in the plants, since sludge, after the treatment process, and control of salmonella, metal, and toxic products, was often used in agriculture. Most antibiotics coming to the wastewater treatment plant stick to the sludge, said informants, and were thus separated from the water. Monitoring was also conducted at city wastewater treatment plants, informants said. In one treatment plant, follow-ups focused on known toxic compounds and on bacteria. The other treatment plant had decided to study pharmaceutical residues with the highest concentration levels in wastewater, the informant reported. However, this did not include antibiotics.

3.2. Informants' Perceptions of Factors Influencing Work

3.2.1. Organisational and Personal Engagement

All informants stated that they or their organisation had a role to play in containing antibiotic resistance. However, many highlighted that Strama (the Swedish strategic programme against antibiotic resistance) was more directly involved in work against antibiotic resistance than their own organisation. A few talked about their personal engagement. One was very frustrated about the low activity to contain antibiotic resistance in Sweden and at the global level.

3.2.2. Legislation, Governance, and Resources

Legislation to protect development of antibiotic resistance in the environment was not an option according to the informants. Legislation was not possible because we do not know which measures to take, said the Environmental Protection Agency informant. The researcher informant did not believe that new regulations were necessary, because factors in society that are important to contain antibiotic resistance, such as functioning healthcare and functioning infrastructure, already existed in Sweden, although they can be improved.

There were different views among the informants on who governs or should govern work to contain antibiotic resistance. One said that healthcare and some social institutions should control the work, whereas another could not see who should be responsible. One informant concluded that there was no central governance in how to conduct the work in wastewater treatment plants. Many had, however, a clear belief that the issue must be on the national agenda. The national government has the resources and must decide what to do, said one informant.

Several of the informants said it was difficult to determine whether enough resources were available for work to contain antibiotic resistance. One informant observed that pharmaceutical companies needed extra resources for development of new antibiotics, and another informant lifted the necessity of long-term funding to preserve existing antibiotics which were no longer profitable.

Furthermore, financing was a factor that could affect the work of many informants. The researcher was dependent on funding for the research group. Informants from wastewater treatment plants applied for funding for monitoring and developing new treatment techniques. According to the informants, the funders were often national authorities and institutions, which in turn were funded by the government.

3.2.3. Cooperation and One Health

All informants thought cooperation was important, and it was mentioned as a facilitating factor in work to combat antibiotic resistance. Reasons for wanting to cooperate were many, e.g., limited resources, the broadness of the issue and involvement of several sectors, or the fact that when working together, organizations could become stronger and were in a better position to make demands. Some informants emphasized the importance of international cooperation and said it was necessary because problems with antibiotic resistance were greater outside Sweden.

Only a few informants knew about the One Health concept. The government authority informant had a general understanding of the concept, and the researcher informant was familiar with the concept. However, the concept One Health was not known among the rest of the informants.

3.3. Informants' Perceptions of Factors Hindering Work

3.3.1. Difficulties in Setting Environmental Requirements

Setting environmental requirements on pharmaceutical production when purchasing drugs for hospitals, as well as for pharmacies, could be difficult according to informants working in these areas.

> "As I have understood it, so this with procurements is quite tricky when it comes to drugs because it is difficult, there is not always good transparency so that you know how this is manufactured [...] As I have understood it the pharmaceutical companies are quite like, it's a bit difficult to get insight into what is done." (M4)

Pharmacy chains cannot influence the production of prescription drugs, informants from this area noted, because Swedish pharmacies must dispense the "product of the period" (i.e., the cheapest available generic of the prescribed drug, decided by the National Dental and Pharmaceutical Benefits Agency, TLV). One pharmacy informant said that the pharmacy chain had tried to influence a national authority to set environmental requirements on prescription medications the pharmacy was required to deliver, but this had failed.

> "They [TLV] refuse and say that we do what the state has ordered from us, that, they are a state authority, and they try to follow the guidelines and requirements that they have from the state." (M7)

Nearly all informants remembered and mentioned the detection of high levels of antibiotics in a river close to a pharmaceutical manufacturing plant in India. The pharmaceutical company informant, reflecting on this from a supplier's perspective, said that a single company cannot make demands on the production of the drugs they buy, and all companies must have the same requirements for this to work. There were two possible options, the informant continued: an alliance of all companies with common agreements, or demands of transparency set by a national authority. According to this informant, the company monitors what is financially feasible to implement and then balances the costs of production with the price they can negotiate with the benefits agency in Sweden.

Maintaining a wide assortment of antibiotics was another challenge. The pharmaceutical company informant explained how the company tried hard to keep the assortment, but this could be difficult due to the fact that the market was shrinking.

> "For this, is the challenge, one of the challenges with existing antibiotics that you have to keep them, they have to exist, there is like no future with them because you want to, you will have reduced use, no money for companies that want to make money." (M10)

3.3.2. Lack of Knowledge

A general problem mentioned by the informants was that knowledge was lacking and it was therefore hard to know which measures to take. For instance, the Environmental Protection Agency had discovered antibiotics in water after treatment in treatment plants, and the researcher informant had been involved in detecting resistant bacteria in water and soil. However, as the informant from the Environmental Protection Agency expressed, we do not know what this means.

> " ... [antibiotics] is one of several chemicals, then you see it as a chemical substance. And if it comes out in water and sludge, then you have a cocktail of everything possible, it's not certain that it is only the antibiotics that play a role, but rather that they interact with everything else that is there [...] So it is very difficult to say which role antibiotics play there." (M2)

3.3.3. Lack of Action

Several informants called for actions from the politicians. Political actions were, for instance, requested to influence the pharmaceutical production sites to reduce pollution of antibiotics. Another suggestion was action from the government to initiate drug treatment at wastewater treatment plants.

3.3.4. Conflicting Priorities

Two informants mentioned how different disciplines sometimes have conflicting priorities. One example was that the hospital hygiene department recommended the hospital to use disposable equipment to reduce infection, whereas the environmental department recommended the hospital to use less disposable equipment for environmental reasons. Another conflict reported by the researcher informant was between physicians and pre-clinical researchers. Physicians want to treat their patients with antibiotics, whereas researchers emphasize the importance of avoiding antibiotics as much as possible. This conflict was also mentioned by the informants from environmental departments.

3.4. Development after the Interviews Were Conducted in 2018

There were four informants who answered the questions. They represented a pharmacy chain, a wastewater treatment plant, the pharmaceutical company, and the Swedish Environmental Agency. Three informants were the same informants that had taken part in the interviews conducted in 2018. The Environmental Agency had a new representative in the cooperation platform against antibiotic resistance, and this person answered the questions.

The informant from the wastewater treatment plant noted that ozone technology had been developed further and the antibiotic residues which were analysed were effectively removed. However, according to this informant, coordination and cooperation in work to contain antibiotic resistance in the environment had not changed since 2018.

In the field of pharmaceutical products, new activities were mentioned. The work at the pharmacy had not changed, wrote the pharmacy chain informant, and the pharmaceutical company informant reported that the company had continued its work to keeping the broad assortment of narrow-spectrum antibiotic products in Sweden. Other engagements which were mentioned in 2018 had grown. The pharmacy chain had continued its engagement for transparency in pharmaceutical production and was now working together with all Swedish pharmacy chains in achieving transparency in the production of non-prescription drugs. The pharmaceutical company informant reported that the cooperative platform, which had recently been initiated in 2018, now gathered more partners, and the informant was now in the management team. The two informants mentioned new measures taken at policy level. These included governmental assignments for the Swedish Medical Products Agency (MPA) and for the National Dental and Pharmaceutical Benefits Agency (TLV), e.g., to organize an environmental premium for procurement of antibiotics, to strengthen access to older antibiotics, and to open a new knowledge centre for pharmaceutics in the environment, with the aim to spreading knowledge and stimulating measures and development in the area.

The informant from the Environmental Protection Agency said that there was no major difference in how the agency was monitoring the environment compared to the year 2018. However, the antibiotic resistance issue had started to reach networks and platforms where the Agency was involved, and during 2018 to 2023, the agency will be distributing grants for drug treatment at wastewater treatment plants. The Swedish platform for agencies has a role to coordinate the work to combat antibiotic resistance, but the antibiotic resistance issue was still no big question at any environment agency, reported the informant.

4. Discussion

This study explored how a selected number of stakeholders from six different health and public service sectors and areas looked upon their role in combating antibiotic resistance. We found that all of them thought they had a role to play, and that their actions can be described in five subcategories: monitoring environment; developing knowledge; spreading knowledge; reducing antibiotics and bacteria reaching the environment; and activities for restrictive antibiotic use. Many informants were active in more than one of these subcategories. Another finding was that most of them felt a lack of governance in this work. In spite of this, their actions were in accordance with measures suggested in the Swedish national action plan. The One Health approach was only known by the policymaker informant and the medical microbiology researcher, but not among informants at the practical level.

Bloomer and McKee [20] suggest four actions to reduce antibiotic resistance in the environment. The first is prevention to reduce the need for and use of antimicrobials. The other three are different actions to prevent or reduce antimicrobials contaminating the environment: improved/alternative wastewater treatment processes; reduced API (active pharmaceutical ingredient) emissions by manufacturers; and management of manure. The stakeholders in the present study were active in all these suggested activities except the management of manure.

This is the third interview study from our research group exploring how stakeholders from different sectors and areas, and from various levels, perceive their role and how they can contribute to containing antibiotic resistance. In total, 34 interviews were performed during a period of six months in the year 2018. At the time of analysis, interviews were divided into three parts: the human sector; the animal sector, and the environment sector. The rational for this was our perception that the work to contain antibiotic resistance were mainly going on in the sectors separately. Our first two studies focused on human medicine and animal production, respectively [18,19]. In both these areas, work to contain antibiotic resistance had started early [21], and extensive efforts within the sectors had resulted in well informed practitioners and low levels of antibiotic resistance in an international perspective [22]. Further similar findings in both studies were the common belief among stakeholders that antibiotics should be used restrictively, and that there were obvious leaders in each sector which were known by stakeholders at the practical level [18,19]. The leaders they identified represented the national level, and their methods were to provide information and the best available knowledge on how to act to combat antibiotic resistance, i.e., using non-authoritative networks to reach stakeholders to gain change.

Our findings in the present study were different. All informants thought they had a role to play to combat antibiotic resistance and talked about activities they were involved in. However, they did not see any leadership of actions. Some of the stakeholders in our study expressed a personal engagement and they followed new findings from research in their area. This could probably explain why their actions were in line with the recommended actions and appeared to be coordinated according to the national action plan, even though they themselves did not seem to be aware of this plan. These stakeholders seemed to be ahead of the national plan in their requests for actions from authorities. A few years later, some of these requested issues were included in the updated national action plan. Other stakeholders in our study were waiting for information from the policy level. One example was the Swedish Environmental Protection Agency which was awaiting directions from the government to act.

The Swedish Environmental Protection Agency could possibly take a role to lead the activities to combat antibiotic resistance in the environment. However, the agency had at the time of the interview just recently been involved in the national network of agencies against antibiotic resistance, and had not yet found its role. As the informant explained, they needed more knowledge about what it means when antibiotic residues are found in the environment, and about which measures to take before they can act. In the autumn 2021, the agency reported that the issue of antibiotic resistance in the environment still was no big question at environmental agencies, but that this question had started to reach the networks and platforms the agency took part in. Our findings are in accordance to the global situation in general, and less attention has been given to antibiotic contamination of the environment [20,23].

A common finding in the three interview studies was that the One Health approach, with few exceptions, was only known at the policymaker level. Swedish agencies have worked together since an intersectoral coordinating mechanism was initiated in 2012 [21]. This means that One Health at the policy level can be perceived as implemented in Sweden. In contrast, professionals at the practical level of the three sectors we have studied were not at all familiar with the concept. Although the Swedish national strategies adopted cross-sectorial work at an early stage in the year 2000 [21], this strategy has not reached the practical level. However, it is possible that practitioners do not have to know about One Health to be successful in their own field to combat antibiotic resistance, as long as they know what measures to take. It is most likely therefore that cooperation between sectors is necessary at the policy level.

Cooperation between stakeholders at different levels was seen in our study in the animal production sector [19]. To involve different stakeholders at practical levels in the environmental sector, with all the diverse areas that are must be involved, coordination is necessary. Gulati et al. [24] define coordination as the deliberate and orderly alignment or adjustment of partners' actions to achieve jointly determined goals. Coordination typically involves the specification and operation of information-sharing, decision-making, and feedback mechanisms in the relationship to unify and bring order to partners' efforts, and to combine partners' resources in productive ways [24].

The use of antibiotics is the main driving factor for antibiotic resistance development [11,12]. Thus, using antibiotics restrictively can slow the development of antibiotic resistance. This strategy is useful in all sectors, even the environmental sector. Many of our informants in the present study worked actively to restrict antibiotic use, for example, through education of medical students and spreading knowledge to the public. Being restrictive includes using narrow-spectrum antibiotics when possible, a perception shared by several informants, and in general accepted in Sweden, where narrow-spectrum penicillin is effective, and thus is often used [25]. Access to narrow-spectrum penicillin is therefore important in Sweden. However, there are large global differences in antibiotic prescribing by doctors, drug dispensing by pharmacists, as well as expectations from the public regarding antibiotics. Promoting restrictive antibiotic use, and making sure the quantity of prescribed antibiotics does not exceed treatment duration, may be hard to accept in countries where patients self-medicate, or are able to purchase antibiotics without prescription [26].

Informants representing wastewater plants, environmental departments at hospitals, and pharmacies appeared to have a role in reducing pollution of antibiotics and other chemicals in the environment. Even here, collection of pharmaceutical waste can differ globally. A study in Ghana revealed that four out of five hospitals were without separate collection and disposal programs for waste management, and that large parts of the population had unused, leftover or expired medicines at home [27,28]. Rules and regulations for waste management exist in many countries, but little appears to be known about how these rules are followed by healthcare facilities [27]. Wastewater treatment systems also differ globally. Many treatment systems in developing countries are neither successful nor sustainable, mainly because they are copies of Western treatment systems, where no consideration has been taken as to the appropriateness of the technology for the culture, land and climate of the country in question [29].

The Environmental Agency monitored toxic compounds in water and soil. However, the identification of antibiotics in treated water by the Environment Agency did not always lead to any action, the argument being that the board needed more knowledge about effective measures before actions could be taken. It is interesting to note that, in this manner, the Environmental Agency appeared to have the least engagement in work to contain antibiotic resistance in the environment.

Lack of knowledge, and not knowing what measures to take, was considered problematic by other informants as well. Other problems included the inability to set environmental requirements when the pharmacies and hospital purchased medications, and the lack of central governance in how to conduct the work. These findings suggest the need for some sort of governance in work to contain antibiotic resistance in the environment. The

Swedish strategic programme against antibiotic resistance (Strama) has played a central role in providing surveillance of antibiotic use and antibiotic resistance in Sweden since 1995. However, as long as there is a lack of knowledge about which methods have the best effect, it is difficult for an organization to lead the work to limit antibiotic resistance in the environment.

Lack of resources and financing could affect the antibiotic resistance work of informants representing pharmaceutical companies and medical research. The pharmaceutical industry is slowly being incorporated into public health efforts regarding which products and how much of them are used [30]. As noted in our findings, there was preservation of existing antibiotics which were no longer profitable and which can affect the spread of antibiotic resistance, and pharmaceutical companies needed extra resources for development of new antibiotics. The medical research informant depended on funding for the research group, a problem that is not unique for just researchers in Sweden. A recent observational analysis of antibacterial research funding in JPIAMR countries (Canada, Czech Republic, Finland, France, Germany, Israel, Italy, Latvia, The Netherlands, Norway, Poland, Romania, South Africa, Spain and Sweden) showed that only 3% of research projects on antibiotic resistance proposed to tackle issues related to the environment [31].

The first Swedish national action plan with a One Health approach was launched in 2016 [9]. However, the need for multisectoral collaboration in work to contain antibiotic resistance was not new at that time. Cross-sectorial work was mentioned in 2000 in a proposal for a Swedish national action plan [32]. A proposition presented in 2005 included work in human medicine and veterinary medicine, agriculture and food production, and proposed the mapping of environmental effects of antibiotic use in order to learn more about consequences of antibiotic pollution [33]. Still, in the national plan from 2016, focus was set on gaining more knowledge [9]. The plan concluded that knowledge was incomplete, but data indicated that antibiotics and other antibacterial agents in the environment could give rise to antibiotic resistance. Technology for the cleaning of pharmaceutical residues and other substances in water treatment plants should be tested and evaluated. Furthermore, the plan included development of support for county councils' procurement processes in order to move towards minimizing releases of antibiotics into the environment during the production of pharmaceuticals.

Strategies were further developed in the updated Swedish national plan from 2020, and issues that the informants in our study asked for have now been included [10]. Now the plan concludes that knowledge of the role of the environment in the development and spread of antibiotic resistance is increasing. Examples of proposed actions include advanced treatment of wastewater, and that Sweden pushes for the development of regulations to steer towards minimized emissions of antibiotics to the environment in pharmaceutical production. According to the updated information given by informants in autumn 2021, some of these proposals have been developed into action by new governmental assignments to the Swedish Medical Products Agency (MPA) and to the National Dental and Pharmaceutical Benefits Agency (TLV).

Strengths and Limitations

The main contribution of this qualitative study is its insight into the unique perspectives and perceptions of work to contain antibiotic resistance in the environment among a select number of informants working in areas that were supposed to have impact on environmental issues in Sweden. All informants perceived they had a role to play in containing antibiotic resistance in the environment. Our intention was not to present a representative survey of all stakeholders' perceptions of work to contain antibiotic resistance in the environment. Our findings are thus based on the perceptions of a small sample size of informants and cannot be generalized. It was beyond the scope of this study to include perceptions of other stakeholders in other regulatory bodies or sectors also involved in work to contain antibiotic resistance in the environment. For example, there were no stakeholders from the animal sector included in this study. If other sectors than the chosen had been included, we would probably have identified other activities to reduce antibiotic resistance and resistant bacteria in the environment. A strength of the study is the qualitative design with interviews that allowed the informant to speak freely around the subject. This design gave us a rich material from each of the informants and good insights into their work from their perspective. The analysis was careful and structured to ensure trustworthiness, and was performed by two experienced qualitative researchers. The findings were further strengthened by the follow-up questions sent to the informants and the answers that were given from informants from four different areas.

5. Conclusions

A One Health approach to contain antibiotic resistance means to simultaneously work to reduce the development and spread of antibiotic resistance in humans, animals, and in the environment. So far, there appears to be little coordination in the work to contain antibiotic resistance in the environment in Sweden. The stakeholders at the practical level were involved in activities in their own area which they perceived could have an impact on antibiotic resistance, but did not feel that they were included in a common program. Their actions seemed to be coordinated, but this was, according to the stakeholders, based on findings from research in their area rather than on strategies developed by national authorities. The One Health approach has been implemented and was known at the policy level in Sweden, but was not established at the practical level.

Supplementary Materials: The following are available online at https://www.mdpi.com/article/10.3390/antibiotics11050646/s1, File S1: Swedish Interview Guide for policy level and professional level.

Author Contributions: Conceptualization, J.E. and C.S.L.; Formal analysis, I.B. and M.R.; Funding acquisition, J.E. and C.S.L.; Writing—original draft, I.B. and M.R.; Writing—review and editing, I.B., M.R., J.E. and C.S.L. All authors have read and agreed to the published version of the manuscript.

Funding: This research was funded by the SAMRC-FORTE Collaborative Research Programme: SAMRC/FORTE-RFA-01-2016, reference number 2017-02174.

Institutional Review Board Statement: The study was conducted according to the guidelines of the Declaration of Helsinki, and approved by the Regional Ethics Board in Stockholm, Reg number: 2017/1999-31.

Informed Consent Statement: Informed consent was obtained from all subjects involved in the study.

Data Availability Statement: The datasets presented in this article are not readily available because they consist of in-depth key informant interviews containing sensitive participant information. Due to the small number of persons in this field in Sweden, it may be possible to deduce the identity of the interviewee, which would violate the anonymity agreement with the participants. Requests to access the datasets should be directed to Jaran Eriksen, jaran.eriksen@ki.se.

Acknowledgments: The authors thank all the informants for taking the time to participate in this study.

Conflicts of Interest: The authors declare no conflict of interest.

References

1. World Health Organization. *Antimicrobial Resistance: Global Report on Surveillance*; World Health Organization: Geneva, Switzerland, 2014; 232p.
2. Ferri, M.; Ranucci, E.; Romagnoli, P.; Giaccone, V. Antimicrobial resistance: A global emerging threat to public health systems. *Crit. Rev. Food Sci. Nutr.* **2017**, *13*, 2857–2876. [CrossRef] [PubMed]
3. Murray, C.J.; Ikuta, K.S.; Sharara, F.; Swetschinski, L.; Aguilar, G.R.; Gray, A.; Han, C.; Bisignano, C.; Rao, P.; Wool, E.; et al. Global burden of bacterial antimicrobial resistance in 2019: A systematic analysis. *Lancet* **2022**, *399*, 629–655. [CrossRef]
4. Jonas, O.B.; Irwin, A.; Berthe, F.C.J.; Le Gall, F.G.; Marquez, P.V. Drug-Resistant Infections: A Threat to Our Economic Future (Vol. 2): Final Report (English). World Bank. 2017. Available online: http://documents.worldbank.org/curated/en/323311493396993758/final-report (accessed on 4 October 2020).
5. Laxminarayan, R.; Duse, A.; Wattal, C.; Zaidi, A.K.M.; Wertheim, H.F.L.; Sumpradit, N.; Vlieghe, E.; Hara, G.L.; Gould, I.M.; Goossens, H.; et al. Antibiotic resistance—the need for global solutions. *Lancet Infect. Dis.* **2013**, *12*, 1057–1098. [CrossRef]

1. WHO. Global Action Plan on Antimicrobial Resistance. World Health Organization: WHO. Antimicrobial Resistance. World Health Organization: Geneva, Switzerland. Available online: https://www.who.int/publications/i/item/9789241509763 (accessed on 15 June 2019).
2. WHO. Antimicrobial Resistance. World Health Organization: Geneva, Switzerland, 2020. Available online: https://www.who.int/news-room/fact-sheets/detail/antimicrobial-resistance (accessed on 4 October 2020).
3. Wernli, D.; Jørgensen, P.S.; Morel, C.M.; Carroll, S.; Harbarth, S.; Levrat, N.; Pittet, D. Mapping global policy discourse on antimicrobial resistance. *BMJ Glob Health* **2017**, *2*, e000378. [CrossRef] [PubMed]
4. Swedish Strategy to Combat Antibiotic Resistance. Swedish Government. Regeringen och Regeringskansliet. 2016. Available online: https://www.government.se/information-material/2016/05/swedish-strategy-to-combat-antibiotic-resistance/ (accessed on 20 September 2020).
5. Updated Swedish Strategy to Combat Antibiotic Resistance. Swedish Government. Regeringen och Regeringskansliet. 2020. Available online: https://www.government.se/articles/2020/04/updated-swedish-strategy-to-combat-antibiotic-resistance/ (accessed on 6 September 2020).
6. Martinez, J.L. The role of natural environments in the evolution of resistance traits in pathogenic bacteria. *Proc. R. Soc. B Biol. Sci.* **2009**, *276*, 2521–2530. [CrossRef] [PubMed]
7. Bengtsson-Palme, J.; Kristiansson, E.; Larsson, D.G.J. Environmental factors influencing the development and spread of antibiotic resistance. *FEMS Microbiol. Rev.* **2018**, *42*, fux053. Available online: https://www.ncbi.nlm.nih.gov/pmc/articles/PMC5812547/ (accessed on 4 October 2020). [CrossRef]
8. Tackling Drug-Resistant Infections Globally: Final Report and Recommendations. 2016. Available online: https://amr-review.org/sites/default/files/160518_Final%20paper_with%20cover.pdf (accessed on 6 October 2020).
9. Bengtsson-Palme, J.; Boulund, F.; Fick, J.; Kristiansson, E.; Larsson, D.G.J. Shotgun metagenomics reveals a wide array of antibiotic resistance genes and mobile elements in a polluted lake in India. *Front. Microbiol.* **2014**, *5*, 648. Available online: http://journal.frontiersin.org/article/10.3389/fmicb.2014.00648/abstract (accessed on 25 October 2020). [CrossRef]
10. Malterud, K. Qualitative research: Standards, challenges, and guidelines. *Lancet* **2001**, *358*, 483–488. [CrossRef]
11. Patton, M.Q. *Qualitative Research & Evaluation Methods*, 4th ed.; Sage Publications, Inc.: Los Angeles, CA, USA, 2015.
12. Hsieh, H.-F.; Shannon, S.E. Three Approaches to Qualitative Content Analysis. *Qual. Health Res.* **2005**, *15*, 1277–1288. [CrossRef]
13. Röing, M.; Björkman, I.; Eriksen, J.; Stålsby Lundborg, C. The challenges of implementing national policies to contain antibiotic resistance in Swedish healthcare—A qualitative study of perceptions among healthcare professionals. *PLoS ONE* **2020**, *15*, e0233236. [CrossRef]
14. Björkman, I.; Röing, M.; Sternberg Lewerin, S.; Stålsby Lundborg, C.; Eriksen, J. Animal Production with Restrictive Use of Antibiotics to Contain Antimicrobial Resistance in Sweden—A Qualitative Study. *Front. Vet. Sci.* **2021**, *15*, 619030. [CrossRef] [PubMed]
15. Bloomer, E.; McKee, M. Policy options for reducing antibiotics and antibiotic-resistant genes in the environment. *J. Public Health Policy* **2018**, *39*, 389–406. [CrossRef] [PubMed]
16. Eriksen, J.; Björkman, I.; Röing, M.; Essack, S.Y.; Stålsby Lundborg, C. Exploring the One Health Perspective in Sweden's Policies for Containing Antibiotic Resistance. *Antibiotics* **2021**, *10*, 526. [CrossRef] [PubMed]
17. European Centre for Disease Prevention and Control. *Antimicrobial Consumption in the EU/EEA, Annual Epidemiological Report for 2018*; European Centre for Disease Prevention and Control: Stockholm, Sweden, 2019.
18. Hanna, N. Integrated Assessment of Environmental and Human Health Risks of Antibiotic Residues and Resistance for Environmental and Health Policy. Ph.D. Thesis, Department of Global Public Health, Karolinska Institutet, Stockholm, Sweden, 2021.
19. Gulati, R.; Wohlgezogen, F.; Zhelyazkov, P. The Two Facets of Collaboration: Cooperation and Coordination in Strategic Alliances. *Acad. Manag. Ann.* **2012**, *6*, 531–583. [CrossRef]
20. Swedres-Svarm. *Sales of Antibiotics and Occurrence of Resistance in Sweden*; Public Health Agency Swed Natl Vet Inst.: Solna/Uppsala, Sweden, 2019; ISSN 1650-6332.
21. Kotwani, A.; Wattal, C.; Joshi, P.C.; Holloway, K. Irrational use of antibiotics and role of the pharmacist: An insight from a qualitative study in New Delhi, India. *J. Clin. Pharm. Ther.* **2012**, *37*, 308–312. [CrossRef] [PubMed]
22. Pore, S.M. Pharmaceutical waste from hospitals and homes: Need for better strategies. *Indian J. Pharmacol.* **2014**, *46*, 459–460. [CrossRef] [PubMed]
23. Sasu, S.; Kümmerer, K.; Kranert, M. Assessment of pharmaceutical waste management at selected hospitals and homes in Ghana. *Waste Manag. Res.* **2012**, *30*, 625–630. [CrossRef] [PubMed]
24. Abdel-Halim, W.; Weichgrebe, D.; Rosenwinkel, K.-H.; Verink, J. Sustainable Sewage Treatment and Re-Use in Developing Countries. Available online: https://www.researchgate.net/publication/228468236_Sustainable_Sewage_Treatment_and_Re-use_in_Developing_Countries#fullTextFileContent (accessed on 12 November 2020).
25. Morel, C.M.; Lindahl, O.; Harbarth, S.; de Kraker, M.E.A.; Edwards, S.; Hollis, A. Industry incentives and antibiotic resistance: An introduction to the antibiotic susceptibility bonus. *J. Antibiot.* **2020**, *73*, 421–428. [CrossRef] [PubMed]
26. Singer, A.C.; Shaw, H.; Rhodes, V.; Hart, A. Review of Antimicrobial Resistance in the Environment and Its Relevance to Environmental Regulators. *Front. Microbiol.* **2016**, *7*, 1728. [CrossRef] [PubMed]

32. Public Health Agency of Sweden. Svenskt Arbete mot Antibiotikaresistens. Verktyg, Arbetssätt och Erfarenheter. [Swedish Work against Antibiotic Resistance. Tools, Measures and Experiences]. 2014. Available online: https://www.folkhalsomyndigheten.se/contentassets/8b846784d2f040648905052438067c75/svenskt-arbete-mot-antibiotikaresistens.pdf (accessed on 6 January 2022). (In Swedish, Abstract in English).
33. Swedish Government. Proportition 2005/06:50. Strategi för ett Samordnat Arbete mot Antibiotikaresistens och Vårdrelaterade Sjukdomar [Strategy for Coordinated Work against Antibiotic Resistance and Health Care Related Diseases]. Available online: https://data.riksdagen.se/fil/E7711022-5A78-4842-988D-10780E89E8D4 (accessed on 25 October 2020). (In Swedish).

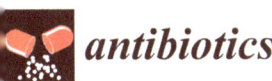

Article

Awareness of Antimicrobial Resistance and Associated Factors among Layer Poultry Farmers in Zambia: Implications for Surveillance and Antimicrobial Stewardship Programs

Steward Mudenda [1,2,*], Sydney Malama [2,3], Musso Munyeme [2], Bernard Mudenda Hang'ombe [4], Geoffrey Mainda [5], Otridah Kapona [6], Moses Mukosha [1], Kaunda Yamba [2,7], Flavien Nsoni Bumbangi [2,8], Ruth Lindizyani Mfune [2,9], Victor Daka [2,9], Darlington Mwenya [2,10], Prudence Mpundu [2,11], Godfrey Siluchali [2,12] and John Bwalya Muma [2]

1. Department of Pharmacy, School of Health Sciences, University of Zambia, Lusaka P.O. Box 50110, Zambia; mukoshamoses@yahoo.com
2. Department of Disease Control, School of Veterinary Medicine, University of Zambia, Lusaka P.O. Box 32379, Zambia; sydneymalama1971@gmail.com (S.M.); mussomunyeme@gmail.com (M.M.); kaundayamba@gmail.com (K.Y.); bnflavien@gmail.com (F.N.B.); lindizyani@gmail.com (R.L.M.); dakavictorm@gmail.com (V.D.); dmmwenya@yahoo.com (D.M.); prudencezimba@gmail.com (P.M.); lifecare346@gmail.com (G.S.); jmuma@unza.zm (J.B.M.)
3. Department of Biological Sciences, School of Natural Sciences, University of Zambia, Lusaka P.O. Box 32379, Zambia
4. Department of Paraclinical Studies, School of Veterinary Medicine, University of Zambia, Lusaka P.O. Box 32379, Zambia; mudenda68@yahoo.com
5. Department of Veterinary Services, Central Veterinary Research Institute, Ministry of Fisheries and Livestock, Lusaka P.O. Box 50060, Zambia; gmainda@hotmail.com
6. Zambia National Public Health, Institute Ministry of Health, Ndeke House, Haile Selassie Avenue, Lusaka P.O. Box 30205, Zambia; otimy1@yahoo.com
7. Department of Pathology and Microbiology, University Teaching Hospitals, Lusaka P.O. Box 50110, Zambia
8. School of Medicine and Health Sciences, Eden University, Lusaka P.O Box 37727, Zambia
9. Michael Chilufya Sata School of Medicine, Copperbelt University, Ndola P.O. Box 21692, Zambia
10. Department of Pathology and Microbiology, School of Medicine, University of Zambia, Lusaka P.O. Box 32379, Zambia
11. Department of Environmental and Occupational Health, School of Health Sciences, Levy Mwanawasa Medical University, Lusaka P.O. Box 33991, Zambia
12. Department of Physiological Sciences, School of Health Sciences, Levy Mwanawasa Medical University, Lusaka P.O. Box 33991, Zambia

* Correspondence: freshsteward@gmail.com; Tel.: +260-977549974

Abstract: Antimicrobial resistance (AMR) is a global public health problem affecting animal and human medicine. Poultry production is among the primary sources of income for many Zambians. However, the increased demand for poultry products has led to a subsequent increase in antimicrobial use. This study assessed the awareness of AMR and associated factors among layer poultry farmers in Zambia. A cross-sectional study was conducted among 77 participants from September 2020 to April 2021. Data was analysed using Stata version 16.1. The overall awareness of AMR among the farmers was 47% (n = 36). The usage of antibiotics in layer poultry production was high at 86% (n = 66). Most antibiotics were accessed from agrovets (31%, n = 24) and pharmacies (21%, n = 16) without prescriptions. Commercial farmers were more likely to be aware of AMR compared to medium-scale farmers (OR = 14.07, 95% CI: 2.09–94.70), as were farmers who used prescriptions to access antibiotics compared to those who did not (OR = 99.66, 95% CI: 7.14–1391.65), and farmers who did not treat market-ready birds with antibiotics compared to those who did (OR = 41.92, 95% CI: 1.26–1396.36). The awareness of AMR among some layer farmers was low. Therefore, policies that promote the rational use of antibiotics need to be implemented together with heightened surveillance activities aimed at curbing AMR.

Keywords: awareness; antimicrobial resistance; antimicrobial stewardship; layer poultry farms; one health; surveillance

1. Introduction

The use of antimicrobials in layer poultry production has continued to increase significantly in the recent past as the demand for poultry meat and eggs increases due to improvements in the social and economic lives of people [1]. Antimicrobial drugs effectively treat infectious diseases caused by pathogenic bacteria that usually affect egg production [2]. However, their increased use for disease prevention and treatment to sustain improved egg production has contributed to escalating antimicrobial resistance (AMR) [3–6]. AMR is a global health problem that continues to negatively affect the health of humans and animals [7–9]. This phenomenon has continued to burden the healthcare system, leading to prolonged hospital admissions, difficulty in treating infections, increased medical bills and increased morbidity and mortality [10,11]. If left unmanaged, AMR will cause more than 10 million deaths by 2050 [12]. AMR awareness among layer poultry farmers is cardinal in curbing this global problem. However, most poultry farmers have been reported to be less aware of AMR and the contributing factors [13].

Humans can contract antimicrobial-resistant microorganisms from animals through the food chain [14–16]. Equally, humans may transmit antimicrobial-resistant microorganisms to animals and the environment [17]. Therefore, this highlights the importance of adherence to biosecurity measures among layer poultry farmers and their workers. Many microorganisms have become resistant to commonly used antimicrobials in livestock production [17]. *Escherichia coli* is one of the highly antimicrobial-resistant pathogens in livestock [18–22]. Equally, antimicrobial-resistant *Enterococcus* and *Salmonella* have been reported in livestock production [16,19,23–25]. Besides, *Staphylococcus aureus* and *Listeria species* have developed resistance to antimicrobials that are commonly used in poultry and humans [23,26–28]. These antimicrobial-resistant pathogens can be transmitted to humans through the food chain and cause disease in humans [24].

Many poultry farmers have access to antibiotics without prescription [29–33]. This means they can easily access antibiotics and administer them to their birds without consulting experts such as veterinarians and pharmaceutical personnel [34]. Hence, the farmers may fail to consistently follow the recommended antibiotic dosage or consider the required withdrawal period before selling their birds. Evidence has shown a link between antibiotic consumption and AMR development [1,3,35]. This implies that the use, misuse, and overuse of antimicrobials have been among the factors contributing to the development of AMR [36,37]. Antimicrobials have been misused in poultry feed and drinking water for growth promotion, egg production, disease prevention or prophylaxis, and empirical treatment [38]. This presents a greater risk for AMR development in poultry flocks and products.

Since AMR has been shown to affect animals, humans and the environment, there is a need to address this problem using the "One Health Approach" [5]. Under the One Health Approach, the focus is on the interaction between animals and humans in the environment and the use of antimicrobials in this interaction [39]. Antimicrobial use (AMU) in animals, humans, and the environment must be monitored and controlled [40]. Therefore, there is a need for continuous monitoring and surveillance of AMU and AMR in poultry farming [41].

At a global level, a lack of awareness of AMR and associated factors among poultry farmers has been reported to be among the factors that exacerbate AMR [42]. Poultry farmers who are not aware of AMR tend to access antimicrobials without prescriptions and use them irrationally and excessively without advice from animal experts [43]. Besides, such poultry farmers do not practise the biosecurity measures that are recommended to help prevent infections in birds. In Africa, a lack of awareness of AMR among poultry farmers has been reported [44]. This has contributed to the rise of AMR because the farmers usually access antimicrobials from unregistered outlets without prescriptions and use them for growth promotion, disease prevention and improving production [44]. This arbitrary use of antimicrobials is a problem that requires urgent attention.

In Zambia, poultry production is a source of income for many farmers and contributes to the country's food security [45]. There has been an increase in the demand for poultry products (eggs and chicken meat) among the Zambian people [45,46]. The increase in the demand for poultry products has led to poultry farmers increasing the use of antibiotics to promote growth and increase the production of eggs [47]. Besides, there is evidence of isolation, identification, and confirmation of antimicrobial-resistant pathogens from Zambian poultry [18,48]. Much of the work on AMR in Zambia has been conducted in regard to broilers, and less in layers. Hence, there is a paucity of information on AMR awareness and associated factors among layer poultry farmers in Zambia.

This study was conducted to assess the awareness of AMR and associated factors among layer poultry farmers in Zambia.

2. Results

2.1. Study Participant Characteristics

Of the 77 layer farmers interviewed, the majority (70; 90.9%) were male. About 22 (28.6%) were from Kitwe, and 24 (31.2%) sourced antibiotics from agrovet shops. A total of 39 (50.7%) participants were commercial farmers (>10,000 birds), 66 (85.7%) used antibiotics, 39 (50.6%) used a prescription to access antibiotics, 45 (58.5%) used antibiotics for the prevention of infections, 66 (85.7%) consulted a veterinary doctor before using antibiotics, and 48 (62.3%) observed the antibiotic withdrawal period. Additionally, 55 (71.4%) farmers did not treat market-ready birds with antibiotics, and 70 (90.1%) practised biosecurity. There was evidence of an association between awareness of AMR and district of residence, type of farmer, source of antibiotics, use of a prescription to access antibiotics, consultation of a veterinary doctor before using antibiotics, knowledge of the observation period, treatment of market-ready birds and biosecurity practice. The overall awareness of AMR among study participants was 46.8% (n = 36), as shown in Table 1.

Table 1. Study characteristics of participants by awareness of AMR in Lusaka and Copperbelt provinces of Zambia.

Factor	Attribute	Total Population (N = 77) n, (%)	Not Aware of AMR (n = 41) {53.3%}	Aware of AMR (n = 36) {46.8%}	p-Value
Sex of farm owner	Female	7 (9.1)	2 (4.9)	5 (13.9)	0.170 [a]
	Male	70 (90.9)	39 (95.1)	31 (86.1)	
District	Chongwe	17 (22.1)	11 (26.8)	6 (16.7)	0.025 [a]
	Kafue	20 (25.9)	9 (21.9)	11 (30.6)	
	Kitwe	22 (28.6)	14 (34.12)	8 (22.2)	
	Lusaka	5 (6.5)	-	5 (13.9)	
	Ndola	10 (12.9)	7 (17.1)	3 (8.3)	
	Rufunsa	3 (3.9)	-	3 (8.3)	
Type of farmer	Commercial	39 (50.7)	14 (34.2)	25 (69.4)	0.004 [b]
	Medium-scale	20 (25.9)	16 (39.0)	4 (11.1)	
	Small-scale	18 (23.4)	11 (26.8)	7 (19.4)	
Antibiotic use	No	11 (14.3)	6 (14.6)	5 (13.9)	0.926 [b]
	Yes	66 (85.7)	35 (85.4)	31 (86.1)	
Source of antibiotics	Agrovet/Pharmacy	16 (20.8)	8 (19.5)	8 (22.2)	0.023 [a]
	Agrovet	24 (31.2)	8 (19.5)	16 (44.4)	
	Pharmacy	7 (9.1)	7 (17.1)	-	
	Not accessed	11 (14.3)	6 (14.6)	5 (13.9)	
	Veterinarian/agrovet	19 (24.7)	12 (29.3)	7 (19.4)	
Use of prescription	No	39 (50.7)	31 (75.6)	8 (22.2)	<0.001 [b]
	Sometimes	15 (19.5)	6 (14.6)	9 (25.0)	
	Yes	23 (29.9)	4 (9.8)	19 (52.8)	

Table 1. Cont.

Factor	Attribute	Total Population (N = 77) n, (%)	Not Aware of AMR (n = 41 {53.3%})	Aware of AMR (n = 36 {46.8%})	p-Value
Prevention of diseases using antibiotics	No	32 (41.6)	13 (31.7)	19 (52.8)	0.061 [b]
	Yes	45 (58.4)	28 (68.3)	17 (47.2)	
Improving production using antibiotics	No	40 (51.9)	19 (46.3)	21 (58.3)	0.293 [b]
	Yes	37 (48.1)	22 (53.7)	15 (41.7)	
Consultation of Veterinarian	No	11 (14.3)	9 (21.9)	2 (5.6)	0.040 [b]
	Yes	66 (85.7)	32 (78.1)	34 (94.4)	
Knowledge of observation period	No	29 (37.7)	25 (60.9)	4 (11.1)	<0.001 [b]
	Yes	48 (62.3)	16 (39.0)	32 (88.9)	
Treatment of market-ready birds	No	55 (71.4)	20 (48.8)	35 (97.2)	<0.001 [b]
	Yes	22 (28.6)	21 (51.2)	1 (2.8)	
Biosecurity practices	No	7 (9.1)	7 (17.1)	-	0.013 [a]
	Yes	70 (90.9)	34 (82.9)	36 (100)	

[a] Fisher's exact test, [b] Pearson Chi-square test, biosecurity practices (fencing of poultry, footbaths at the farm and poultry entrance, restrictions on poultry entrance, limited access to poultry by other animals and isolation of sick birds).

2.2. Factors Associated with Awareness of AMR in Layer Poultry Farms

The results from a multivariable analysis of factors associated with awareness of AMR are shown in Table 2. In the adjusted model, factors associated with awareness of AMR were: the farmer type, source of antibiotics, use of prescriptions to access antibiotics, and treatment of market-ready birds with antibiotics. The analysis revealed that commercial farmers were more likely to be aware of AMR than medium-scale farmers (OR = 14.07, 95% CI: 2.09–94.70). Additionally, farmers who used prescriptions to access antibiotics were more likely to be aware of AMR than those who did not (OR = 99.66, 95% CI: 7.14–1391.65). Furthermore, farmers who sourced antibiotics from agrovets only were more likely to be aware of AMR than those who did not or sourced antibiotics from other sources (OR = 1.38, 95% CI: 0.11–18.20). Besides, farmers who did not treat market-ready birds with antibiotics (OR = 41.92, 95% CI: 1.26–1396.36) compared to than those who did and female farmers (OR= 17.14, 95% CI: 1.02, 286.74) were associated with higher odds of AMR awareness.

Table 2. Multivariable logistic regression model of factors associated with AMR awareness.

Factor	Attribute	Crude Estimates		Adjusted Estimates	
		OR	95% CI	OR	95% CI
Sex of farm owner	Male	Ref		Ref	
	Female	3.14	0.57, 17.33	17.14	1.02, 286.74 [a]
Type of farmer	Medium	Ref		Ref	
	Commercial	7.14	1.99, 25.59	14.07	2.09, 94.70 [b]
	Small scale	2.55	0.60, 10.84	9.26	0.76, 112.69
Source of antibiotics	Agrovet/pharmacy	Ref		Ref	
	Agrovet only	3.75	0.55, 7.31 a	1.38	0.11, 18.20
	Not accessed	1.56	0.36, 6.76	1.10	0.04, 27.58
	Veterinarian/Agrovet	1.09	0.31, 3.88	0.07	0.01, 1.31
Use of prescription	No	Ref		Ref	
	Sometimes	5.81	1.60, 21.17 [b]	5.25	0.48, 57.49
	Yes	18.40	4.87, 69.54 [b]	99.66	7.14, 1391.65 [b]
Treatment of market-ready birds	Yes	Ref		Ref	
	No	36.75	4.59, 294.15 [b]	41.92	1.26, 1396.36 [a]

Key: OR—odds ratio, 95% CI—95% confidence intervals, [a] $p < 0.05$, [b] $p < 0.01$.

3. Discussion

This study aimed to assess antimicrobial resistance (AMR) awareness and the associated factors among layer poultry farmers in Zambia. The overall awareness of AMR among the layer poultry farmers was 46.8%. Factors associated with awareness of AMR in our study included type of farmer (i.e., being a commercial farmer rather than a medium-scale farmer), source of antibiotics (i.e., sourcing antibiotics from agrovet shops rather than general pharmacies or veterinarians), use of prescriptions to access antibiotics and avoiding the use of antibiotics to treat market-ready birds.

Less than 50% of the participants in the current study were aware of AMR and the associated factors. These results corroborate the findings in similar studies conducted in low- and medium-income countries, where the majority of the participants were not aware of AMR and the associated factors [13,42,49]. A lack of AMR awareness and associated factors has been linked to the development of antimicrobial-resistant pathogens [50]. The lack of awareness of AMR and associated factors by poultry farmers is mainly due to a lack of training or education on antimicrobials [50]. Besides, poultry farmers who are not aware of AMR tend to misuse antimicrobials, leading to the exacerbation of AMR and its consequences, such as increased morbidity in both animals and humans [51]. Therefore, there is a need to provide adequate and appropriate information to poultry farmers on antibiotics and the possible consequences of their inappropriate use. The appropriate information can be conveyed to layer poultry farmers through the extension of veterinarian support services or visitation, training, and educational programs on the use of antimicrobials and the factors that can lead to AMR [52,53]. This can eventually lead to increased awareness of AMR and its associated risk factors among the layer poultry farmers.

Commercial farmers from different districts were more aware of AMR than medium-scale and small-scale farmers. Similarly, a study in Ghana reported that commercial farmers tend to be more aware of AMR and antibiotic use than medium and small-scale farmers [54]. In low- and medium-income countries (LMICs), small-scale farmers have been reported to have limited information about AMR and are more likely to misuse antibiotics compared to medium-scale and commercial layer farmers [54,55]. This could be because commercial farmers keep more birds than medium-scale and small-scale farmers. Hence, they are concerned about the ease of disease transmission from one bird to another and huge business losses due to high mortality [44]. Commercial farmers tend to have a better awareness of AMR and associated factors because they can afford to pay for the services of the veterinarians who usually visit their farms compared to medium- and small-scale poultry farmers [44,54]. Such farm visits also translate into opportunities to offer some extension services. Additionally, commercial farmers tend to engage or employ more skilled and qualified workers who are aware of AMR, compared to medium- and small-scale poultry farmers.

Our study found that farmers who accessed antibiotics from agrovets were more likely to be aware of AMR than those who only went to the veterinarian or general pharmacies. This could be because agrovets are more accessible than veterinarians and general pharmacies and there are more agrovets in many areas than veterinarians and general pharmacies [56]. Similarly, in Bangladesh, many poultry farmers accessed antibiotics for their birds from agrovets due to ease of access to these premises [1]. According to another study, many African poultry farmers obtained antibiotics from agrovet stores without consulting pharmaceutical or veterinary experts [57]. In Vietnam, livestock farmers sourced antibiotics from local drug vendors and depended on information regarding antimicrobial use and AMR provided by unqualified personnel [58]. Sourcing antibiotics from feed and chick sellers alone may prevent poultry farmers from getting advice from pharmaceutical and veterinary experts regarding antibiotic use and AMR. Accessing antibiotics from privately owned shops, such as unregistered local drug vendors, hinders access to expert input from animal health professionals [44,57,58]. This calls for the implementation of antimicrobial stewardship (AMS) programs and the strengthening of surveillance systems for monitoring AMR and AMU in poultry production. Further, there is a need for strict regulation of poultry antibiotic prescribing and dispensing by pharmaceutical and veterinary experts. Furthermore, providers of antibiotics such as general pharmacies and veterinarians need to undergo continuous AMR training programs so that they can educate poultry farmers on the prudent use of antibiotics [56]. There is a need to increase access to animal specialist personnel who can provide essential information on AMR and associated factors to the poultry farmers.

Antibiotics were used by 86% of the layer poultry farmers and were mainly accessed through agrovet shops and veterinarians without using a prescription. Similar findings have been observed in some studies conducted in other countries, including Ghana, Kenya and Grenada [44,49,59]. In a study conducted in Ghana, the use of antibiotics in poultry was high, and antibiotics were mainly obtained without prescriptions from agrovet shops [44]. In Kenya, the use of antibiotics in poultry was high, with antibiotics mainly obtained without prescriptions from veterinary offices [49]. Similarly, a high rate of use of antibiotics that were accessible without a prescription was reported in Grenada [59]. Many poultry farmers use antibiotics because of the enormous demand for poultry products such as eggs and chicken meat [1]. We speculate that this could be because many poultry farmers depend on their personal experience, peer-to-peer advice, and information from feed sellers regarding disease prevention and treatment using antibiotics. The use of farmers' personal experience and information gathered from feed sellers have been among the causes of inappropriate use of antibiotics and a contributing factor to the rise of AMR [43,50,59]. Studies conducted in Ghana and Nigeria reported lower use of antibiotics in poultry at approximately 43% and 8%, respectively [54,60]. The current study found that most poultry farmers used antibiotics for prophylaxis against infections and to improve poultry production. Similarly, layer farmers in Bangladesh and Ghana used antibiotics for prophylaxis and growth promotion [1,54]. This usage is inappropriate because it can lead to the development of AMR across common pathogens found in poultry.

Our study found that most layer poultry farmers consulted veterinarians on antibiotics in poultry. Despite accessing antibiotics from various sources, the participants reported that they consulted veterinarians on antibiotics used in poultry. Similarly, a study conducted in Ghana showed that many poultry farmers consulted veterinary officers on antibiotics [61]. Consulting veterinarians is essential because they can provide expert and necessary information to the poultry farmers about the antibiotics used to treat animal diseases [55]. In the current study, the majority of the participants stated that they observed the treatment-withdrawal period and never treated market-ready birds with antibiotics, although this was not verified. These findings are different from the study findings reported in Ghana, where the use of antimicrobials such as tetracyclines was very high with little or no observation of the withdrawal period [62]. Another study in Nepal reported that poultry farmers did not observe the withdrawal period of antibiotics, hence contributing to the global problem of AMR [42]. In Cameroon, poultry farmers did not observe the antibiotic withdrawal period [63]. In Bangladesh, poultry products were sold while antibiotics such as ciprofloxacin, trimethoprim-sulphonamides, and amoxicillin were still being administered [1]. Non-adherence to the withdrawal period exposes consumers of poultry products to antibiotic residues, especially sulphonamide antibiotics [64]. Most farmers are worried about losing money if they adhere to withdrawal periods [44,56]. This is because they would have to get rid of the eggs produced during the period in which they were still administering antibiotics to the birds.

Our study revealed that many farmers implemented and practised suitable biosecurity measures on their farms. This is good for the layer poultry farmers because biosecurity measures help prevent the transmission of infections from humans to animals and vice-versa. The biosecurity measures included the fencing of poultry, footbaths at the gate, restriction on poultry entrance, limited access to poultry by other animals and isolation of sick birds. Biosecurity measures in poultry farming are crucial for disease prevention in poultry and a consequent reduction in the use of antimicrobials [65,66]. However, a study in Ethiopia reported that layer poultry farmers and their employees implemented poor biosecurity measures [67]. The poor biosecurity status among the Ethiopian poultry farmers and their employees was due to a lack of training regarding biosecurity. Poor biosecurity practices can lead to disease transmission from sick birds to those that are not sick, or from people to the birds, or from the environment to the birds, and vice-versa. Therefore, poultry farmers must practice good biosecurity measures that help prevent the spread of infectious diseases around the farm premises and thus reduce the use of antibiotics in poultry [68,69]. Finally, the training of poultry farmers in implementing good biosecurity practices should be encouraged.

This study had some limitations that must be considered when interpreting our findings. The study used a small sample size of the poultry farmers that were registered with the animal health authorities of Lusaka and Copperbelt provinces at the time of the survey. However, to the best of our knowledge, this study was the first to be conducted in Zambia to pave the way for the development and implementation of AMR surveillance strategies in layer poultry farming. Thus, this epidemiological survey will be combined with molecular methods that will help come up with the best ways of monitoring AMR in layer poultry production in Zambia.

4. Materials and Methods

4.1. Study Design and Site

A cross-sectional study was conducted in Zambia's Lusaka and Copperbelt provinces from September 2020 to April 2021. Lusaka, Kafue, Rufunsa, Chongwe, Kitwe, and Ndola cities were purposively selected from the two provinces after considering the similarities in farming activities, practices, and population density based on the Poultry Association of Zambia (PAZ) data for layer poultry farms [70]. The map of Zambia and its respective provinces and the sampled cities are shown in Figure 1.

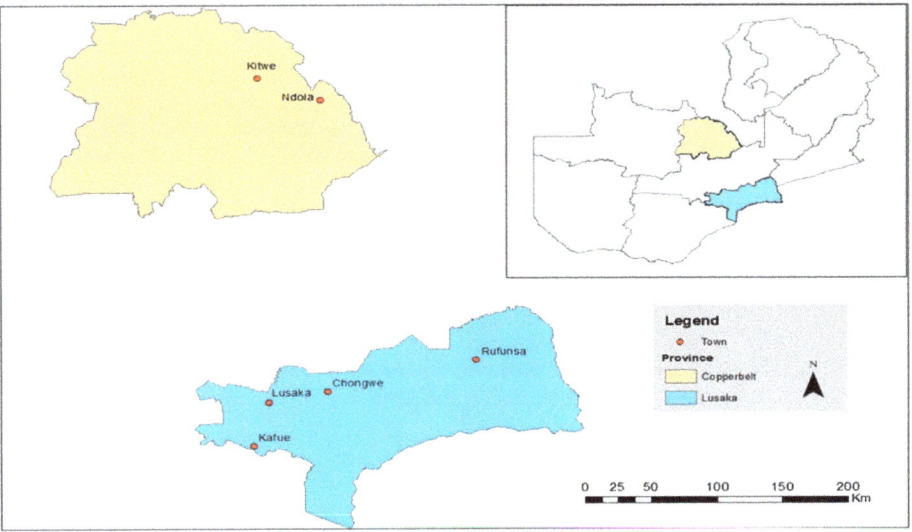

Figure 1. Map of Zambia indicating the sampling sites.

4.2. Study Population

The study was conducted among eligible layer poultry farmers in the study sites. To be eligible, a farmer had to reside in Lusaka or Copperbelt provinces and sign a written consent to be part of the study. All the farmers reared layer chickens in the production stage at the time of data collection. We excluded layer farmers who were not available during the study period and those who were not comfortable being interviewed due to the fear of contracting COVID-19. We also excluded layer farmers who reared layer chickens that were not in the production stage.

A multi-stage sampling procedure was used in this study. The districts in Lusaka and Copperbelt provinces were categorised based on farming activities and practices. Lusaka province had seven (7) districts, while the Copperbelt had 10 districts. Then, we purposively selected a total of six (6) districts from the two (2) provinces. In Lusaka province, the selected districts included Chongwe, Kafue, Lusaka and Rufunsa whereas the selected districts from the Copperbelt province were Kitwe and Ndola. Research assistants were first assigned in each province to identify potential participants from the eligible farms in each selected district. Registers from PAZ and District Veterinary Offices (DVOs) revealed a total of 96 (n = 56 for Lusaka, n = 40 for Copperbelt) layer poultry farms. In each of the selected districts, farms were categorised into three (3) strata, i.e., commercial farms (>10,000 birds), medium-scale farms (1001 to 10,000 birds) and small-scale farms ($\leq$1000 birds). Of the 96 farmers that were identified, 92 met the inclusion criteria. Since the obtained number of layer poultry farms was small, we conducted a complete enumeration. Therefore, we aimed to enrol all the farmers that were identified through the registers and met the inclusion criteria. Overall, 77 eligible layer farmers were included in the study and completed the questionnaire.

4.3. Data Collection Tool

The data were collected using a semi-structured questionnaire adapted from a study by Nkansa and colleagues [44]. Firstly, the questionnaire was circulated to public health and epidemiology experts to allow for face and content validation. The questionnaire was pre-validated for accuracy, simplicity, clarity, relevance, and understandability. The adapted questionnaire had a Cronbach's α-value of 0.78, indicating an acceptable internal consistency. Then, a pilot study was conducted in conjunction with the University of Zambia School of Veterinary Medicine AMR team under the Animal Fleming Fund Project to validate the data collection tool. In the pilot study, 12 farmers were recruited and were excluded from the final analysis. After the pilot study, minor modifications of the questionnaire were done by incorporating the suggestions that came from the farmers. Face-to-face interviews were conducted by the principal investigator and two research assistants. The 20–30 min interviews were conducted in English and local languages, i.e., in Bemba and Chinyanja. The questionnaire was divided into two (2) sections, namely, section A, which contained questions on farm epidemiological data, and section B, which contained questions on antibiotic use, source of antibiotics, use of prescriptions when accessing antibiotics, prevention and treatment of infections using antibiotics, using antibiotics to improve egg production, consulting veterinarians, knowledge of the withdrawal period, treatment of market-ready birds, and biosecurity measures implemented at the farm. Finally, the farmers were asked if they were aware of AMR or not. At the end of the interview, the participants were allowed to ask questions and express any concerns regarding the use of antibiotics, poultry infections, and AMR. See Supplementary Material.

4.4. Statistical Analysis

For statistical analyses, the collected data were entered into Microsoft Excel® and imported into Stata® version 16.1 (Stata Corp., College Station, TX, USA). Categorical variables were expressed as frequencies and percentages. The test of associations was done using the Pearson chi-square test and, where necessary, Fisher's exact value.

For the study outcome (awareness of AMR), univariable logistic regression was performed with the study characteristics to obtain crude odds ratios. Further, a multivariable logistic regression model was fitted, including only variables with a $p < 0.20$ from the univariable analysis to obtain adjusted odds ratios. The multivariable regression model was fitted using a machine-led backward stepwise regression technique. The final model was fitted using robust standard errors to account for clustering among the farmers from similar farming blocks. The Hosmer–Lemeshow goodness-of-fit test was used to assess the predictive ability of the model. Since the model fit was inadequate, we further investigated the possible interactions between significant variables and none were found to reach any statistical significance. Additionally, we assessed for multicollinearity using the variance inflated factor (VIF), and the highest value was 3.54, suggesting that multicollinearity was not a problem. All statistical tests were done at a 5% significance level and a 95% confidence level.

5. Conclusions

The study found low awareness of AMR and associated factors among layer poultry farmers in Zambia. These findings indicate the need to provide education to the farmers on AMR and associated factors. There is a need to develop and implement AMR surveillance and antimicrobial stewardship programs in layer poultry production in Zambia.

Supplementary Materials: The following are available online at https://www.mdpi.com/article/10.3390/antibiotics11030383/s1, Table S1. Questionnaire.

Author Contributions: Conceptualisation, S.M. (Steward Mudenda) and J.B.M.; methodology, S.M. (Steward Mudenda), S.M. (Sydney Malama), M.M. (Musso Munyeme), G.S. and J.B.M.; software, S.M. (Steward Mudenda), M.M. (Moses Mukosha) and J.B.M.; validation, S.M. (Steward Mudenda), G.M. and J.B.M.; formal analysis, S.M. (Steward Mudenda), M.M. (Moses Mukosha) and J.B.M.; investigation, S.M. (Steward Mudenda), D.M. and G.S.; resources, S.M. (Steward Mudenda), B.M.H.; G.M., O.K. and J.B.M.; data curation, S.M. (Steward Mudenda) and J.B.M.; writing—original draft preparation, S.M. (Steward Mudenda); writing—review and editing, S.M. (Steward Mudenda), S.M. (Sydney Malama), M.M. (Musso Munyeme), B.M.H., G.M., O.K., M.M. (Moses Mukosha), K.Y., F.N.B., R.L.M., V.D., D.M., P.M., G.S. and J.B.M.; visualization, S.M. (Steward Mudenda); supervision, S.M. (Sydney Malama), M.M. (Musso Munyeme) and J.B.M.; project administration, S.M. (Steward Mudenda); funding acquisition, J.B.M. All authors have read and agreed to the published version of the manuscript.

Funding: This study was funded by the African Centre for Infectious Diseases in Humans and Animals in conjunction with the University of Zambia (ACEIDHA-UNZA).

Institutional Review Board Statement: The study was conducted according to the guidelines of the Declaration of Helsinki and approved by the ERES CONVERGE Ethics Committee (Ref No. 2019-Dec-004) in December 2019. After IRB ethical approval, regulatory approval was obtained from the National Health Research Authority (NHRA).

Informed Consent Statement: Informed consent was obtained from the layer poultry farmers.

Data Availability Statement: The data supporting the reported results can be made available on request from the corresponding author.

Acknowledgments: We would like to acknowledge the Lusaka and Copperbelt Provincial and District Veterinary Offices and officers for offering support during data collection. We are grateful to all the layer poultry farmers that participated in the survey. We acknowledge the Lusaka, Kitwe and Ndola District Veterinary Offices for their assistance during data collection. We give many thanks to our sponsor, ACEIDHA, in conjunction with UNZA for providing financial and resource support. We also want to thank the Fleming Fund Project-UNZA for their support.

Conflicts of Interest: The authors declare no conflict of interest. The funders had no role in the study's design, in the collection, analyses, or interpretation of data, in the writing of the manuscript, or in the decision to publish the results.

References

1. Imam, T.; Gibson, J.S.; Foysal, M.; Das, S.B.; Gupta, S.D.; Fournié, G.; Hoque, M.A.; Henning, J. A Cross-Sectional Study of Antimicrobial Usage on Commercial Broiler and Layer Chicken Farms in Bangladesh. *Front. Vet. Sci.* **2020**, *7*, 576113. [CrossRef] [PubMed]
2. Wall, S. Prevention of antibiotic resistance—An epidemiological scoping review to identify research categories and knowledge gaps. *Glob. Health Action* **2019**, *12*, 1756191. [CrossRef] [PubMed]
3. Agyare, C.; Etsiapa Boamah, V.; Ngofi Zumbi, C.; Boateng Osei, F. Antibiotic Use in Poultry Production and Its Effects on Bacterial Resistance. In *Antimicrobial Resistance—A Global Threat*; IntechOpen: London, UK, 2018; ISBN 978-1-78985-784-9.

4. Carrique-Mas, J.; Van, N.T.B.; Van Cuong, N.; Truong, B.D.; Kiet, B.T.; Thanh, P.T.H.; Lon, N.N.; Giao, V.T.Q.; Hien, V.B.; Padungtod, P.; et al. Mortality, disease and associated antimicrobial use in commercial small-scale chicken flocks in the Mekong Delta of Vietnam. *Prev. Vet. Med.* **2019**, *165*, 15–22. [CrossRef]
5. Pokharel, S.; Shrestha, P.; Adhikari, B. Antimicrobial use in food animals and human health: Time to implement 'One Health' approach. *Antimicrob. Resist. Infect. Control* **2020**, *9*, 181. [CrossRef] [PubMed]
6. Caudell, M.A.; Quinlan, M.B.; Subbiah, M.; Call, D.R.; Roulette, C.J.; Roulette, J.W.; Roth, A.; Matthews, L.; Quinlan, R.J. Antimicrobial Use and Veterinary Care among Agro-Pastoralists in Northern Tanzania. *PLoS ONE* **2017**, *12*, e0170328. [CrossRef]
7. Prestinaci, F.; Pezzotti, P.; Pantosti, A. Antimicrobial resistance: A global multifaceted phenomenon. *Pathog. Glob. Health* **2015**, *109*, 309. [CrossRef]
8. Gray, P.; Jenner, R.; Norris, J.; Page, S.; Browning, G. Antimicrobial prescribing guidelines for poultry. *Aust. Vet. J.* **2021**, *99*, 181–235. [CrossRef]
9. Davies, J.; Davies, D. Origins and Evolution of Antibiotic Resistance. *Microbiol. Mol. Biol. Rev.* **2010**, *74*, 417. [CrossRef]
10. Dadgostar, P. Antimicrobial resistance: Implications and costs. *Infect. Drug Resist.* **2019**, *12*, 3903–3910. [CrossRef]
11. Michael, C.A.; Dominey-Howes, D.; Labbate, M. The Antimicrobial Resistance Crisis: Causes, Consequences, and Management. *Front. Public Health* **2014**, *2*, 145. [CrossRef]
12. de Kraker, M.E.A.; Stewardson, A.J.; Harbarth, S. Will 10 Million People Die a Year due to Antimicrobial Resistance by 2050? *PLoS Med.* **2016**, *13*, 1002184. [CrossRef] [PubMed]
13. Geta, K.; Kibret, M. Knowledge, attitudes and practices of animal farm owners/workers on antibiotic use and resistance in Amhara region, north western Ethiopia. *Sci. Rep.* **2021**, *11*, 21211. [CrossRef] [PubMed]
14. Verraes, C.; Van Boxstael, S.; Van Meervenne, E.; Van Coillie, E.; Butaye, P.; Catry, B.; de Schaetzen, M.A.; Van Huffel, X.; Imberechts, H.; Dierick, K.; et al. Antimicrobial resistance in the food chain: A review. *Int. J. Environ. Res. Public Health* **2013**, *10*, 2643–2669. [CrossRef] [PubMed]
15. Hassell, J.M.; Ward, M.J.; Muloi, D.; Bettridge, J.M.; Robinson, T.P.; Kariuki, S.; Ogendo, A.; Kiiru, J.; Imboma, T.; Kang'ethe, E.K.; et al. Clinically relevant antimicrobial resistance at the wildlife–livestock–human interface in Nairobi: An epidemiological study. *Lancet Planet. Health* **2019**, *3*, e259–e269. [CrossRef]
16. Nulty, K.M.; Soon, J.M.; Wallace, C.A.; Nastasijevic, I. Antimicrobial resistance monitoring and surveillance in the meat chain: A report from five countries in the European Union and European Economic Area. *Trends Food Sci. Technol.* **2016**, *58*, 1–13. [CrossRef]
17. Woolhouse, M.; Ward, M.; van Bunnik, B.; Farrar, J. Antimicrobial resistance in humans, livestock and the wider environment. *Philos. Trans. R. Soc. B Biol. Sci.* **2015**, *370*, 20140083. [CrossRef]
18. Chishimba, K.; Hang'ombe, B.M.; Muzandu, K.; Mshana, S.E.; Matee, M.I.; Nakajima, C.; Suzuki, Y. Detection of Extended-Spectrum Beta-Lactamase-Producing Escherichia coli in Market-Ready Chickens in Zambia. *Int. J. Microbiol.* **2016**, *2016*, 5275724. [CrossRef]
19. Varga, C.; Guerin, M.T.; Brash, M.L.; Slavic, D.; Boerlin, P.; Susta, L. Antimicrobial resistance in fecal Escherichia coli and Salmonella enterica isolates: A two-year prospective study of small poultry flocks in Ontario, Canada. *BMC Vet. Res.* **2019**, *15*, 464. [CrossRef]
20. Mainda, G.; Bessell, P.B.; Muma, J.B.; McAteer, S.P.; Chase-Topping, M.E.; Gibbons, J.; Stevens, M.P.; Gally, D.L.; Barend, B.M. Prevalence and patterns of antimicrobial resistance among Escherichia coli isolated from Zambian dairy cattle across different production systems. *Sci. Rep.* **2015**, *5*, 26589. [CrossRef]
21. Kabali, E.; Pandey, G.S.; Munyeme, M.; Kapila, P.; Mukubesa, A.N.; Ndebe, J.; Muma, J.B.; Mubita, C.; Muleya, W.; Muonga, E.M.; et al. Identification of Escherichia coli and Related Enterobacteriaceae and Examination of Their Phenotypic Antimicrobial Resistance Patterns: A Pilot Study at A Wildlife–Livestock Interface in Lusaka, Zambia. *Antibiotics* **2021**, *10*, 238. [CrossRef]
22. Muloi, D.; Kiiru, J.; Ward, M.J.; Hassell, J.M.; Bettridge, J.M.; Robinson, T.P.; van Bunnik, B.A.D.; Chase-Topping, M.; Robertson, G.; Pedersen, A.B.; et al. Epidemiology of antimicrobial-resistant Escherichia coli carriage in sympatric humans and livestock in a rapidly urbanizing city. *Int. J. Antimicrob. Agents* **2019**, *54*, 531–537. [CrossRef] [PubMed]
23. Barbour, E.K.; Nabbut, N.H. Isolation of salmonella and some other potential pathogens from two chicken breeding farms in Saudi Arabia. *Avian Dis.* **1982**, *26*, 234–244. [CrossRef] [PubMed]
24. de Jong, A.; Stephan, B.; Silley, P. Fluoroquinolone resistance of Escherichia coli and Salmonella from healthy livestock and poultry in the EU. *J. Appl. Microbiol.* **2012**, *112*, 239–245. [CrossRef]
25. Boulianne, M.; Arsenault, J.; Daignault, D.; Archambault, M.; Letellier, A.; Dutil, L. Drug use and antimicrobial resistance among escherichia coli and enterococcus spp. Isolates from chicken and turkey flocks slaughtered in Quebec, Canada. *Can. J. Vet. Res.* **2016**, *80*, 49–59. [PubMed]
26. Samutela, M.T.; Kalonda, A.; Mwansa, J.; Lukwesa-Musyani, C.; Mwaba, J.; Mumbula, E.M.; Mwenya, D.; Simulundu, E.; Kwenda, G. Molecular characterisation of methicillin-resistant Staphylococcus aureus (MRSA) isolated at a large referral hospital in Zambia. *Pan Afr. Med. J.* **2017**, *26*, 108. [CrossRef]
27. Yehia, H.M.; Elkhadragy, M.F.; Aljahani, A.H.; Alarjani, K.M. Prevalence and antibiotic resistance of Listeria monocytogenes in camel meat. *Biosci. Rep.* **2020**, *40*, 20201062. [CrossRef] [PubMed]

28. Mpundu, P.; Mbewe, A.R.; Muma, J.B.; Mwasinga, W.; Mukumbuta, N.; Munyeme, M. A global perspective of antibiotic-resistant Listeria monocytogenes prevalence in assorted ready to eat foods: A systematic review. *Vet. World* **2021**, *14*, 2219–2229. [CrossRef]
29. Albernaz-Gonçalves, R.; Olmos, G.; Hötzel, M.J. Exploring Farmers' Reasons for Antibiotic Use and Misuse in Pig Farms in Brazil. *Antibiotics* **2021**, *10*, 331. [CrossRef]
30. Benavides, J.A.; Streicker, D.G.; Gonzales, M.S.; Rojas-Paniagua, E.; Shiva, C. Knowledge and use of antibiotics among low-income small-scale farmers of Peru. *Prev. Vet. Med.* **2021**, *189*, 105287. [CrossRef]
31. Phares, C.A.; Danquah, A.; Atiah, K.; Agyei, F.K.; Michael, O.-T. Antibiotics utilization and farmers' knowledge of its effects on soil ecosystem in the coastal drylands of Ghana. *PLoS ONE* **2020**, *15*, e0228777. [CrossRef]
32. Chauhan, A.S.; George, M.S.; Chatterjee, P.; Lindahl, J.; Grace, D.; Kakkar, M. The social biography of antibiotic use in smallholder dairy farms in India. *Antimicrob. Resist. Infect. Control* **2018**, *7*, 60. [CrossRef] [PubMed]
33. Xu, J.; Sangthong, R.; McNeil, E.; Tang, R.; Chongsuvivatwong, V. Antibiotic use in chicken farms in northwestern China. *Antimicrob. Resist. Infect. Control* **2020**, *9*, 10. [CrossRef] [PubMed]
34. Redding, L.E.; Barg, F.K.; Smith, G.; Galligan, D.T.; Levy, M.Z.; Hennessy, S. The role of veterinarians and feed-store vendors in the prescription and use of antibiotics on small dairy farms in rural Peru. *J. Dairy Sci.* **2013**, *96*, 7349–7354. [CrossRef] [PubMed]
35. Jibril, A.H.; Okeke, I.N.; Dalsgaard, A.; Olsen, J.E. Association between antimicrobial usage and resistance in Salmonella from poultry farms in Nigeria. *BMC Vet. Res.* **2021**, *17*, 234. [CrossRef] [PubMed]
36. Harbarth, S.; Balkhy, H.H.; Goossens, H.; Jarlier, V.; Kluytmans, J.; Laxminarayan, R.; Saam, M.; Van Belkum, A.; Pittet, D. Antimicrobial resistance: One world, one fight! *Antimicrob. Resist. Infect. Control* **2015**, *4*, 49. [CrossRef]
37. Masud, A.A.; Rousham, E.K.; Islam, M.A.; Alam, M.U.; Rahman, M.; Mamun, A.A.; Sarker, S.; Asaduzzaman, M.; Unicomb, L. Drivers of Antibiotic Use in Poultry Production in Bangladesh: Dependencies and Dynamics of a Patron-Client Relationship. *Front. Vet. Sci.* **2020**, *7*, 78. [CrossRef]
38. Roth, N.; Käsbohrer, A.; Mayrhofer, S.; Zitz, U.; Hofacre, C.; Domig, K.J. The application of antibiotics in broiler production and the resulting antibiotic resistance in Escherichia coli: A global overview. *Poult. Sci.* **2019**, *98*, 1791–1804. [CrossRef]
39. Mackenzie, J.S.; Jeggo, M. The one health approach-why is it so important? *Trop. Med. Infect. Dis.* **2019**, *4*, 88. [CrossRef]
40. Kimera, Z.I.; Mshana, S.E.; Rweyemamu, M.M.; Mboera, L.E.G.; Matee, M.I.N. Antimicrobial use and resistance in food-producing animals and the environment: An African perspective. *Antimicrob. Resist. Infect. Control* **2020**, *9*, 37. [CrossRef]
41. Varona, O.M.; Chaintarli, K.; Muller-Pebody, B.; Anjum, M.F.; Eckmanns, T.; Norström, M.; Boone, I.; Tenhagen, B.A. Monitoring antimicrobial resistance and drug usage in the human and livestock sector and foodborne antimicrobial resistance in six European countries. *Infect. Drug Resist.* **2020**, *13*, 957–993. [CrossRef]
42. Lambrou, A.S.; Innes, G.K.; O'Sullivan, L.; Luitel, H.; Bhattarai, R.K.; Basnet, H.B.; Heaney, C.D. Policy implications for awareness gaps in antimicrobial resistance (AMR) and antimicrobial use among commercial Nepalese poultry producers. *Glob. Health Res. Policy* **2021**, *6*, 6. [CrossRef] [PubMed]
43. Hassan, M.M.; Kalam, M.A.; Alim, M.A.; Shano, S.; Nayem, M.R.K.; Badsha, M.R.; Mamun, M.A.A.; Hoque, A.; Tanzin, A.Z.; Nath, C.; et al. Knowledge, attitude, and practices on antimicrobial use and antimicrobial resistance among commercial poultry farmers in Bangladesh. *Antibiotics* **2021**, *10*, 784. [CrossRef] [PubMed]
44. Nkansa, M.; Agbekpornu, H.; Kikimoto, B.B.; Chandler, C.I. Antibiotic Use Among Poultry Farmers in the Dormaa Municipality, Ghana. Report for Fleming Fund Fellowship Programme. *Rep. Fleming Fund Fellowsh. Program.* **2020**, 1–72. [CrossRef]
45. Dumas, S.E.; Lungu, L.; Mulambya, N.; Daka, W.; McDonald, E.; Steubing, E.; Lewis, T.; Backel, K.; Jange, J.; Lucio-Martinez, B.; et al. Sustainable smallholder poultry interventions to promote food security and social, agricultural, and ecological resilience in the Luangwa Valley, Zambia. *Food Secur.* **2016**, *8*, 507–520. [CrossRef]
46. Samboko, P.C.; Zulu-Mbata, O.; Chapoto, A. Analysis of the animal feed to poultry value chain in Zambia. *Dev. South. Afr.* **2018**, *35*, 351–368. [CrossRef]
47. Munang'andu, H.M.; Kabilika, S.H.; Chibomba, O.; Munyeme, M.; Muuka, G.M. Bacteria Isolations from Broiler and Layer Chicks in Zambia. *J. Pathog.* **2012**, *2012*, 520564. [CrossRef]
48. Mtonga, S.; Nyirenda, S.S.; Mulemba, S.S.; Ziba, M.W.; Muuka, G.M.; Fandamu, P. Epidemiology and antimicrobial resistance of pathogenic E. coli in chickens from selected poultry farms in Zambia. *J. Zoonotic Dis.* **2020**, *2021*, 18–28. [CrossRef]
49. Ndukui, J.G.; Gikunju, J.K.; Aboge, G.O.; Mbaria, J.M. Antimicrobial Use in Commercial Poultry Production Systems in Kiambu County, Kenya: A Cross-Sectional Survey on Knowledge, Attitudes and Practices. *Open J. Anim. Sci.* **2021**, *11*, 658–681. [CrossRef]
50. McKernan, C.; Benson, T.; Farrell, S.; Dean, M. Antimicrobial use in agriculture: Critical review of the factors influencing behaviour. *JAC Antimicrob. Resist.* **2021**, *3*, dlab178. [CrossRef]
51. Nhung, N.T.; Chansiripornchai, N.; Carrique-Mas, J.J. Antimicrobial resistance in bacterial poultry pathogens: A review. *Front. Vet. Sci.* **2017**, *4*, 126. [CrossRef]
52. Moffo, F.; Mouliom Mouiche, M.M.; Kochivi, F.L.; Dongmo, J.B.; Djomgang, H.K.; Tombe, P.; Mbah, C.K.; Mapiefou, N.P.; Mingoas, J.P.K.; Awah-Ndukum, J. Knowledge, attitudes, practices and risk perception of rural poultry farmers in Cameroon to antimicrobial use and resistance. *Prev. Vet. Med.* **2020**, *182*, 105087. [CrossRef]
53. Kramer, T.; Jansen, L.E.; Lipman, L.J.A.; Smit, L.A.M.; Heederik, D.J.J.; Dorado-García, A. Farmers' knowledge and expectations of antimicrobial use and resistance are strongly related to usage in Dutch livestock sectors. *Prev. Vet. Med.* **2017**, *147*, 142–148. [CrossRef] [PubMed]

54. Paintsil, E.K.; Ofori, L.A.; Akenten, C.W.; Fosu, D.; Ofori, S.; Lamshöft, M.; May, J.; Danso, K.O.; Krumkamp, R.; Dekker, D. Antimicrobial usage in commercial and domestic poultry farming in two communities in the ashanti region of ghana. *Antibiotics* **2021**, *10*, 800. [CrossRef] [PubMed]
55. Hedman, H.D.; Vasco, K.A.; Zhang, L. A Review of Antimicrobial Resistance in Poultry Farming within Low-Resource Settings. *Animals* **2020**, *10*, 1264. [CrossRef]
56. Afakye, K.; Kiambi, S.; Koka, E.; Kabali, E.; Dorado-Garcia, A.; Amoah, A.; Kimani, T.; Adjei, B.; Caudell, M.A. The Impacts of Animal Health Service Providers on Antimicrobial Use Attitudes and Practices: An Examination of Poultry Layer Farmers in Ghana and Kenya. *Antibiotics* **2020**, *9*, 554. [CrossRef] [PubMed]
57. Caudell, M.A.; Dorado-Garcia, A.; Eckford, S.; Creese, C.; Byarugaba, D.K.; Afakye, K.; Chansa-Kabali, T.; Fasina, F.O.; Kabali, E.; Kiambi, S.; et al. Towards a bottom-up understanding of antimicrobial use and resistance on the farm: A knowledge, attitudes, and practices survey across livestock systems in five African countries. *PLoS ONE* **2020**, *15*, e0220274. [CrossRef]
58. Pham-Duc, P.; Cook, M.A.; Cong-Hong, H.; Nguyen-Thuy, H.; Padungtod, P.; Nguyen-Thi, H.; Dang-Xuan, S. Knowledge, attitudes and practices of livestock and aquaculture producers regarding antimicrobial use and resistance in Vietnam. *PLoS ONE* **2019**, *14*, e0223115. [CrossRef]
59. Glasgow, L.; Forde, M.; Brow, D.; Mahoney, C.; Fletcher, S.; Rodrigo, S. Antibiotic Use in Poultry Production in Grenada. *Vet. Med. Int.* **2019**, *2019*, 6785195. [CrossRef]
60. Alhaji, N.B.; Haruna, A.E.; Muhammad, B.; Lawan, M.K.; Isola, T.O. Antimicrobials usage assessments in commercial poultry and local birds in North-central Nigeria: Associated pathways and factors for resistance emergence and spread. *Prev. Vet. Med.* **2018**, *154*, 139–147. [CrossRef]
61. Boamah, V.; Agyare, C. Antibiotic Practices and Factors Influencing the Use of Antibiotics in Selected Poultry Farms in Ghana. *J. Antimicro.* **2016**, *2*, 1000120.
62. Johnson, S.; Bugyei, K.; Nortey, P.; Tasiame, W. Antimicrobial drug usage and poultry production: Case study in Ghana. *Anim. Prod. Sci.* **2019**, *59*, 177–182. [CrossRef]
63. Kamini, M.G.; Tatfo Keutchatang, F.; Yangoua Mafo, H.; Kansci, G.; Medoua Nama, G. Antimicrobial usage in the chicken farming in Yaoundé, Cameroon: A cross-sectional study. *Int. J. Food Contam.* **2016**, *3*, 10. [CrossRef]
64. Sasanya, J.J.; Ogawal Okeng, J.W.; Ejobi, F.; Muganwa, M. Use of sulfonamides in layers in Kampala district, Uganda and sulfonamide residues in commercial eggs. *Afr. Health Sci.* **2005**, *5*, 33–39. [CrossRef]
65. Conan, A.; Goutard, F.L.; Sorn, S.; Vong, S. Biosecurity measures for backyard poultry in developing countries: A systematic review. *BMC Vet. Res.* **2012**, *8*, 240. [CrossRef]
66. Scott, A.B.; Singh, M.; Groves, P.; Hernandez-Jover, M.; Barnes, B.; Glass, K.; Moloney, B.; Black, A.; Toribio, J.A. Biosecurity practices on Australian commercial layer and meat chicken farms: Performance and perceptions of farmers. *PLoS ONE* **2018**, *13*, e0195582. [CrossRef]
67. Ismael, A.; Abdella, A.; Shimelis, S.; Tesfaye, A.; Muktar, Y. Assessment of Biosecurity Status in Commercial Chicken Farms Found in Bishoftu Town, Oromia Regional State, Ethiopia. *Vet. Med. Int.* **2021**, *2021*, 5591932. [CrossRef]
68. Maduka, C.V.; Igbokwe, I.O.; Atsanda, N.N. Appraisal of Chicken Production with Associated Biosecurity Practices in Commercial Poultry Farms Located in Jos, Nigeria. *Scientifica* **2016**, *2016*, 1914692. [CrossRef]
69. Hafez, H.M.; Attia, Y.A. Challenges to the Poultry Industry: Current Perspectives and Strategic Future After the COVID-19 Outbreak. *Front. Vet. Sci.* **2020**, *7*, 516. [CrossRef]
70. Krishnan, S.B.; Peterburs, T. *Zambia Jobs in Value Chains: Opportunities in Agribusiness*; World Bank: Washington, DC, USA, 2017.

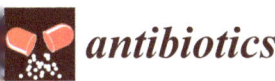

Systematic Review

Systematic Review and Meta-Analysis of Integrated Studies on Salmonella and Campylobacter Prevalence, Serovar, and Phenotyping and Genetic of Antimicrobial Resistance in the Middle East—A One Health Perspective

Said Abukhattab [1,2,*], Haneen Taweel [3], Areen Awad [3], Lisa Crump [1,2], Pascale Vonaesch [4], Jakob Zinsstag [1,2], Jan Hattendorf [1,2] and Niveen M. E. Abu-Rmeileh [3]

1. Swiss Tropical and Public Health Institute, Kreuzstr. 2, CH-4123 Allschwil, Switzerland; lisa.crump@swisstph.ch (L.C.); jakob.zinsstag@swisstph.ch (J.Z.); jan.hattendorf@swisstph.ch (J.H.)
2. University of Basel, Petersplatz 1, CH-4001 Basel, Switzerland
3. Institute of Community and Public Health, Birzeit University, West Bank P.O. Box 14, Palestine; htaweel@birzeit.edu (H.T.); areenjaawwad@gmail.com (A.A.); nrmeileh@birzeit.edu (N.M.E.A.-R.)
4. Department of Fundamental Microbiology, University of Lausanne, Bâtiment Biophore, CH-1015 Lausanne, Switzerland; pascale.vonaesch@unil.ch
* Correspondence: said.abukhattab@swisstph.ch

Abstract: Background: *Campylobacter* and *Salmonella* are the leading causes of foodborne diseases worldwide. Recently, antimicrobial resistance (AMR) has become one of the most critical challenges for public health and food safety. To investigate and detect infections commonly transmitted from animals, food, and the environment to humans, a surveillance–response system integrating human and animal health, the environment, and food production components (iSRS), called a One Health approach, would be optimal. **Objective**: We aimed to identify existing integrated One Health studies on foodborne illnesses in the Middle East and to determine the prevalence, serovars, and antimicrobial resistance phenotypes and genotypes of *Salmonella* and *Campylobacter* strains among humans and food-producing animals. **Methods**: The databases Web of Science, Scopus, and PubMed were searched for literature published from January 2010 until September 2021. Studies meeting inclusion criteria were included and assessed for risk of bias. To assess the temporal and spatial relationship between resistant strains from humans and animals, a statistical random-effects model meta-analysis was performed. **Results**: 41 out of 1610 studies that investigated *Campylobacter* and non-typhoid *Salmonella* (NTS) in the Middle East were included. The NTS prevalence rates among human and food-producing animals were 9% and 13%, respectively. The *Campylobacter* prevalence rates were 22% in humans and 30% in food-producing animals. The most-reported NTS serovars were *Salmonella* Enteritidis and *Salmonella* Typhimurium, while *Campylobacter jejuni* and *Campylobacter coli* were the most prevalent species of *Campylobacter*. NTS isolates were highly resistant to erythromycin, amoxicillin, tetracycline, and ampicillin. *C. jejuni* isolates showed high resistance against amoxicillin, trimethoprim–sulfamethoxazole, nalidixic acid, azithromycin, chloramphenicol, ampicillin, tetracycline, and ciprofloxacin. The most prevalent Antimicrobial Resistance Genes (ARGs) in isolates from humans included tetO (85%), Class 1 Integrons (81%), blaOXA-61 (53%), and cmeB (51%), whereas in food-producing animals, the genes were tetO (77%), Class 1 integrons (69%), blaOXA-61 (35%), and cmeB (35%). The One Health approach was not rigorously applied in the Middle East countries. Furthermore, there was an uneven distribution in the reported data between the countries. **Conclusion**: More studies using a simultaneous approach targeting human, animal health, the environment, and food production components along with a solid epidemiological study design are needed to better understand the drivers for the emergence and spread of foodborne pathogens and AMR in the Middle East.

Keywords: Middle East; One Heath; antimicrobial resistance; foodborne pathogens; *Campylobacter* spp.; *Salmonella* spp.; systematic review; meta-analysis

Citation: Abukhattab, S.; Taweel, H.; Awad, A.; Crump, L.; Vonaesch, P.; Zinsstag, J.; Hattendorf, J.; Abu-Rmeileh, N.M.E. Systematic Review and Meta-Analysis of Integrated Studies on Salmonella and Campylobacter Prevalence, Serovar, and Phenotyping and Genetic of Antimicrobial Resistance in the Middle East—A One Health Perspective. *Antibiotics* 2022, 11, 536. https://doi.org/10.3390/antibiotics11050536

Academic Editor: Piera Anna Martino

Received: 30 March 2022
Accepted: 17 April 2022
Published: 19 April 2022

Publisher's Note: MDPI stays neutral with regard to jurisdictional claims in published maps and institutional affiliations.

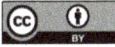

Copyright: © 2022 by the authors. Licensee MDPI, Basel, Switzerland. This article is an open access article distributed under the terms and conditions of the Creative Commons Attribution (CC BY) license (https://creativecommons.org/licenses/by/4.0/).

1. Introduction

Campylobacter spp. and *Salmonella* spp. are the leading causes of foodborne diseases worldwide [1,2]. According to a report published by the World Health Organization (WHO) in 2018, the global burden of food-borne illnesses is 1 in 10 individuals each year [3]. Annually, non-typhoid *Salmonella* (NTS) is responsible for more than 155,000 annual deaths and 94 million annual cases worldwide [4]. *Campylobacter* infection is a public health problem, causing about 8% of global diarrheal cases [5]. Since 2005, *Campylobacter* has been the most reported gastrointestinal bacterial pathogen in humans in the European Union (EU) [6,7].

The Middle East region has the third-highest prevalence of foodborne illness, with 100 million people estimated to be ill from foodborne illnesses each year. Norovirus, *Escherichia coli*, *Campylobacter*, and NTS are responsible for 70% of all foodborne diseases in the Middle East region [8]. The incidence rate of NTS among Jordanians was 124 per 100,000 in 2003–2004 and 30 per 100,000 among Israelis in 2009 [9,10]. In addition, *Campylobacter* was identified in 61% of children with dysentery (63/99) in Israel, 33% (76/230) in Iran 4.7% (7/150) in Palestine, and 3.7% (13/356) in Egypt during the period 2005–2015 [11–14].

Antimicrobial resistance (AMR) is a major public health concern mainly resulting from the use and misuse of antimicrobial agents. AMR occurs when bacteria, fungi, parasites, and viruses change over time and are no longer susceptible to medicines, making infections difficult to treat and increasing the risk of spreading the infection, intensifying the severity of the disease, and raising death rates [15,16]. After the bacteria has acquired resistance, AMR disseminates by clonal spreads of the bacteria and horizontal gene transfer (HGT), that is, by integrons or plasmids, leading to the accumulation of antimicrobial resistance genes (ARGs) in pathogenic and non-pathogenic bacteria within an individual organism [16]. Rising antimicrobial use contributes to the sharing of resistant bacteria and resistance genes between food animals and humans through the food production chain [15]. AMR in *Campylobacter* spp. and *Salmonella* spp. has been shown to be directly associated with antimicrobial use in animal production. Food-borne diseases caused by these resistant bacteria are well documented in humans [15].

Since humans and animals are in close contact and are intricately interconnected, food safety and AMR are fundamental One Health issues [17,18]. However, most of the current research in low- and middle-income countries (LMICs) focuses on human or animal health risks separately and only a few studies have been conducted to understand the problem in an interconnected manner [19,20]. Additional components of human and animal health must be incorporated to make significant progress in reducing many foodborne diseases [19].

The Joint Programming Initiative on Antimicrobial Resistance (JPIAMR) (www.jpiamr.eu, accessed on 19 March 2022) identified several critical knowledge gaps. First, the relative contributions of different sources of antibiotics and antibiotic-resistant bacteria into the environment are unmeasured. Second, the role of the environment, particularly the anthropogenic inputs, on the evolution of resistance is not understood. Third, the overall human and animal health impacts caused by exposure to resistant bacteria from the environment have not been studied. Finally, the efficacy of technological, social, economic, and behavioral interventions to mitigate environmental antibiotic resistance have not been evaluated [21]. A recent review of integrated studies on antimicrobial resistance in Africa concluded that data on AMR from a One Health perspective in Africa are scarce with only 18 studies meeting the minimal standards of addressing simultaneously at least two of the environment–animal–human realms [16].

This systematic review and meta-analysis aims to summarize the scientific literature published between January 2010 and August 2021 on the prevalence, serovars, and antimicrobial resistance phenotypes and genotypes (ARGs) of *Salmonella* and *Campylobacter* strains from integrated studies, studying at the same time humans and food-producing animals and their products in the Middle East region. In addition, it attempts to address the knowledge gap and summarize the available information about the situation by applying the integrated studies to follow up *Salmonella* spp. and *Campylobacter* spp. as the leading foodborne illnesses in the Middle East.

2. Methodology

The protocol for this systematic review was registered in the International Prospective Register of Systematic Reviews (PROSPERO ID: CRD42021277400).

2.1. Search Strategy

We conducted a systematic search on PubMed, Web of Science, and Scopus, limiting the search to the literature published from 2010 until 30 September 2021. Two reviewers performed the initial search, abstract screening, and data extraction, and any discordances were solved by a third reviewer. The exact search strategy used for each database is included in Supplementary Table S1.

2.2. Inclusion and Exclusion Criteria

We aimed to analyze the available information about prevalence, serovar distribution, and antimicrobial resistance phenotypes and genotypes of *Salmonella* and *Campylobacter* strains among humans and food-producing (terrestrial) animals and their products in the Middle East region. It included all peer-reviewed literature published from 1 January 2010, until 30 September 2021. The search included only studies that were published in English. We excluded publications published before 2010, grey literature, non-peer-reviewed literature, and studies with a different design than cross-sectional, cohort studies, and studies using survey system data (Routine data). In addition to information on Salmonella spp. and Campylobacter spp. isolates originating from companion animals, plant-based food, aquatic products (fish), water sources, and concerning *Salmonella* enterica serotypes Typhi and Paratyphi.

2.3. Study Selection

Two independent reviewers used Covidence software (www.covidence.org, accessed on 23 September 2021) for the title and abstract screening. Studies that were eligible for full-text review were further reviewed. Subsequently, risk assessment and data extraction were undertaken. Disagreements between reviewers in the title and abstract screening or full-text review were resolved through consultation with a third reviewer.

2.4. Data Extraction

Two independent reviewers extracted the data for the included papers, and the required data was entered into an Excel (Microsoft Inc.^{TM}, Redmond, WA, USA) sheet. Data included author, publication year, year of data collection, collection country, study outcomes, study design, the validity and reliability of the study methodology, as well as details available regarding analysis, human and animal sample sizes, sample sources, isolated bacteria source, and prevalence. In addition, data regarding serotype prevalence, AMR gene prevalence, and NTS and *Campylobacter* AMR profiles were collected.

2.5. Risk of Bias Assessment

We used the risk of bias tool developed by Hoy et al., 2012 [22] to assess the overall quality of the papers. Two independent reviewers performed the risk of bias assessment and disagreements were solved by consensus.

2.6. Data Synthesis

The number of studies remaining at each stage of the selection process is summarized in the flowchart in Figure 1.

The pooled prevalence rate of *Salmonella* spp. and *Campylobacter* spp. and their main serotypes for human and food-producing animals (live animals and products) were calculated separately based on the following Equation (1):

$$Prevalence\ rate = \frac{No.\ of\ isolated\ bacteria}{Total\ number\ of\ collected\ samples}. \qquad (1)$$

AMR profile among NTS and *C. jejuni* was calculated using Equation (2):

$$Resistance\ rate = \frac{No.\ of\ resistance\ Isolates}{Total\ number\ of\ isoalted\ bacteria}. \qquad (2)$$

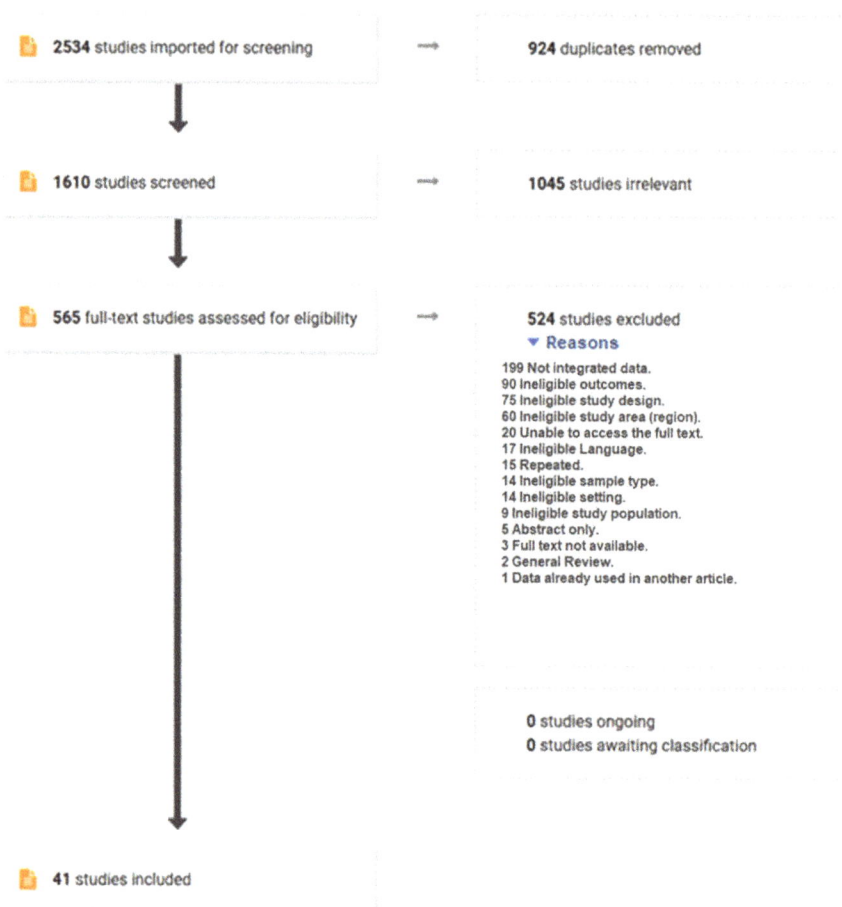

Figure 1. Search strategy and PRISMA flow diagram.

2.7. Statistical Analysis

Relative risks were assessed based on the total number of samples and the number of NTS, *Campylobacter* spp., and AMR positive samples (phenotype and genotype). Studies were stratified by bacterial species and sources. A pooled risk ratio (RR) was calculated separately for each bacterial species. The I^2 and r^2 statistics assessed heterogeneity. We exclusively used the random-effects model, irrespective of the heterogeneity results. For all statistical analyses, we used the R software environment version 4.0.3 and the "meta-package" version 4.14-0. We used the function 'metabin' using the Mantel–Haenszel method with inverse variance weighting for pooling [23].

3. Results

3.1. Studies Identified and Included in the Final Analysis

Based on the eligibility criteria, a total of 2534 publications were identified. After removing duplicates, we screened 1610 abstracts of which 565 were eligible for full-text screening. Out of 565 articles, 41 studies met the inclusion criteria for this meta-analysis (Figure 1). In total, 31 studies used a cross-sectional study design, and 10 studies used routine data (Supplementary Table S2).

The overall result of the risk assessment that was conducted for the included studies indicated that the majority of studies had an overall low risk of bias, and none of the papers had a high risk of bias. This result was based on the risk of bias assessment using the Hoy et al., 2012 tool [22].

3.2. Overview of the Selected Studies

A total of 16 countries were included in this literature review: Qatar, United Arab Emirates, Bahrain, Saudi Arabia, Kuwait, Israel, Oman, Iran, Jordan, Lebanon, Palestine, Syria, Yemen, Turkey, Iraq, and Egypt. Of these, nine countries had no published literature matching the study inclusion criteria available (Qatar, United Arab Emirates, Bahrain, Saudi Arabia, Kuwait, Oman, Syria, Yemen, and Iraq), while seven countries had at least one article available (Egypt, Iran, Turkey, Lebanon, Israel, Jordan, and Palestine).

Of the included studies, 26 (63.41%) were conducted in Egypt, 8 in Iran (19.51%), 2 in Turkey (4.88%), 2 in Lebanon (4.88%), 1 in Israel (2.44%), 1 in Jordan (2.44%), and 1 in Palestine (2.44%) (Figure 2a). Of these, 17 reports (42%) included data about *Salmonella* spp. (the number of reports used for *Salmonella* spp is the same as that used for NTS), and 8 reports (20%) had data about *Campylobacter* spp. In addition, some articles focused on one of *Salmonella* and *Campylobacter* serovars; *Campylobacter jejuni* (nine reports, 22%), *Campylobacter coli* (one report, 2%), *Salmonella* Enteritidis (four reports, 10%), *Salmonella* Typhimurium (one report, 2%), and *Salmonella* Heidelberg (one report, 2%) (Figure 2b) and (Supplementary Table S3).

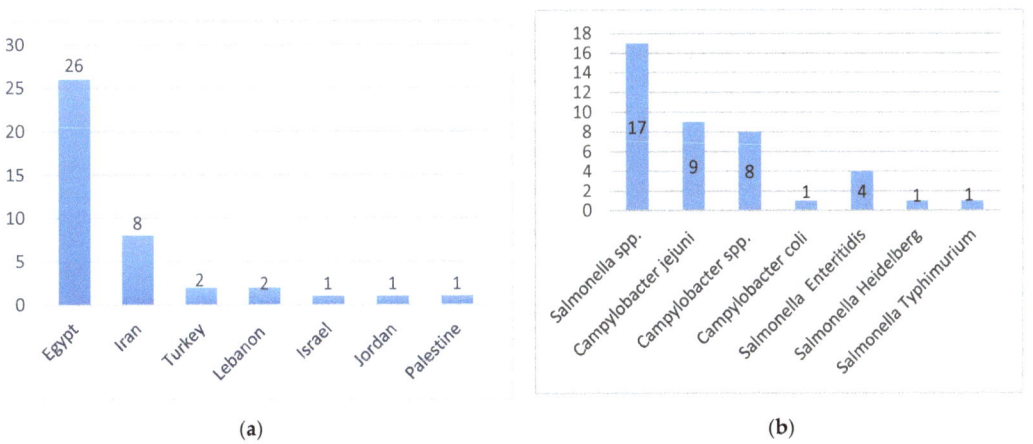

Figure 2. Number of studies (a) per country and (b) per pathogen.

3.3. Prevalence and Serotype Distribution of Salmonella spp. and Campylobacter spp. among Humans and Food-Producing Animals

Out of 41 eligible articles, 31 were cross-sectional studies. We used the cross-sectional data to calculate the prevalence rate for each pathogen separately. Of the 1317 human samples, 167 (13%) were positive for *Salmonella* spp. (14% in diarrhea patients and 9% in high-risk population). In food-producing animals, out of 3520 samples, 585 (17%) were positive for *Salmonella* spp. (31% in poultry and poultry products and 4% in ruminants and ruminant products). Moreover, NTS was reported with a prevalence of 9% (109/1167) in humans (10% in diarrhea patients and 6% in high-risk populations) and 13% (352/2718) in food-producing animals (33% in poultry and poultry products and 4% in ruminants and ruminant products). The two most common NTS serovars were *S.* Typhimurium with a prevalence of 5% (36/780) in humans (4% in diarrhea patients and 6% in high-risk populations) and 3% (91/3038) in food-producing animals (7% in poultry and poultry products and 0.6% in ruminants and ruminant products) and *S.* Enteritidis with a prevalence of 2% (12/585) in humans (2% in diarrhea patients and 2% in high-risk population) and 3% (87/2534) in food-producing animals (9% in poultry and poultry products and 0.3% in ruminants and ruminant products) (Tables 1 and 2).

Campylobacter spp. was reported with a prevalence of 22% (435/2008) in humans (23% in diarrhea patients and 14% in high-risk populations) and 30% (1253/4122) in food-producing animals (39% in poultry and poultry products and 10% in ruminants and ruminant products). The two most commonly detected *Campylobacter* spp. serovars were *C. jejuni* with a prevalence of 16% (422/2693) in humans (16% in diarrhea patients and 9% in high-risk populations) and 22% (1182/5472) in food-producing animals (25% in poultry and poultry products and 14% in ruminants and ruminant products) and *Campylobacter coli* with a prevalence of 4% (72/1938) in humans (3% in diarrhea patients and 8% in high-risk populations) and 9% (367/4037) in food-producing animals (13% in poultry and poultry products and 2% in ruminants and ruminant products) (Tables 1 and 2).

3.4. Microbial Resistance Patterns Detected by Phenotypic Screening

Based on the prevalence rate results and the number of eligible articles included in this review, NTS and *C. jejuni* were the two most prevalent representatives of *Salmonella* spp. and *Campylobacter* spp., respectively. The average resistance of NTS and *C. jejuni* was calculated for each pathogen separately depending on the source of the isolated bacteria (human or food-producing animals) (Supplementary Table S4).

For NTS, information on 13 different antibiotics was available and is summarized in Table 3. NTS isolated from humans showed resistance against erythromycin (100%), amoxicillin (71%), tetracycline (62%), ampicillin (52%), azithromycin (43%), amoxicillin–clavulanic acid (42%), streptomycin (40%), cefotaxime (31%), trimethoprim–sulfamethoxazole (24%), chloramphenicol (15%), ciprofloxacin (9%), imipenem (2%), and ceftriaxone (1%). NTS isolated from food-producing animals showed resistance against erythromycin (100%), amoxicillin (91%), tetracycline (50%), ampicillin (69%), azithromycin (9%), amoxicillin–clavulanic acid (70%), streptomycin (43%), cefotaxime (63%), trimethoprim–sulfamethoxazole (8%), chloramphenicol (12%), ciprofloxacin (17%), and ceftriaxone (7%). Amoxicillin–clavulanic acid was used more frequently in animal isolates (70%), with a pooled risk ratio (RR) of 1.09 (95% confidence interval (CI): 1.01–1.18) and with a heterogeneity of $I^2 = 34\%$ and $r^2 \leq 0.001$, while the pooled RR close to 1 in ampicillin and streptomycin suggests a similar probability of occurrence in humans and animals. For the other antibiotics, no clear pattern was detected (Table 3).

For *C. jejuni*, we had data on 11 antibiotics. The phenotypic resistance results are summarized in (Table 4). *C. jejuni* isolated from humans showed resistance against amoxicillin (100%), trimethoprim–sulfamethoxazole (93%), nalidixic acid (89%), azithromycin (88%), chloramphenicol (82%), ampicillin (81%), tetracycline (75%), ciprofloxacin (73%), amoxicillin–clavulanic acid (68%), erythromycin (65%), and streptomycin (39%). *C. jejuni* isolated from food-producing animals showed complete resistance against amoxicillin (100%) and azithromycin (100%) and to a lesser extent resistance against trimethoprim–sulfamethoxazole (83%), nalidixic acid (76%), chloramphenicol (69%), ampicillin (64%), tetracycline (56%), ciprofloxacin (71%), amoxicillin–clavulanic acid (32%), erythromycin (38%), and streptomycin (21%).

Table 1. Overall prevalence of *Salmonella* and *Campylobacter* and main serotypes.

Pathogens	No. of Isolated Bacteria from Humans	Total Number of Collected Samples from Humans	The Pooled Prevalence Rate among Humans (%)	No. of Isolated Bacteria from Animals	Total Number of Collected Samples from Animals	The Pooled Prevalence Rate among Animals (%)
Salmonella spp. nontyphoidal	167	1317	13	585	3520	17
Salmonella	109	1167	9	352	2718	13
S. typhimurium	36	780	5	91	3038	3
S. enteritidis	12	585	2	87	2534	3
Campylobacter	435	2008	22	1253	4122	30
C. jejuni	422	2693	16	1182	5472	22
C. coli	72	1938	4	367	4037	9

Table 2. Prevalence of *Salmonella* and *Campylobacter* and main serotypes based on the samples sources.

Pathogens	N (%) Isolated Bacteria from Asymptomatic Humans	Total Number of Asymptomatic Humans Samples	N (%) Isolated Bacteria from Symptomatic Humans	Total Number of Symptomatic Humans Samples	N (%) Isolated Bacteria from Poultry and Poultry Products	Total Number of Poultry and Poultry Product Samples	N (%) Isolated Bacteria from Ruminants and Ruminant Products	Total Number of Ruminants and Ruminant Products Samples
Salmonella spp. Nontyphoidal	29 (9%)	342	138 (14%)	975	492 (31%)	1597	76 (4%)	1717
Salmonella	11 (6%)	192	98 (10%)	975	259 (33%)	795	76 (4%)	1717
S. typhimurium	13 (6%)	205	23 (4%)	575	80 (7%)	1195	9 (0.6)	1637
S. enteritidis	1 (2%)	60	11 (2%)	525	82 (9%)	897	5 (0.3)	1637
Campylobacter	28 (14%)	206	407 (23%)	1802	1048 (39%)	2695	205 (10%)	1427
C. jejuni	21 (9%)	226	401 (16%)	2467	968 (25%)	3894	214 (14%)	1578
C. coli	18 (8%)	236	54 (3%)	1702	341 (13%)	2610	26 (2%)	1427

Table 3. Microbial resistance patterns detected by phenotypic screening among non-typhoidal *Salmonella*.

Antibiotic	No. of Resistance Human Isolates	Human Isolates	Resistance Ratio/Human Isolates	No. of Resistance Animal Isolates	Animal Isolates	Resistance Ratio/Animal Isolates	Relative Risk	95%CI
Amoxicillin–Clavulanic acid	53	126	42%	62	88	70%	1.09	[1.01; 1.18]
Amoxicillin	50	70	71%	64	70	91%	4.02	[0.16; 103.61]
Ampicillin	97	186	52%	96	139	69%	1.10	[0.92; 1.31]
Azithromycin	32	75	43%	2	22	9%	0.21	[0.06; 0.82]
Cefotaxime	45	145	31%	58	92	63%	3	[0.23; 39.38]
Ceftriaxone	2	231	1%	9	131	7%	4.33	[0.93; 20.26]
Chloramphenicol	42	281	15%	21	181	12%	1.29	[0.86; 1.96]
Ciprofloxacin	26	281	9%	30	181	17%	1.36	[0.73; 2.51]
Erythromycin	57	57	100%	52	52	100%	1	[0.96; 1.04]
Imipenem	3	194	2%	0	108	0%	0.45	[0.05; 4.02]
Streptomycin	50	126	40%	38	88	43%	1.09	[0.80; 1.49]
Tetracycline	142	231	62%	66	131	50%	0.79	[0.59; 1.06]
Trimethoprim–sulfamethoxazole	67	281	24%	15	181	8%	0.57	[0.18; 1.80]

Table 4. Microbial resistance patterns detected by phenotypic screening among *Campylobacter jejuni*.

Antibiotic	Campylobacter jejuni						
	No. of Resistance Human Isolates	Human Isolates	Resistance Ratio/Human Isolates	No. of Resistance Animal Isolates	Animal Isolates	Resistance Ratio/Animal Isolates	Relative Risk	95%CI
Amoxicillin–Clavulanic acid	283	416	68%	56	173	32%	0.79	[0.67; 0.95]
Amoxicillin	297	297	100%	52	52	100%	1	[0.96; 1.04]
Ampicillin	466	579	81%	142	223	65%	1	[0.97; 1.03]
Azithromycin	261	297	88%	52	52	100%	1.13	[1.04; 1.24]
Chloramphenicol	258	316	82%	50	73	68%	1.01	[0.89; 1.14]
Ciprofloxacin	460	627	73%	187	265	71%	0.92	[0.84; 1.01]
Erythromycin	393	608	65%	92	244	37%	1	[0.97; 1.03]
Nalidixic acid	558	627	89%	201	265	76%	0.89	[0.77; 1.02]
Streptomycin	213	544	39%	50	235	21%	1.02	[0.83; 1.26]
Tetracycline	248	330	75%	119	213	55%	0.94	[0.84; 1.05]
Trimethoprim–sulfamethoxazole	371	399	93%	85	103	82%	1.01	[0.97; 1.04]

Azithromycin was detected more frequently in animal isolates, with a pooled risk ratio (RR) of 1.13 (95% confidence interval (CI): 1.04–1.24) and a heterogeneity of $I^2 = 72\%$ and $r^2 = 0.033$. Amoxicillin–clavulanic acid was detected more frequently in human isolates, with a pooled risk ratio (RR) of 0.79 (95% confidence interval (CI): 0.67–0.95) and heterogeneity of $I^2 = 53\%$ and $r^2 \leq 0.001$. For the other antibiotics, no clear pattern was detected. Most phenotypic resistance had a pooled RR close to 1, suggesting a similar probability of occurrence in humans and animals (Table 4).

3.5. Assessment of Shared Antimicrobial Resistance Genes

Only six studies reported resistance genes targeted at three serovars of *Salmonella* spp. and *Campylobacter* spp. These serovars were *C. jejuni* (three studies), NTS (two studies), and *Salmonella* Heidelberg (one study). We calculated the average prevalence for every single resistance gene from food-producing animals and human sources separately. For human isolates, *tetO* was the gene with the highest prevalence (85%), followed by Class 1 Integrons (81%), *blaOXA-61* (53%), *cmeB* (51%), *blaCMY-2* (38%), Class 2 integrons (29%), *tetA* (21%), *blaOXA* (21%), *blaSHV* (19%), *AAC(6')-Ib* (16%), *blaCTXM-1* (16%), *blaAMPc* (13%), and *blaTEM* (13%). For food-producing animals, tetO was the most prevalent gene (77%), followed by Class 1 Integrons (69%), *blaOXA-61* (35%), *cmeB* (35%), *tetA* (30%), Class 2 integrons (27%), *blaCTXM-1* (22%), *AAC(6')-Ib* (22%), *blaSHV* (20%), *blaTEM* (15%), *blaCMY-2* (11%), *blaOXA* (11%), and *blaAMPc* (3%) (Table 5) (Supplementary Table S5a–c).

Resistance in *Campylobacter* spp. was exclusively reported as data for *C. jejuni* isolates. The three studies reporting data on resistance compromised 274 isolates (232 human isolates and 42 food-producing animals and their products). The most frequent genes were Class 1 Integrons (96%), *tetO* (85%), *blaOXA-61* (53%), *cmeB* (51%), and *tetA* (17%). For food-producing animals and their product isolates, the most frequently detected genes were Class 1 Integrons (100%), *tetO* (77%), *blaOXA-61* (35%), *cmeB* (35%), and *tetA* (30%). There was no evidence for a significant difference in the occurrence of the genes between human and food-producing animals and their products (Table 5) except for Class 1 integrons, which were detected more frequently in food-producing animals, with a risk ratio (RR) of 1.04 (95% confidence interval (CI): 1.01; 1.08) (Table 5). No clear pattern was detected for the other genes, with most of the genes having a pooled RR close to 1, suggesting a similar probability of occurrence in humans and animals (Table 5) (Supplementary Table S5a).

The two studies on NTS compromised 197 isolates (125 human isolate and 72 food-producing animals and their products). The most frequent genes were Class 1 Integrons (51%), Class 2 Integrons (29%), *blaSHV* (16%), *blaCTXM-1* (16%), *AAC(6')-Ib* (16%), *blaTEM* (10%), and blaAMPc (1%). For food-producing animal isolates, the most frequently detected genes were Class 1 Integrons (41%), Class 2 Integrons (27%), *blaSHV* (22%), *blaCTXM-1* (22%), *AAC(6')-Ib* (22%), and *blaTEM* (15%). No clear pattern emerged for the majority of the genes in the random effect models comparing frequencies in humans and animals (Table 5), suggesting there was no evidence for a significant difference in the occurrence of the genes between humans and food-producing animals (Table 5) (Supplementary Table S5b).

The single study including *Salmonella* Enterica Serovar Heidelberg compromised 33 isolates (24 human isolates and 9 food-producing animals and their products). In isolates from human sources, the most frequent genes were *blaAMPc* (50%), *blaCMY-2* (38%), *blaTEM* (29%), blaSHV (25%), and blaOXA (20%). For food-producing animal isolates, the most frequently detected genes were *blaAMPc* (11%), *blaCMY-2* (11%), *blaTEM* (11%), *blaSHV* (11%), and *blaOXA* (11%). There was no evidence of a significant difference in the occurrence of the genes between humans and food-producing animals (Supplementary Table S5c).

Table 5. Prevalence of AMR genes found in non-typhoidal *Salmonella* spp. and *Campylobacter jejuni*.

AMR Gen	Study ID	Pathogen	HN	HI	Prevalance_H	AN	AI	Prevalnce_A_	RR	95%CI	Lab Technique
blaAMPc	Besharati et al., 2020 and Elhariri et al., 2020	NTS and S. H	99	13	13.13%	31	1	3.23%	0.34	[0.07; 1.72]	PCR
AAC(6')-1b	Youssef et al., 2021	NTS	50	8	16.00%	50	11	22.00%	1.38	[0.6; 3.13]	PCR
bla CMY-2	Elhariri et al., 2020	S. H	24	9	37.50%	9	1	11.11%	0.3	[0.04; 2.02]	PCR
bla CTXM-1	Youssef et al., 2021	NTS	50	8	16.00%	50	11	22.00%	1.38	[0.6; 3.13]	PCR
bla OXA	Elhariri et al., 2020	S. H	24	5	20.83%	9	1	11.11%	0.53	[0.07; 3.96]	PCR
											PCR
bla OXA-61	Divsalar et al., 2019	*C. jejuni*	80	42	52.50%	20	7	35.00%	0.67	[0.35; 1.25]	PCR
bla SHV	Youssef et al., 2021 and Elhariri et al., 2020 Youssef et al., 2021,	NTS and S. H	74	14	18.92%	59	12	20.34%	1.13	[0.49; 2.61]	PCR
blaTEM	Besharati et al., 2020 and Elhariri et al., 2020	NTS, NTS, and S. H	149	19	12.75%	81	12	14.81%	0.91	[0.34; 2.44]	PCR
Class 1 Integrons	Besharati et al., 2020 and AbdEl-Aziz et al., 2020	NTS and *C. jejuni*	223	180	80.72%	42	29	69.05%	1.04	[1.01; 1.08]	PCR
class 2 Integrons	Besharati et al., 2020	NTS	75	22	29.33%	22	6	27.27%	0.93	[0.43; 2]	PCR
cme B	Divsalar et al., 2019	*C. jejuni*	80	41	51.25%	20	7	35.00%	0.68	[0.36; 1.29]	PCR
tet(A)	Divsalar et al., 2019	*C. jejuni*	80	17	21.25%	20	6	30.00%	1.41	[0.64; 3.11]	PCR
tet(O)	Divsalar et al., 2019 and Ghoneim et al., 2020	*C. jejuni*	84	71	84.52%	22	17	77.27%	0.92	[0.73; 1.16]	PCR

HN: Number of human isolates; HI: human isolates that have this gene; prevalance_H: prevalence among human isolates; AN: number of animal isolates; AI: animal isolates that have this gene; prevalance_A: prevalence among animal isolates; RR: relative risk; NTS: non-typhoidal *Salmonella*; S.H: *Salmonella* Heidelberg; *C. jejuni*: *Campylobacter jejuni*.

4. Discussion

Although 41 articles were eligible for inclusion in this systematic review and meta-analysis, there is an uneven distribution of the sources of the studies included. The majority (63%) of eligible studies were from Egypt and 20% from Iran. On the other hand, there are no published papers on applying a comprehensive One Health approach to study one of the two major foodborne diseases (*Salmonella* and *Campylobacter*) in 9 counties from the 16 Middle Eastern countries, and none came from those high-income countries members of the Gulf Cooperation Council.

Of the 41 studies included in this review, 31 were cross-sectional, and 10 were routine data studies. Studies allow a comparison between human and animal sources; they do not evaluate actual transmission methods because the few studies eligible for inclusion in this review suffered from insufficient statistical data on foodborne pathogens and AMR and assess only selected sections of the social ecosystem.

Furthermore, our systematic review and meta-analysis showed the prevalence of *Salmonella* spp. and *Campylobacter* spp., resistance rates, and antimicrobial resistance genes circulating in the Middle East region by using the random-effects model. The model showed high heterogeneity results, which indicate variability in the study data. This might be due to the study design (epidemiological study vs. routine data) or due to diverse sample types. The human isolates used in the studies were from different sources (symptomatic and asymptomatic participants), and the animal isolates used were from various sources (live animals and products). Finally, the small sample size in each study and, in particular, the human sample size could influence the results when measuring the prevalence and the relationship between the humans and animal settings. The heterogeneity might explain the insignificant relationship between animals and humans.

The low quantity (low sample size), uneven distribution in the reported data, and weak epidemiological study designs from a One Health methodological perspective [24] in the studies that targeted foodborne illness and antimicrobial resistance in the Middle East can be explained by the food safety system's challenges in this region. These challenges are the lack of epidemiological and disease ecological capacity, diagnostic tools, and laboratory facilities. Moreover, there is a lack of quality control and standardization of microbiological identification and susceptibility testing techniques [15].

Our review demonstrates the prevalence of NTS and *Campylobacter* spp. and their serovars circulating in the Middle East. The pooled prevalence of *Campylobacter* spp. among humans was close to the higher estimate for the ranges reported in Sub-Saharan Africa: and Northern Africa (2–27.5%) and more than the ranges reported in Southeast Asia (8%) [25–27]. Additionally, the results show the prevalence of *Campylobacter* spp. in food-producing animals and their products (30%). For *Campylobacter* spp., the prevalence rate is similar to the systematic review and meta-analysis results that targeted *Campylobacter* spp. globally, with approximately 30% of animal food products analyzed reporting *Campylobacter* spp. [28]. Additionally, we looked at which *Campylobacter* serovars are circulating in the Middle East and found *C. jejuni* and *C. coli* to be the predominant serovars, similar to results that targeted *Campylobacter* in Africa as the *C. jejuni* and *C. coli* predominates in Sub-Saharan Africa [29].

We identified two systematic reviews conducted by Al-Rifai and his colleagues that targeted the Middle East and South African countries in 2019 and 2020; we will compare our results with these relevant studies. In this review, the pooled prevalence rates of NTS were 9% and 13% among humans and animals and their products, respectively. The pooled prevalence in humans is higher than the results in the Al-Rifai study (2019) which was 7% [30]. In addition, the prevalence of the food-producing animals in this review is more than the results of the Al-Rifai (2020) study, which was 9% [31]. Our findings are similar to Al-Rifai's studies of NTS serovars, in which *S.* Typhimurium and *S.* Enteritidis were the main NTS serovars reported in this region [30,31].

Furthermore, this systematic review showed *Campylobacter* and *Salmonella* serovars are highly prevalent in poultry and poultry products in the Middle East. The Campylobacter prevalence in animals was less than the prevalence reported in broiler meat in Poland, Slovenia, Spain, and Austria. Conversely, more than reported in Denmark and Finland [32]. The *Salmonella* prevalence in animals showed results less than the prevalence reported in raw chicken at retail markets in China and more than reported in chicken carcasses in Spain [33,34]. This endemic *Campylobacter* and *Salmonella* bacteria in animal food products can be explained, at least partially, by the changes in animal production systems that have tended to be more intense over the past decades [28]. These findings are essential because transmission along the production chain is generally established as the most common pathway used by *Campylobacter* and *Salmonella* to generate human infection [29].

AMR is a transboundary public health problem. New types of AMR strains can expand worldwide following initial endemic emergence, as demonstrated by several resistant pathogens that spread globally [35]. Our meta-analysis revealed a high NTS resistance against erythromycin, amoxicillin, tetracycline, and ampicillin for isolates from humans and food-producing animals. The isolates have similar resistance rates between humans and animals in erythromycin but are higher in isolates from animal sources for amoxicillin and ampicillin and higher in isolates from human sources in tetracycline. These results are close to those reported by Alsayeqh's systematic review in the Middle East region [15]. In addition, the most recent report on AMR in the EU in 2019–2020 found that resistance of NTS to sulfonamides, ampicillin, and tetracycline was high in human isolates, while it ranged from moderate to very high in animal isolates [36].

AMR phenotypic results for *C. jejuni* isolates (human and food-producing animals) showed high resistance against amoxicillin, trimethoprim–sulfamethoxazole, nalidixic acid, azithromycin, chloramphenicol, ampicillin, tetracycline, and ciprofloxacin. These findings were close to Alsayeqh's systematic review for trimethoprim–sulfamethoxazole, nalidixic acid, and tetracycline. In comparison, it has a lower resistance rate for amoxicillin, chloramphenicol, ampicillin, and ciprofloxacin [15]. Our results show that *C. jejuni* isolated from humans has a phenotypical resistance rate against nalidixic acid and tetracycline more than that reported in Italy and less against ciprofloxacin based on the same study results [37]. At the same time, our results show that *C. jejuni* isolated from animals has a phenotypical resistance rate against nalidixic acid, ciprofloxacin, and tetracycline more than that reported in broiler chicken in Belgium [38]. This systematic review demonstrated moderate to high resistance of *C. jejuni* to erythromycin. Conversely, the recent EU report on AMR found that *C. jejuni* resistance to erythromycin was either undetected or detected at very low levels in *C. jejuni* from food-producing animals and humans [36].

The WHO, Food and Agriculture Organization of the United Nations (FAO), and World Organization for Animal Health (OIE) recommend reducing antibiotic use in animal husbandry, particularly for those known to cause cross-resistance [39–41]. However, some antimicrobials traditionally used in animal production as growth promoters and/or for treating gastrointestinal infections are also used to control human infectious diseases (e.g., tetracycline and quinolones) [42]. The misuse and overuse of antimicrobials in clinical and veterinary medicine and agriculture have increased antimicrobial resistance pathogens, including *Campylobacter* and *Salmonella* [43]. For instance, the Quesada study showed that *Salmonella* isolated from animal food has significant antibiotic resistance in Latin American countries [44]. The therapeutic and prophylactic use of antibiotics in animal production for long periods is likely contributing to the widespread resistance against antibiotics [43]. More integrated environmental–animal–human studies are needed in the region to ascertain its effect on public health. This way, microbiological and clinical evidence on the transmission of AMR between animals and humans can be ascertained in Middle Eastern countries [43–45].

Data on antimicrobial resistance genes (ARGs) among *Salmonella* spp. and *Campylobacter* spp. in the Middle East is limited. However, based on the reported information, we can argue that food-producing animals and their products in the Middle East are not the main drivers for the emergence of ARGs.

Based on our eligibility criteria, six studies targeted ARGs among *Salmonella* and *Campylobacter* as foodborne illnesses in the Middle East region [46–51]. Besharati's study and Youssef's study were two studies that reported the ARGs among NTS. Besharati's study shows an association between the AMR phenotype results and ARGs results in Integron 1 and 2 classes and trimethoprim/sulfamethoxazole in Iran. Conversely, in Youssef's study, results from Egypt revealed no association between AMR phenotype results and ARGS.

Three studies reported the ARGs among *C. jejuni* (Abd-El-Aziz, Divsalar, and Ghoneim) [46–48]. The results in Divsalar and Ghoneim could not show a significant association between the targeted ARGs and the AMR phenotype results. In turn, Abd-El-Aziz found an association between Class 1 integrons and aminoglycoside resistance.

We identified small-scale studies with a small sample size for the ARGs in the NTS and *C. jejuni*. The small sample size in the eligible studies might be responsible for the insignificant difference in the occurrence of the genes between humans and food-producing animals. Our results agreed with Escher's systematic review that targeted ARGs in Africa and found eligible studies characterized by small-scale studies and with a small sample size [16]. Therefore, future studies should have an integrated approach to assess the ARGs and should have a suitable sample size.

Partial sequencing of *C. jejuni* and NTS were performed using conventional PCR to extract the ARGs. Therefore, there is a lack of laboratory techniques that determine the order of bases in an organism's genome in one process such as with Whole-genome sequencing (WGS), to follow the foodborne illnesses and ARGs. Undertaking WGS of isolates, especially those with high-level antibiotic resistance, is strongly encouraged to demonstrate the involved ARGs and their genetic localization (plasmid, chromosome, genomic islands, integrative and conjugative element, and transposon) as well as to detect the most prevalent resistant serovars [36,52,53], detail their potential of horizontal transmission, and evaluate the different sources and comparison of human and animal isolates [54].

5. Conclusions

To the best of our knowledge, this is the first systematic review assessing integrated environment–animal–human studies using a One Health approach in the Middle East to pursue foodborne illnesses and antimicrobial resistance. The One Health approach was not rigorously applied in the Middle East countries. In addition to weak epidemiological study designs from a One Health methodological perspective, there is an uneven distribution in the reported data with about 60% of Middle Eastern countries having no published papers included in this review. More research on foodborne illnesses and AMR in the Middle East is urgently needed. The AMR phenotype results showed a high prevalence of resistance rate for the isolated bacteria that highlights the importance of antimicrobial stewardship in humans and animals in tandem. Furthermore, introducing new laboratory techniques that determine the order of bases in an organism's genome is essential to follow up the foodborne illness outbreak and ARGs.

A simultaneous approach that targets human and animal health in tandem with a solid epidemiological study design has a high potential to provide evidence for understanding the drivers for the emergence and spread of foodborne pathogens and AMR. A comprehensive One Health approach, integrating by a sound epidemiological design the spatio-temporal relationship of humans, animals, and their environment, will allow us to identify key transmission pathways, which are essential for designing more efficient food safety systems and AMR control policies.

Supplementary Materials: The following supporting information can be downloaded at: https://www.mdpi.com/article/10.3390/antibiotics11050536/s1, Supplementary Table S1: The search strategy used for each database., Supplementary Table S2: Overview of the selected studies, Supplementary Table S3: Summary of the selected studies showing the country and pathogens together, Supplementary Table S4: Phenotypic resistance to antibiotics for all isolated serovars, Supplementary Table S5. a, b, and c: Genotypic resistance to antibiotics for all isolated serovars.

Author Contributions: S.A., H.T., L.C., J.Z., P.V. and N.M.E.A.-R., designed the search strategy and data-extraction form; S.A. and H.T. screened studies for selection; S.A., H.T. and A.A. extracted the data; S.A. and J.H. managed and analyzed the data; P.V. provided expert microbiological and antimicrobial resistance advice; J.Z. provided expert One Health and epidemiology advice; N.M.E.A.-R. provided expert epidemiology advice; S.A. and H.T. wrote the first draft of the manuscript; A.A., L.C., J.Z., P.V., J.H. and N.M.E.A.-R. critically revised and finalized the manuscript. All authors have read and agreed to the published version of the manuscript.

Funding: This research received no external funding.

Institutional Review Board Statement: Not applicable.

Informed Consent Statement: Not applicable.

Data Availability Statement: The datasets generated during the current meta-analysis are available from the corresponding author upon reasonable request. All data analyzed for meta-analysis are included in the corresponding published articles, as reported in Supplementary Table S2.

Conflicts of Interest: The authors declare no conflict of interest.

References

1. Devleesschauwer, B.; Bouwknegt, M.; Mangen, M.-J.J.; Havelaar, A.H. Health and economic burden of Campylobacter. In *Campylobacter*; Elsevier: Amsterdam, The Netherlands, 2017; pp. 27–40.
2. Ferrari, R.G.; Rosario, D.K.; Cunha-Neto, A.; Mano, S.B.; Figueiredo, E.E.; Conte-Junior, C.A. Worldwide epidemiology of Salmonella serovars in animal-based foods: A meta-analysis. *Appl. Environ. Microbiol.* **2019**, *85*, e00591-19. [CrossRef] [PubMed]
3. Amuasi, J.H.; May, J. Non-typhoidal salmonella: Invasive, lethal, and on the loose. *Lancet Infect. Dis.* **2019**, *19*, 1267–1269. [CrossRef]
4. Majowicz, S.E.; Scallan, E.; Jones-Bitton, A.; Sargeant, J.M.; Stapleton, J.; Angulo, F.J.; Yeung, D.H.; Kirk, M.D. Global incidence of human Shiga toxin–producing Escherichia coli infections and deaths: A systematic review and knowledge synthesis. *Foodborne Pathog. Dis.* **2014**, *11*, 447–455. [CrossRef]
5. Connerton, I.; Connerton, P. Campylobacter foodborne disease. In *Foodborne Diseases*; Elsevier: Amsterdam, The Netherlands, 2017; pp. 209–221.
6. Kaakoush, N.O.; Castaño-Rodríguez, N.; Mitchell, H.M.; Man, S.M. Global epidemiology of Campylobacter infection. *Clin. Microbiol. Rev.* **2015**, *28*, 687–720. [CrossRef]
7. Authority, E.F.S. The European Union summary report on trends and sources of zoonoses, zoonotic agents and food-borne outbreaks in 2017. *EFSA J.* **2018**, *16*, e05500.
8. WHO's First Ever Global Estimates of Foodborne Diseases Find Children under 5 Account for Almost One Third of Deaths. 2015. Available online: https://www.who.int/news/item/03-12-2015-who-s-first-ever-global-estimates-of-foodborne-diseases-find-children-under-5-account-for-almost-one-third-of-deaths (accessed on 20 February 2022).
9. Cohen, D.; Gargouri, N.; Ramlawi, A.; Abdeen, Z.; Belbesi, A.; Al Hijawi, B.; Haddadin, A.; Ali, S.S.; Al Shuaibi, N.; Bassal, R. A Middle East subregional laboratory-based surveillance network on foodborne diseases established by Jordan, Israel, and the Palestinian Authority. *Epidemiol. Infect.* **2010**, *138*, 1443–1448. [CrossRef]
10. Bassal, R.; Reisfeld, A.; Andorn, N.; Yishai, R.; Nissan, I.; Agmon, V.; Peled, N.; Block, C.; Keller, N.; Kenes, Y. Recent trends in the epidemiology of non-typhoidal Salmonella in Israel, 1999–2009. *Epidemiol. Infect.* **2012**, *140*, 1446–1453. [CrossRef]
11. El-Shabrawi, M.; Salem, M.; Abou-Zekri, M.; El-Naghi, S.; Hassanin, F.; El-Adly, T.; El-Shamy, A. The burden of different pathogens in acute diarrhoeal episodes among a cohort of Egyptian children less than five years old. *Prz. Gastroenterol.* **2015**, *10*, 173–180. [CrossRef]
12. Dayan, N.; Revivo, D.; Even, L.; Elkayam, O.; Glikman, D. Campylobacter is the leading cause of bacterial gastroenteritis and dysentery in hospitalized children in the Western Galilee Region in Israel. *Epidemiol. Infect.* **2010**, *138*, 1405–1406. [CrossRef]
13. Feizabadi, M.M.; Dolatabadi, S.; Zali, M.R. Isolation and drug-resistant patterns of Campylobacter strains cultured from diarrheic children in Tehran. *Jpn. J. Infect. Dis.* **2007**, *60*, 217–219.
14. Elamreen, F.H.A.; Abed, A.A.; Sharif, F.A. Detection and identification of bacterial enteropathogens by polymerase chain reaction and conventional techniques in childhood acute gastroenteritis in Gaza, Palestine. *Int. J. Infect. Dis.* **2007**, *11*, 501–507. [CrossRef] [PubMed]
15. Alsayeqh, A.F.; Baz, A.H.A.; Darwish, W.S. Antimicrobial-resistant foodborne pathogens in the Middle East: A systematic review. *Environ. Sci. Pollut. Res.* **2021**, *28*, 68111–68133. [CrossRef] [PubMed]
16. Escher, N.A.; Muhummed, A.M.; Hattendorf, J.; Vonaesch, P.; Zinsstag, J. Systematic review and meta-analysis of integrated studies on antimicrobial resistance genes in Africa—A One Health perspective. *Trop. Med. Int. Health* **2021**, *26*, 1153–1163. [CrossRef] [PubMed]
17. Garcia, S.N.; Osburn, B.I.; Jay-Russell, M.T. One health for food safety, food security, and sustainable food production. *Front. Sustain. Food Syst.* **2020**, *4*. [CrossRef]

18. Racloz, V.; Waltner-Toews, D.; DC, K.S. 8 Integrated Risk Assessment–Foodborne Diseases. In *One Health: The Theory and Practice of Integrated Health Approaches*; CABI: Wallingford, UK, 2015; p. 85.
19. King, L.J. Combating the triple threat: The need for a One Health approach. *Microbiol. Spectr.* **2013**, *1*. [CrossRef]
20. Paul, R.J.; Varghese, D. AMR in Animal Health: Issues and One Health Solutions for LMICs. In *Antimicrobial Resistance*; Springer: Berlin, Germany, 2020; pp. 135–149.
21. Larsson, D.J.; Andremont, A.; Bengtsson-Palme, J.; Brandt, K.K.; de Roda Husman, A.M.; Fagerstedt, P.; Fick, J.; Flach, C.-F.; Gaze, W.H.; Kuroda, M. Critical knowledge gaps and research needs related to the environmental dimensions of antibiotic resistance. *Environ. Int.* **2018**, *117*, 132–138. [CrossRef]
22. Hoy, D.; Brooks, P.; Woolf, A.; Blyth, F.; March, L.; Bain, C.; Baker, P.; Smith, E.; Buchbinder, R. Assessing risk of bias in prevalence studies: Modification of an existing tool and evidence of interrater agreement. *J. Clin. Epidemiol.* **2012**, *65*, 934–939. [CrossRef]
23. Mantel, N.; Haenszel, W. Statistical aspects of the analysis of data from retrospective studies of disease. *J. Natl. Cancer Inst.* **1959**, *22*, 719–748.
24. Zinsstag, J.; Schelling, E.; Crump, L.; Whittaker, M.; Tanner, M.; Stephen, C. *One Health: The theory and Practice of Integrated Health Approaches*; CABI: Wallingford, UK, 2020.
25. Gahamanyi, N.; Mboera, L.E.; Matee, M.I.; Mutangana, D.; Komba, E.V. Prevalence, risk factors, and antimicrobial resistance profiles of thermophilic Campylobacter species in humans and animals in sub-saharan Africa: A systematic review. *Int. J. Microbiol.* **2020**, *2020*, 2092478. [CrossRef]
26. Asuming-Bediako, N.; Parry-Hanson Kunadu, A.; Abraham, S.; Habib, I. Campylobacter at the human–food interface: The african perspective. *Pathogens* **2019**, *8*, 87. [CrossRef]
27. Wada, Y.; Abdul-Rahman, Z. Human Campylobacteriosis in Southeast Asia: A Meta-Analysis and Systematic Review. *Int. J. Infect. Dis.* **2022**, *116*, S75. [CrossRef]
28. Zbrun, M.V.; Rossler, E.; Romero-Scharpen, A.; Soto, L.P.; Berisvil, A.; Zimmermann, J.A.; Fusari, M.L.; Signorini, M.; Frizzo, L.S. Worldwide meta-analysis of the prevalence of Campylobacter in animal food products. *Res. Vet. Sci.* **2020**, *132*, 69–77. [CrossRef] [PubMed]
29. Hlashwayo, D.F.; Sigaúque, B.; Noormahomed, E.V.; Afonso, S.M.; Mandomando, I.M.; Bila, C.G. A systematic review and meta-analysis reveal that Campylobacter spp. and antibiotic resistance are widespread in humans in sub-Saharan Africa. *PLoS ONE* **2021**, *16*, e0245951. [CrossRef] [PubMed]
30. Al-Rifai, R.H.; Chaabna, K.; Denagamage, T.; Alali, W.Q. Prevalence of enteric non-typhoidal Salmonella in humans in the Middle East and North Africa: A systematic review and meta-analysis. *Zoonoses Public Health* **2019**, *66*, 701–728. [CrossRef]
31. Al-Rifai, R.H.; Chaabna, K.; Denagamage, T.; Alali, W.Q. Prevalence of non-typhoidal Salmonella enterica in food products in the Middle East and North Africa: A systematic review and meta-analysis. *Food Control* **2020**, *109*, 106908. [CrossRef]
32. Skarp, C.; Hänninen, M.-L.; Rautelin, H. Campylobacteriosis: The role of poultry meat. *Clin. Microbiol. Infect.* **2016**, *22*, 103–109. [CrossRef]
33. Capita, R.; Alonso-Calleja, C.; Prieto, M. Prevalence of Salmonella enterica serovars and genovars from chicken carcasses in slaughterhouses in Spain. *J. Appl. Microbiol.* **2007**, *103*, 1366–1375. [CrossRef]
34. Yang, B.; Xi, M.; Wang, X.; Cui, S.; Yue, T.; Hao, H.; Wang, Y.; Cui, Y.; Alali, W.; Meng, J. Prevalence of Salmonella on raw poultry at retail markets in China. *J. Food Prot.* **2011**, *74*, 1724–1728. [CrossRef]
35. Cave, R.; Cole, J.; Mkrtchyan, H.V. Surveillance and prevalence of antimicrobial resistant bacteria from public settings within urban built environments: Challenges and opportunities for hygiene and infection control. *Environ. Int.* **2021**, *157*, 106836. [CrossRef]
36. Authority, E.F.S. The European Union Summary Report on Antimicrobial Resistance in zoonotic and indicator bacteria from humans, animals and food in 2019–2020. *EFSA J.* **2022**, *20*. [CrossRef]
37. Marotta, F.; Garofolo, G.; Di Marcantonio, L.; Di Serafino, G.; Neri, D.; Romantini, R.; Sacchini, L.; Alessiani, A.; Di Donato, G.; Nuvoloni, R. Antimicrobial resistance genotypes and phenotypes of Campylobacter jejuni isolated in Italy from humans, birds from wild and urban habitats, and poultry. *PLoS ONE* **2019**, *14*, e0223804. [CrossRef] [PubMed]
38. Elhadidy, M.; Miller, W.G.; Arguello, H.; Álvarez-Ordóñez, A.; Duarte, A.; Dierick, K.; Botteldoorn, N. Genetic basis and clonal population structure of antibiotic resistance in Campylobacter jejuni isolated from broiler carcasses in Belgium. *Front. Microbiol.* **2018**, *9*, 1014. [CrossRef] [PubMed]
39. WHO. *WHO Guidelines on Use of Medically Important Antimicrobials in Food-Producing Animals: Web Annex A: Evidence Base*; World Health Organization: Geneva, Switzerland, 2017.
40. Antimicrobial Resistance: FAO. 2021. Available online: https://www.fao.org/antimicrobial-resistance/world-antimicrobial-awareness-week/en/ (accessed on 20 February 2022).
41. Antimicrobial Resistance: OIE. Available online: https://www.oie.int/en/what-we-do/global-initiatives/antimicrobial-resistance/ (accessed on 20 February 2022).
42. Rodrigues, G.L.; Panzenhagen, P.; Ferrari, R.G.; Paschoalin, V.M.F.; Conte-Junior, C.A. Antimicrobial resistance in nontyphoidal Salmonella isolates from human and swine sources in brazil: A systematic review of the past three decades. *Microb. Drug Resist.* **2020**, *26*, 1260–1270. [CrossRef] [PubMed]
43. Economou, V.; Gousia, P. Agriculture and food animals as a source of antimicrobial-resistant bacteria. *Infect. Drug Resist.* **2015**, *8*, 49–61. [CrossRef]

44. Quesada, A.; Reginatto, G.A.; Ruiz Español, A.; Colantonio, L.D.; Burrone, M.S. Antimicrobial resistance of Salmonella spp. isolated animal food for human consumption. *Rev. Peru. Med. Exp. Salud Publica* **2016**, *33*, 32–44. [CrossRef]
45. Kim, D.-W.; Cha, C.-J. Antibiotic resistome from the One-Health perspective: Understanding and controlling antimicrobial resistance transmission. *Exp. Mol. Med.* **2021**, *53*, 301–309. [CrossRef]
46. El-Aziz, A.; Norhan, K.; Ammar, A.M.; Hamdy, M.M.; Gobouri, A.A.; Azab, E.; Sewid, A.H. First report of aacC5-aadA7Δ4 Gene Cassette array and phage tail tape measure protein on Class 1 Integrons of Campylobacter Species isolated from animal and human sources in Egypt. *Animals* **2020**, *10*, 2067. [CrossRef]
47. Ghoneim, N.H.; Sabry, M.A.; Ahmed, Z.S.; Elshafiee, E.A. Campylobacter Species Isolated from Chickens in Egypt: Molecular Epidemiology and Antimicrobial Resistance. *Pak. J. Zool.* **2020**, *52*, 917–926. [CrossRef]
48. Divsalar, G.; Kaboosi, H.; Khoshbakht, R.; Shirzad-Aski, H.; Ghadikolaii, F.P. Antimicrobial resistances, and molecular typing of Campylobacter jejuni isolates, separated from food-producing animals and diarrhea patients in Iran. *Comp. Immunol. Microbiol. Infect. Dis.* **2019**, *65*, 194–200. [CrossRef]
49. Besharati, S.; Sadeghi, A.; Ahmadi, F.; Tajeddin, E.; Salehi, R.M.; Fani, F.; Pouladfar, G.; Nikmanesh, B.; Majidpour, A.; Moghadam, S.S. Serogroups, and drug resistance of nontyphoidal Salmonella in symptomatic patients with community-acquired diarrhea and chicken meat samples in Tehran. *Iran. J. Vet. Res.* **2020**, *21*, 269–278.
50. Elhariri, M.; Elhelw, R.; Selim, S.; Ibrahim, M.; Hamza, D.; Hamza, E. Virulence and antibiotic resistance patterns of extended-spectrum beta-lactamase-producing Salmonella enterica serovar Heidelberg isolated from broiler chickens and poultry workers: A potential hazard. *Foodborne Pathog. Dis.* **2020**, *17*, 373–381. [CrossRef] [PubMed]
51. Youssef, R.A.; Abbas, A.M.; El-Shehawi, A.M.; Mabrouk, M.I.; Aboshanab, K.M. Serotyping and Antimicrobial Resistance Profile of Enteric Nontyphoidal Salmonella Recovered from Febrile Neutropenic Patients and Poultry in Egypt. *Antibiotics* **2021**, *10*, 493. [CrossRef] [PubMed]
52. Mouftah, S.F.; Cobo-Díaz, J.F.; Álvarez-Ordóñez, A.; Elserafy, M.; Saif, N.A.; Sadat, A.; El-Shibiny, A.; Elhadidy, M. High-throughput sequencing reveals genetic determinants associated with antibiotic resistance in *Campylobacter* spp. from farm-to-fork. *PLoS ONE* **2021**, *16*, e0253797. [CrossRef]
53. Collineau, L.; Boerlin, P.; Carson, C.A.; Chapman, B.; Fazil, A.; Hetman, B.; McEwen, S.A.; Parmley, E.J.; Reid-Smith, R.J.; Taboada, E.N. Integrating whole-genome sequencing data into quantitative risk assessment of foodborne antimicrobial resistance: A review of opportunities and challenges. *Front. Microbiol.* **2019**, *10*, 1107. [CrossRef] [PubMed]
54. Mourkas, E.; Florez-Cuadrado, D.; Pascoe, B.; Calland, J.K.; Bayliss, S.C.; Mageiros, L.; Méric, G.; Hitchings, M.D.; Quesada, A.; Porrero, C. Gene pool transmission of multidrug resistance among Campylobacter from livestock, sewage and human disease. *Environ. Microbiol.* **2019**, *21*, 4597–4613. [CrossRef] [PubMed]

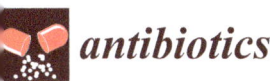

Article

Salmonella in Pig Farms and on Pig Meat in Suriname

Patrick Butaye [1,2,*], Iona Halliday-Simmonds [1] and Astrid Van Sauers [3]

1. Department of Biosciences, School of Veterinary Medicine, Ross University, Basseterre 00334, Saint Kitts and Nevis; IHalliday-Simmonds@rossvet.edu.kn
2. Department of Pathobiology, Pharmacology and Zoological Medicine, Faculty of Veterinary Medicine, Ghent University, B-9820 Merelbeke, Belgium
3. The Veterinary Services, Ministry of Agriculture, Paramaribo, Suriname; astrid.vansauers@gmail.com
* Correspondence: pabuta@gmail.com

Abstract: *Salmonella* is one of the most important food borne zoonotic pathogens. While mainly associated with poultry, it has also been associated with pigs. Compared to the high-income countries, there is much less known on the prevalence of *Salmonella* in low- and middle-income countries, especially in the Caribbean area. Therefore, we investigated the prevalence of *Salmonella* in pigs and pig meat in Suriname. A total of 53 farms and 53 meat samples were included, and *Salmonella* was isolated using standard protocols. Strains were subjected to whole genome sequencing. No *Salmonella* was found on pig meat. Five farms were found to be positive for *Salmonella*, and a total of eight different strains were obtained. Serotypes were *S*. Anatum ($n = 1$), *S*. Ohio ($n = 2$), a monophasic variant of *S*. Typhimurium ($n = 3$), one *S*. Brandenburg, and one *S*. Javaniana. The monophasic variant of *S*. Typhimurium belonged to the ST34 pandemic clone, and the three strains were very similar. A few resistance genes, located on mobile genetic elements, were found. Several plasmids were detected, though only one was carrying resistance genes. This is the first study on the prevalence of *Salmonella* in pigs in the Caribbean and that used whole genome sequencing for characterization. The strains were rather susceptible. Local comparison of similar serotypes showed a mainly clonal spread of certain serotypes.

Keywords: *Salmonella enterica*; pigs; Suriname; whole genome sequencing

1. Introduction

Few studies have been performed on *Salmonella* in the Caribbean region, and those mainly dealt with the prevalence in poultry. Prevalences were very variable depending on the study. Moreover, most studies were performed in Trinidad and were mainly on food products, both fresh and ready to eat. The prevalence on those products varied between 0% (mainly ready to eat) and 7%. Several serotypes were isolated, including *S*. Agona *S*. Kiambu, *S*. Kentucky, *S*. Derby, and *S*. Mbandaka as the most reported. The few studies in the Caribbean that have been performed on live animals dealt with layer chickens, and apart from one study, all were on eggs. Eggs have been a major focus for the Caribbean. Prevalence on eggs varied from 1 to 13%, and a multicountry study in 2014 showed that 3% of the layer farms were positive. Prevalence in Barbados on layer farms was the highest, with 73% of the farms being positive. It should be noted that for the different studies, different sampling and isolation methods were used, and as such, comparisons are difficult [1,2].

Several studies were performed on pet animals and mainly wildlife. In dogs, eight *Salmonella* strains were recovered [3]; in iguanas, mongooses, tree boa, leatherback turtles, blue land crabs, and toads, a few strains were found, though it should be noted that the serotypes were very different, and that the iguanas had to be regarded as wildlife. These strains in general carried few resistances [4–10].

There are very few studies on pork or pigs in the Caribbean region. An old study in Trinidad and Tobago showed that about 18% of the swine carcasses sampled were positive

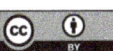

Citation: Butaye, P.; Halliday-Simmonds, I.; Van Sauers, A. *Salmonella* in Pig Farms and on Pig Meat in Suriname. *Antibiotics* **2021**, *10*, 1495. https://doi.org/10.3390/antibiotics10121495

Academic Editor: Piera Anna Martino

Received: 11 November 2021
Accepted: 3 December 2021
Published: 6 December 2021

Publisher's Note: MDPI stays neutral with regard to jurisdictional claims in published maps and institutional affiliations.

Copyright: © 2021 by the authors. Licensee MDPI, Basel, Switzerland. This article is an open access article distributed under the terms and conditions of the Creative Commons Attribution (CC BY) license (https://creativecommons.org/licenses/by/4.0/).

for *Salmonella* [11], while a small-scale baseline study in the Bahamas showed that 8/42 of the retail meat samples were positive for *Salmonella*. At a pig slaughter plant, 44.1% (15/34) and 2.9% (1/34) were found positive at the beginning and the end of the slaughter process, respectively [12]. In both diarrheic and non-diarrheic pigs of different ages from Trinidad, a prevalence between 3 and 4.5% was recorded. A more recent study in Cuba demonstrated a prevalence of 2.2% in weaned piglets [13]. Apart from those studies, we found no other studies in live pigs.

In humans, there is no systematic surveillance of nontyphoid *Salmonella* infections, and as such, the incidence is unknown. However, the incidence has been estimated at an annual rate of over five cases per 100,000 persons in Trinidad and Tobago [6,14].

Pig production is important in the food supply in Suriname. In 2018, 208 farms were active, with a total of 21,362 pigs divided over the different farms. Since pig meat can also be a major source of *Salmonella* infections in humans, we investigated the prevalence, as well as the types of *Salmonella* in pigs in Suriname.

2. Materials and Methods

2.1. Sampling

Samples from pigs were taken at the only pork slaughterhouse in Paramaribo, Suriname in 2018. Farms were located in the districts of Paramaribo, Wanica Saramacca, and Coronie. Pigs were mixed breed pigs, with breeds involved being the Dutch Landrace, Yorkshire, Pietrain, and Duroc. Pigs originated from 53 farms in the central part of Suriname that were delivering pork to the slaughterhouse. One pig per farm was sampled except for two farms; from one of these, two pigs were sampled on the same day; and from another farm, two pigs were sampled, but on different sampling days. A sample was taken from the cecum and ileocecal lymph node of each pig.

Meat samples were obtained from 53 retail stores in Paramaribo and Wanica. Most retail stores are in Paramaribo, which contains about half of the population of Suriname. Per retail store, one piece of fresh pork chop sample was obtained. There is no food tracing system in Surname, and as such, the slaughter date nor origin of the meats could be traced.

2.2. Isolation and Identification

Salmonella was isolated using the ISO 6579 annex D. Briefly, after homogenization, the sample (25 g) was inoculated in Buffered Peptone Water (BPW, Bio-Rad, Hercules, CA, USA) (1:10, W/V) and incubated for 16–20 h at 37 °C. Of this, 0.1 mL was inoculated on a Modified Semisolid Rappaport Vassiliadis agar plate (MSRV, Bio-Rad, Hercules, CA, USA) and incubated for 21–27 h at 41 °C. Positive samples were inoculated on Xylose Lysine Deoxycholaat agar plate (XLD, Bio-Rad, Hercules, CA, USA) and a nalidixine-BGA plate and incubated for 21–27 h at 37 °C. Suspected colonies were inoculated on Triple Sugar Iron agar (TSI, Bio-Rad, Hercules, CA, USA) and lysine decarboxylase broth (Thermo Fisher Scientific, Waltham, MA, USA) and incubated for 18–24 h at 37 °C for presumptive identification. Further identification was performed using the Gram-Negative ID Plate (Sensititre GNID, TREK Diagnostic Systems, Cleveland, OH, USA), using the protocols provided by the supplier, and using a Sensititre OptiRead analyzer (TREK Diagnostic Systems, Cleveland, OH, USA). *Salmonella* isolates were then serogrouped using the Wellcolex Color *Salmonella* Rapid Latex Agglutination Test Kit (Thermo Fisher Scientific, Waltham, MA, USA). Strains that could serogrouped were selected for whole genome sequencing.

2.3. Whole Genome Sequencing

Purified strains were sent to Macrogen (Seoul, Korea) for DNA extraction and sequencing on an Illumina platform using a TruSeq Babi DNA kit and 151 bp long paired-end sequencing.

Raw sequences (fastq files) were submitted to the NCBI database under PRJNA751882 with SAMN20584910, SAMN20584911, SAMN20584912, SAMN20584913. SAMN20584914, SAMN20584915, SAMN20584916, and SAMN20584917.

Sequences were trimmed and assembled using SKESA [15]. Annotation was done with PROKKA [16] and RAST [17]. The serotype was determined with Sistr [18]. The MLST profile was determined using 'mlst' [19]. Phylogenetic analysis of the isolates of a same serotype was done with NASP [20]. Further analysis of the strains was done using ARIBA against the plasmid finder [21], ARg-ANNOT [22], and ResFinder [23,24]. Plasmids were confirmed with Platon [25]. Using RAST analysis, we located the different associated genes.

2.4. Statistical Analysis

Confidence intervals of the prevalence of *Salmonella* on farms in Suriname were calculated using exact binomials in an Excel file.

3. Results

3.1. Prevalence, Serotyes, and Epidemiology

Salmonella could not be isolated from any of the food samples. Of the 53 farms investigated, a total of eight strains were isolated. Strains originated from five different farms (9%, of the farms were positive, confidence interval 3.1–21%) and seven different animals. Five different serotypes were isolated, including one *S.* Anatum, *S.* Ohio ($n = 2$), a monophasic variant of *S.* Typhimurium ($n = 3$), one *S.* Brandenburg, and one *S.* Javaniana (Table 1).

Table 1. Isolation and serotype results and origin of the strains.

Isolate	Farm	Origin	Serotype	MLST
173	B	Cecal	Anatum	ST64
174 *	X	Cecal	Ohio	ST329
175 *	X	Cecal	Monophasic variant of Typhimurium	ST34
179	X	Lymph node	Monophasic variant of Typhimurium	ST34
180	P	Lymph node	Monophasic variant of Typhimurium	ST34
222	E	Cecal	Brandenburg	ST65
250	X	Lymph node	Javaniana	ST1674
543	F	Lymph node	Ohio	ST329

* Strains from the same animal.

3.2. Antimicrobial Resistance Genes

All strains had at least one resistance gene (Table 2), though it should be taken into account that all *Salmonella* have the $aac(6')$ gene in their chromosome [26]. As such, three strains did not show any additional resistance gene. A total of five out of eight strains were resistant to penicillins, mediated by the bla_{TEM-1} gene. All strains had at least one resistance gene for aminoglycosides, and some strains had up to four different aminoglycoside resistance genes. Four strains carried the *sul2* gene, indicating sulfonamide resistance. Only two strains carried the tetracycline resistance gene, *tet*(B), and one strain carried a trimethoprim resistance gene, *dfrAB*. However, the latter strain was susceptible to sulfonamide.

Table 2. T Antimicrobial resistance and plasmids associated with the different isolates.

Isolate	Serotype	β-Lactam	Aminoglycoside	Sulphonamide	Tetracycline	Trimethoprim	Plasmids
173	Anatum		aac(6′)				ColpVC_
174	Ohio		aac(6′)				
175	Monophasic variant of Typhimurium	bla$_{TEM-1}$	aac(6′), aph(6)-Id, aph(3″)-Ib, aph(3′)-Ia	sul2			IncQ1_1
179	Monophasic variant of Typhimurium	bla$_{TEM-1}$	aac(6′), aph(6)-Id, aph(3″)-Ib, aph(3′)-Ia	sul2			IncQ1_1, IncI1_1_Alpha
180	Monophasic variant of Typhimurium	bla$_{TEM-1}$	aac(6′), aph(6)-Id, aph(3″)-Ib, aph(3′)-Ia	sul2			IncQ1_1
222	Brandenburg	bla$_{TEM-1}$	aac(6′), aph(6)-Id, aph(3″)-Ib	sul2	tet(B)		IncFIA(HI1)_1_HI1, IncH1A/B, ColRNAI_1, Col440I_1
250	Javaniana		aac(6′)				
543	Ohio	bla$_{TEM-1}$	aac(6′), aph(6)-Id, aph(3″)-Ib	sul2	tet(B)	dfrAB	IncFIA(HI1)_1_HI1, IncHI1B(R27)_1_R27, Col440I_1

3.3. Plasmids

Two strains did not carry any plasmids (strain 174, S. Ohio; and 250, S. Javaniana). Five different Inc plasmids were detected: IncQ1_1, IncI1_1_Alpha, IncFIA(HI1)_1_HI1, IncH1A/B, and IncHI1B(R27)_1_R27.

Three different colicin plasmids were found. The full sequence of a small plasmid ColpVC_1 was found by Platon in strain 173, and this plasmid was nearly similar to earlier described plasmids in E. coli and Salmonella (NCBI BLAST result). The Col440I_1 plasmid from the S. Brandenburg and S. Ohio strain were identical. It was a small circular plasmid of 1748 bp and contained four genes. The ColRNAI_1 plasmid from the S. Brandenburg strain was 4597 bp and had seven genes.

3.4. Association of Resistance Genes with Mobile Genetic Elements

The aph(6)-Id (strB), aph(3″)-Ib (strA) genes in the three monophasic S. Typhimurium strains were located on a same contig together with a sul2. However, there were no other genes on that contig, making its location speculative. In the S. Brandenburg strain, this same gene cluster was located on a 63,539 pb contig that also contained the bla$_{TEM-1}$ gene, downstream of the sul2 gene. In the S. Ohio strain 543, the aph(6)-Id, aph(3″)-Ib, bla$_{TEM-1}$, and sul2 genes were located as one cluster with a similar structure to the S. Typhimurium and S. Brandenburg strains, and associated with the IS1 gene InsB, though the downstream part associated with Tn7 was missing on the contig. In addition, copper and zinc resistance genes were present in this cluster. This gene cluster most likely was associated with a mobile Tn7-like transposon.

The aph(3′)-Ia gene was typically located on the InQ1_1 plasmid in the three monophasic S. Typhimurium strains.

The tetracycline resistance genes found in the strains of this collection were located on the same structure; however, the contig containing the tet(B) gene was too small to determine the exact location Blast analysis of the whole contig showed that it was similar to a chromosomal location in the bacterial species Glasseralla parasuis, E. coli, and Shigella flexneri.

4. Discussion

This is one of the few more systematic investigations on Salmonella in pigs in the Caribbean. Though few samples per farm could be tested, when lowering the sensitivity for detecting positive farms, we found 5/53 farms positive, which was close to 10% of the farms being positive. This was higher than what has been found in Cuba, though it should be noted that this study was conducted on weaned pigs, while our study was conducted on pigs at slaughter [13]. Our findings were lower than what was found on pig carcasses in Trinidad in 1978, while higher than what was found in the same country in fecal material of pigs in 1993 (4.1% of the 294 pigs) and in 1994, with 4.5% of the diarrheic pigs and 3.4% (n = 179) of the non-diarrheic pigs (n = 117) originating from 25 farms sampled at different ages being positive [1,27]. The variations can also be explained by the age or carcass contamination, as it is known that older pigs are in general more prone to be positive than piglets [28], while contamination at the slaughter line may increase the apparent prevalence [29].

In this study, we found five different serotypes. The most commonly found in the European Union and the US are S. Typhimurium, S. 1,4,[5],12:i:-, S. Derby, and S. Rissen, though this varies in time and space [29,30]. While the monophasic variant of S. Typhimurium is one of the most commonly found serotypes in pigs worldwide, and S. Brandenburg is less commonly found, the other serotypes, S. Ohio, S. Anatum, and S. Javaniana, are more rarely reported. This may indicate that there may be some differences in the epidemiology of Salmonella in the Caribbean; however, due to the low numbers of strains recovered, this should be interpreted with care. Two of the monophasic S. Typhimurium strains were the same based on the NASP SNP analysis, as they had no SNPs in the core genome, while the other strain had only 235 SNPs different. It was striking that the two equal monophasic S. Typhimurium strains were from two different farms. Unfortunately, we could not determine whether those two farms had epidemiological connections. The two different monophasic S. Typhimurium strains came from the same farm, but from different pigs, indicating several different clones were circulating in that farm. All the monophasic Typhimurium strains were ST 34, an epidemic clone in Europe [31] and other parts of the world that is to be regarded as a pandemic strain [32–34]. Compared to other S. Typhimurium ST34 strains, the Caribbean clone was remarkably susceptible. This may be due to the limited availability of antimicrobials in Suriname. S. Anatum ST64 has been reported as one of the most prevalent strains on retail pork in Juiangsu China [35]; however, few data are available on this clone. The two S. Ohio strains originated from different farms and had 716 SNPs different, indicating that they were unrelated strains.

We could not find a single study on antimicrobial resistance genes in *Salmonella* from pigs in the Caribbean, and only few on *Salmonella* as a whole in the Caribbean. In poultry strains in Trinidad, a quite higher prevalence of resistance was found compared to our study, and this included plasmid-mediated colistin resistance [36–38].

All monophasic S. Typhimurium strains carried the IncQ1_1 plasmid. The full sequence of 6644 bp of this mobilizable plasmid was obtained. This plasmid also has been found in other *Salmonella* and *E. coli* (BLAST search 2/2021), as well as in *Aeromonas hydrophila* isolated from swine [39]. The IncI1 plasmid, found in one of the monophasic S. Typimurium strains, is a conjugative plasmid frequently associated with antimicrobial resistance genes, though here we could not identify any. However, since the sequence was not closed or complete (though it consisted of 68,689 bp), we could not confirm this. Nevertheless, we found genes associated with heavy metal resistance: there was a silver and copper resistance gene cluster on this plasmid. Copper is used in swine rearing, and this use might have selected for this resistance.

The two IncHI1A_1 and IncHI1B_1 sequences were found on the same contig, indicating this was a hybrid plasmid with two different replicons. Most likely, the IncFIA(HI1)_1_HI1 replicon was also on this plasmid, as this rep protein was on a single gene contig, and has been reported before on the same plasmid in other different serotypes of *Salmonella* worldwide [40]. This combination of replicons, together with an IncN replicon, has also been found in *E. coli*. This plasmid carried an *mcr*-gene encoding colistin resistance [41]. A plasmid with exactly the same sequences was found in S. Brandenburg and S. Ohio from two different farms, indicating its spread amongst *Salmonella* in Suriname. Using BLAST on the NCBI database, a similar plasmid, though with lower coverage and similarity, was found in a *Klebsiella* strain. Similarly, the ColpVC_1 plasmid was found worldwide in different bacterial species [42]. It is clear that all the col plasmids spread between the different Salmonella serotypes in Suriname.

It was somehow difficult to locate all resistance genes, as Illumina sequencing, also depending on the sequence depth, created several contigs that cannot be linked. Nevertheless, on bigger contigs as well, it is not always evident to link to structures. We could link the cluster encoding aminoglycoside, sulphomamide, and β-lactam ($aph(6)$-Id ($strB$), $aph(3'')$-Ib ($strA$), $sul2$, bla_{TEM-1}) resistance to an Tn7-like structure, also indicating its mobility, as it was present in several strains and moving around as coresistances. This means when one of the antimicrobials was used, it selected for all the resistance genes, and thus created a larger problem. Moreover, we also had to take into account the use of heavy metals such as zinc and copper in veterinary medicine. Resistance genes against these metals are also located on this mobile genetic element (data not shown). The $aph(3')$-Ia gene could not be linked to any mobile structure. The location of the $tet(B)$ gene could not really be determined; however, through BLAST analysis, the same genes in the contig were also present in *Glasseralla parasuis*, *E. coli*, and *Shigella flexneri*, which indicated the mobility or preferential location of this gene.

5. Conclusions

In conclusion, this was the first study on the prevalence of *Salmonella* in pigs in the Caribbean. About 25 of all the farms in Suriname were sampled, and prevalence was 9% (CI 3.1–21%). Few strains were isolated, although they included the pandemic monophasic S. Typhimurium ST34. Fewer resistances were found compared to other monophasic S. Typhimurium ST34 strains isolated in other countries. In general, the strains were rather susceptible, except for aminoglycoside resistance. Most resistances could be located on mobile genetic elements, with a multi-resistant, Tn7-like element spreading. Local comparison of similar serotypes showed a rather clonal spread of certain serotypes. More strains should be analyzed to determine the local epidemiology of *Salmonella* in pigs in Suriname. The fact that no strains could be isolated from meat samples showed that food safety is not hampered very much by the presence of *Salmonella* in pigs.

Author Contributions: Conceptualization, P.B. and A.V.S.; methodology, P.B. and A.V.S.; software, P.B.; validation, P.B., A.V.S. and I.H.-S.; formal analysis, P.B.; investigation, P.B.; resources, P.B. and A.V.S.; data curation, P.B. and A.V.S.; writing—original draft preparation, P.B.; writing—review and editing, P.B., A.V.S. and I.H.-S.; supervision, P.B.; project administration, P.B.; funding acquisition, P.B. and A.V.S. All authors have read and agreed to the published version of the manuscript.

Funding: This research was funded by WHO AGISAR, under grant number "Focused project, Determination of the transfer of Salmonella from pigs to food in Suriname" 2017/725664-0.

Institutional Review Board Statement: Not applicable.

Informed Consent Statement: Not applicable.

Data Availability Statement: Raw sequences (fastq files) were submitted to the NCBI database under PRJNA751882 with SAMN20584910, SAMN20584911, SAMN20584912, SAMN20584913. SAMN205849 SAMN20584915, SAMN20584916, and SAMN20584917.

Conflicts of Interest: The authors declare no conflict of interest. The funders had no role in the design of the study; in the collection, analyses, or interpretation of data; in the writing of the manuscript; or in the decision to publish the results.

References

1. Adesiyun, A.; Webb, L.; Musai, L.; Louison, B.; Joseph, G.; Stewart-Johnson, A.; Samlal, S.; Rodrigo, S. Survey of *Salmonella* contamination in chicken layer farms in three Caribbean countries. *J. Food Prot.* **2014**, *77*, 1471–1480. [CrossRef]
2. Guerra, M.M.; de Almeida, A.M.; Willingham, A.L. An overview of food safety and bacterial foodborne zoonoses in food production animals in the Caribbean region. *Trop. Anim. Health Prod.* **2016**, *48*, 1095–1108. [CrossRef]
3. Amadi, V.A.; Hariharan, H.; Arya, G.; Matthew-Belmar, V.; Nicholas-Thomas, R.; Pinckney, R.; Sharma, R.; Johnson, R. Serovars and antimicrobial resistance of non-typhoidal *Salmonella* isolated from non-diarrhoeic dogs in Grenada, West Indies. *Vet. Med. Sci.* **2017**, *4*, 26–34. [CrossRef]

4. Miller, S.; Zieger, U.; Ganser, C.; Satterlee, S.A.; Bankovich, B.; Amadi, V.; Hariharan, H.; Stone, D.; Wisely, S.M.J. Influence of land use and climate on *Salmonella* carrier status in the small Indian mongoose (*Herpestes auropunctatus*) in Grenada, West Indies. *J. Wildl. Dis.* **2015**, *51*, 60–68. [CrossRef]
5. Sylvester, W.R.; Amadi, V.; Pinckney, R.; Macpherson, C.N.; McKibben, J.S.; Bruhl-Day, R.; Johnson, R.; Hariharan, H. Prevalence, serovars and antimicrobial susceptibility of *Salmonella* spp. from wild and domestic green iguanas (*Iguana iguana*) in Grenada, West Indies. *Zoonoses Public Health* **2014**, *61*, 436–441. [CrossRef]
6. Peterson, R.; Hariharan, H.; Matthew, V.; Chappell, S.; Davies, R.; Parker, R.; Sharma, R. Prevalence, serovars, and antimicrobial susceptibility of *Salmonella* isolated from blue land crabs (*Cardisoma guanhumi*) in Grenada, West Indies. *J. Food Prot.* **2013**, *76*, 1270–1273. [CrossRef]
7. Drake, M.; Amadi, V.; Zieger, U.; Johnson, R.; Hariharan, H. Prevalence of *Salmonella* spp. in cane toads (*Bufo marinus*) from Grenada, West Indies, and their antimicrobial susceptibility. *Zoonoses Public Health* **2013**, *60*, 437–441. [CrossRef]
8. Rush, E.M.; Amadi, V.A.; Johnson, R.; Lonce, N.; Hariharan, H. *Salmonella* serovars associated with Grenadian tree boa (*Corallus grenadensis*) and their antimicrobial susceptibility. *Vet. Med. Sci.* **2020**, *6*, 565–569. [CrossRef]
9. Prud'homme, Y.; Burton, F.J.; McClave, C.; Calle, P.P. Prevalence, incidence, and identification of *Salmonella enterica* from wild and captive grand cayman iguanas (*cyclura lewisi*). *J. Zoo Wildl. Med.* **2018**, *49*, 959–966. [CrossRef]
10. Dutton, C.S.; Revan, F.; Wang, C.; Xu, C.; Norton, T.M.; Stewart, K.M.; Kaltenboeck, B.; Soto, E. *Salmonella enterica* prevalence in leatherback sea turtles (*Dermochelys coriacea*) in St. Kitts, West Indies. *J. Zoo Wildl. Med.* **2013**, *44*, 765–768. [CrossRef]
11. Cazabon, E.; Berment, M.; Supersad, N. *Salmonella* infection in market swine, Trinidad and Tobago. *Bull. Pan Am. Health Organ.* **1978**, *12*, 51–54.
12. Hanlon, K.E.; Echeverry, A.; Miller, M.F.; Brashears, M.M. Establishment of a preliminary baseline of *Salmonella* presence on pork and goat carcasses harvested in the Bahamas to address food and nutritional security interventions. *Anim. Front.* **2018**, *8*, 26–32. [CrossRef]
13. de la Fé Rodríguez, P.Y.; Martin, L.O.; Muñoz, E.C.; Imberechts, H.; Butaye, P.; Goddeeris, B.M.; Cox, E. Several enteropathogens are circulating in suckling and newly weaned piglets suffering from diarrhea in the province of Villa Clara, Cuba. *Trop. Anim. Health Prod.* **2013**, *45*, 435–440. [CrossRef]
14. Persad, A.K.; LeJeune, J. A Review of Current Research and Knowledge Gaps in the Epidemiology of Shiga Toxin-Producing *Escherichia coli* and *Salmonella* spp. in Trinidad and Tobago. *Vet. Sci.* **2018**, *5*, 42. [CrossRef]
15. Souvorov, A.; Agarwala, R.; Lipman, D.J. SKESA: Strategic k-mer extension for scrupulous assemblies. *Genom. Biol.* **2018**, *19*, 153. [CrossRef]
16. Seemann, T. Prokka: Rapid prokaryotic genome annotation. *Bioinformatics* **2014**, *30*, 2068–2069. [CrossRef]
17. Aziz, R.K.; Bartels, D.; Best, A.A.; DeJongh, M.; Disz, T.; Edwards, R.A.; Formsma, K.; Gerdes, S.; Glass, E.M.; Kubal, M.; et al. The RAST Server: Rapid annotations using subsystems technology. *BMC Genom.* **2008**, *9*, 75. [CrossRef]
18. Yoshida, C.; Kruczkiewicz, P.; Laing, C.R.; Lingohr, E.J.; Gannon, V.P.J.; Nash, J.H.E.; Taboada, E.N. The *Salmonella* In Silico Typing Resource (SISTR): An open web-accessible tool for rapidly typing and subtyping draft *Salmonella* genome assemblies. *PLoS ONE* **2016**, *11*, e0147101. [CrossRef]
19. Larsen, M.V.; Cosentino, S.; Rasmussen, S.; Friis, C.; Hasman, H.; Marvig, R.L.; Jelsbak, L.; Sicheritz-Pontén, T.; Ussery, D.W.; Aarestrup, F.M.; et al. Multilocus Sequence Typing of Total Genome Sequenced Bacteria. *J. Clin. Microbiol.* **2012**, *50*, 1355–1361. [CrossRef]
20. Sahl, J.W.; Lemmer, D.; Travis, J.; Schupp, J.M.; Gillece, J.D.; Aziz, M.; Driebe, E.M.; Drees, K.P.; Hicks, N.D.; Williamson, C.H.D.; et al. NASP: An accurate, rapid method for the identification of SNPs in WGS datasets that supports flexible input and output formats. *Microb. Genom.* **2016**, *2*, e000074. [CrossRef]
21. Carattoli, A.; Zankari, E.; García-Fernández, A.; Voldby Larsen, M.; Lund, O.; Villa, L.; Møller Aarestrup, F.; Hasman, H. In silico detection and typing of plasmids using PlasmidFinder and plasmid multilocus sequence typing. *Antimicrob. Agents Chemother.* **2014**, *58*, 3895–3903. [CrossRef]
22. Gupta, S.K.; Padmanabhan, B.R.; Diene, S.M.; Lopez-Rojas, R.; Kempf, M.; Landraud, L.; Rolain, J.M. ARG-ANNOT, a new bioinformatic tool to discover antibiotic resistance genes in bacterial genomes. *Antimicrob. Agents Chemother.* **2014**, *58*, 212–220. [CrossRef] [PubMed]
23. Bortolaia, V.; Kaas, R.F.; Ruppe, E.; Roberts, M.C.; Schwarz, S.; Cattoir, V.; Philippon, A.; Allesoe, R.L.; Rebelo, A.R.; Florensa, A.R.; et al. ResFinder 4.0 for predictions of phenotypes from genotypes. *J. Antimicrob. Chemother.* **2020**, *75*, 3491–3500. [CrossRef]
24. Zankari, E.; Allesøe, R.; Joensen, K.G.; Cavaco, L.M.; Lund, O.; Aarestrup, F.M. PointFinder: A novel web tool for WGS-based detection of antimicrobial resistance associated with chromosomal point mutations in bacterial pathogens. *J. Antimicrob. Chemother.* **2017**, *72*, 2764–2768. [CrossRef] [PubMed]
25. Schwengers, O.; Barth, P.; Falgenhauer, L.; Hain, T.; Chakraborty, T.; Goesmann, A. Platon: Identification and characterization of bacterial plasmid contigs in short-read draft assemblies exploiting protein sequence-based replicon distribution scores. *Microb. Genom.* **2020**, *6*, mgen000398. [CrossRef]
26. Neuert, S.; Nair, S.; Day, M.R.; Doumith, M.; Ashton, P.M.; Mellor, K.C.; Jenkins, C.; Hopkins, K.L.; Woodford, N.; de Pinna, E.; et al. Prediction of phenotypic antimicrobial resistance profiles from Whole Genome Sequences of Non-typhoidal *Salmonella enterica*. *Front. Microbiol.* **2018**, *9*, 592. [CrossRef] [PubMed]

27. Adesiyun, A.A.; Kaminjolo, J.S.; Loregnard, R.; Kitson-Piggott, W. Epidemiology of *Salmonella* infections in Trinidadian livestock farms. *Rev. Elev. Med. Vet. Pays Trop.* **1993**, *46*, 435–437. [CrossRef] [PubMed]
28. Rasschaert, G.; Michiels, J.; Arijs, D.; Wildemauwe, C.; De Smet, S.; Heyndrickx, M. Effect of farm type on within-herd *Salmonella* prevalence, serovar distribution, and antimicrobial resistance. *J. Food Prot.* **2012**, *75*, 859–866. [CrossRef]
29. Bonardi, S. *Salmonella* in the pork production chain and its impact on human health in the European Union. *Epidemiol. Infect.* **2017**, *145*, 1513–1526. [CrossRef] [PubMed]
30. Campos, J.; Mourão, J.; Peixe, L.; Antunes, P. Non-typhoidal *Salmonella* in the pig production chain: A comprehensive analysis of its impact on human health. *Pathogens* **2019**, *8*, 19. [CrossRef] [PubMed]
31. Cadel-Six, S.; Cherchame, E.; Douarre, P.E.; Tang, Y.; Felten, A.; Barbet, P.; Litrup, E.; Banerji, S.; Simon, S.; Pasquali, F.; et al. The spatiotemporal dynamics and microevolution events that favored the success of the highly clonal multidrug-resistant monophasic *Salmonella* Typhimurium circulating in Europe. *Front. Microbiol.* **2021**, *12*, 651124. [CrossRef]
32. Tassinari, E.; Bawn, M.; Thilliez, G.; Charity, O.; Acton, L.; Kirkwood, M.; Petrovska, L.; Dallman, T.; Burgess, C.M.; Hall, N.; et al. Whole-genome epidemiology links phage-mediated acquisition of a virulence gene to the clonal expansion of a pandemic *Salmonella enterica* serovar Typhimurium clone. *Microb. Genom.* **2020**, *6*, mgen000456. [CrossRef] [PubMed]
33. Al-Gallas, N.; Khadraoui, N.; Hotzel, H.; Tomaso, H.; El-Adawy, H.; Neubauer, H.; Belghouthi, K.; Ghedira, K.; Gautam, H.K.; Kumar, B.; et al. Quinolone resistance among *Salmonella* Kentucky and Typhimurium isolates in Tunisia: First report of *Salmonella* Typhimurium ST34 in Africa and *qnrB19* in Tunisia. *J. Appl. Microbiol.* **2021**, *130*, 807–818. [CrossRef] [PubMed]
34. Elbediwi, M.; Beibei, W.; Pan, H.; Jiang, Z.; Biswas, S.; Li, Y.; Yue, M. Genomic characterization of *mcr-1*-carrying *Salmonella enterica* Serovar 4,[5],12:i:- ST 34 clone isolated from pigs in China. *Front. Bioeng. Biotechnol.* **2020**, *8*, 663. [CrossRef] [PubMed]
35. Li, Y.C.; Pan, Z.M.; Kang, X.L.; Geng, S.Z.; Liu, Z.Y.; Cai, Y.Q.; Jiao, X.A. Prevalence, characteristics, and antimicrobial resistance patterns of *Salmonella* in retail pork in Jiangsu province, eastern China. *J. Food Prot.* **2014**, *77*, 236–245. [CrossRef] [PubMed]
36. Khan, A.S.; Georges, K.; Rahaman, S.; Abebe, W.; Adesiyun, A.A. Characterization of *Salmonella* isolates recovered from stages of the processing lines at four broiler processing plants in Trinidad and Tobago. *Microorganisms* **2021**, *9*, 1048. [CrossRef]
37. Maguire, M.; Khan, A.S.; Adesiyun, A.A.; Georges, K.; Gonzalez-Escalona, N. Closed genome sequence of a *Salmonella enterica* Serotype Senftenberg strain carrying the *mcr-9* gene isolated from broken chicken eggshells in Trinidad and Tobago. *Microbiol. Resour. Announc.* **2021**, *10*, e0146520. [CrossRef] [PubMed]
38. Kumar, N.; Mohan, K.; Georges, K.; Dziva, F.; Adesiyun, A.A. Occurrence of virulence and resistance genes in *Salmonella* in cloacae of slaughtered chickens and ducks at pluck shops in Trinidad. *J. Food Prot.* **2021**, *84*, 39–46. [CrossRef]
39. Poole, T.L.; Schlosser, W.D.; Anderson, R.C.; Norman, K.N.; Beier, R.C.; Nisbet, D.J. Whole-Genome Sequence of *Aeromonas hydrophila* CVM861 isolated from diarrhetic neonatal Swine. *Microorganisms* **2020**, *8*, 1648. [CrossRef] [PubMed]
40. Shigemura, H.; Sakatsume, E.; Sekizuka, T.; Yokoyama, H.; Hamada, K.; Etoh, Y.; Carle, Y.; Mizumoto, S.; Hirai, S.; Matsui, M.; et al. Food workers as a reservoir of extended-spectrum-cephalosporin-resistant *Salmonella* strains in Japan. *Appl. Environ. Microbiol.* **2020**, *86*, e00072-20. [CrossRef]
41. Li, R.; Zhang, P.; Yang, X.; Wang, Z.; Fanning, S.; Wang, J.; Du, P.; Bai, L. Identification of a novel hybrid plasmid coproducing MCR-1 and MCR-3 variant from an *Escherichia coli* strain. *J. Antimicrob. Chemother.* **2019**, *74*, 1517–1520. [CrossRef] [PubMed]
42. van den Berg, R.R.; Dissel, S.; Rapallini, M.L.B.A.; van der Weijden, C.C.; Wit, B.; Heymans, R. Characterization and whole genome sequencing of closely related multidrug-resistant *Salmonella enterica* serovar Heidelberg isolates from imported poultry meat in the Netherlands. *PLoS ONE* **2019**, *14*, e0219795. [CrossRef]

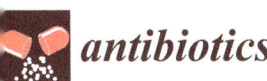

Article

Multi-Drug Resistance to *Salmonella* spp. When Isolated from Raw Meat Products

Joanna Pławińska-Czarnak [1,*], Karolina Wódz [2], Magdalena Kizerwetter-Świda [3], Janusz Bogdan [1], Piotr Kwieciński [2], Tomasz Nowak [2], Zuzanna Strzałkowska [1] and Krzysztof Anusz [1]

1. Department of Food Hygiene and Public Health Protection, Institute of Veterinary Medicine, Warsaw University of Life Sciences, Nowoursynowska 159, 02-776 Warsaw, Poland; janusz_bogdan@sggw.edu.pl (J.B.); z.strzalkowska@gmail.com (Z.S.); krzysztof_anusz@sggw.edu.pl (K.A.)
2. Laboratory of Molecular Biology, Vet-Lab Brudzew, Ul. Turkowska 58c, 62-720 Brudzew, Poland; karolina.wodz@labbrudzew.pl (K.W.); vetlab@interia.pl (P.K.); tomasz@labbrudzew.pl (T.N.)
3. Department of Preclinical Sciences, Institute of Veterinary Medicine, Warsaw University of Life Sciences-SGGW, Ciszewskiego Str. 8, 02-786 Warsaw, Poland; magdalena_kizerwetter_swida@sggw.edu.pl
* Correspondence: joanna_plawinska_czarnak@sggw.edu.pl

Abstract: *Salmonella* spp. is the most frequent cause of foodborne diseases, and the increasing occurrence of MDR strains is an additional and increasing problem. We collected *Salmonella* spp. strains isolated from meat (poultry and pork) and analysed their antibiotic susceptibility profiles and the occurrence of resistance genes. To determine the susceptibility profiles and identify MDR strains, we used two MIC methods (MICRONAUT and VITEC2 Compact) and 25 antibiotics. Phenotypic tests showed that 53.84% strains were MDR. Finally, molecular analysis strains revealed the presence of bla_{SHV}, bla_{PSE-1}, bla_{TEM}, but not bla_{CTX-M} genes. Moreover, several genes were associated with resistance to aminoglycosides, cephalosporins, fluorochinolones, sulfonamides, and tetracyclines. This suggests that further research on the prevalence of antibiotic resistance genes (ARGs) in foodborne strains is needed, especially from a One Health perspective.

Keywords: *Salmonella enterica*; Enteritidis; multidrug-resistant; Derby; foodborne pathogens

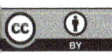

1. Introduction

The annual report on trends and sources of zoonoses published in December 2021 by the European Food Safety Authority (EFSA) and the European Centre for Disease Prevention and Control (ECDC) shows that nearly one in four foodborne outbreaks in the European Union (EU) in 2020 were caused by *Salmonella* spp., which makes this bacteria the most frequently reported causative agent for foodborne outbreaks (694 foodborne outbreaks in 2020) [1].

In the EU 52,702 confirmed cases of salmonellosis in humans were reported and salmonellosis remains the second most commonly reported zoonosis in humans after campylobacteriosis. The three most commonly reported *Salmonella enterica* subsp. *Enterica* serovars in 2020 were *S. enteritidis*, *S. typhimurium*, and monophasic *S. typhimurium*, representing 72.2% of confirmed human cases with known serovar in 2020. Most of the reported salmonellosis foodborne outbreaks were caused by *S. enteritidis* serovar (57.9%). *S. enteritidis* was the predominant serovar in both human salmonellosis cases and reported foodborne outbreaks. Due to the COVID-19 pandemic, total numbers of reported salmonellosis cases as well as foodborne outbreaks are lower compared to previous years' data. Increased use of hygiene equipment, reduced exposure to food served in restaurants and canteens, and more frequent cleaning during domestic food preparations might have had an impact on reported data on salmonellosis. Despite the facts above, trends in salmonellosis occurrence since 2016 data did not reveal statistically significant changes (EFSA December 2021) [1].

Bacteria of the genus *Salmonella* are gram-negative, mostly motile rods, belonging to the *Enterobacteriaceae* family. *Salmonella* spp. is well-established as a pathogen causing gastrointestinal diseases in humans and animals all over the world. Two species are included in the genus *Salmonella*: *Salmonella enterica* spp. and *Salmonella bongori* spp. Almost 99% of the *Salmonella* strains that cause infections in humans or other warm-blooded animals belong to the species *S. enterica*, which includes six subspecies and >2587 serovars [2].

Salmonella enterica subsp. *Enterica* includes approximately 1547 serotypes which can cause infections in animals and humans [2]. *Salmonella* infections in humans are usually caused by eating food of animal origin, mostly eggs, poultry meat, or pork [3,4]. The analysis by Gutema et al. (2019) shows that beef and veal can also be a source of *Salmonella* spp. infection due to these animals being potential asymptomatic carriers [3].

Currently, one of the most important health problems in the world is the antimicrobial resistance of *Salmonella* spp. [4,5]. Data from the EU show that the occurrence of resistance in *Salmonella* from pigs, cattle, and broiler chickens largely resembles the appearance of resistance reported for *Salmonella* in various foodstuffs and in people (EFSA [4]).

Multi-drug resistant *Salmonella* constitutes a serious threat to public health through food-borne infections [6–8]. Currently, such multi-drug resistant strains are increasingly isolated from beef and pork [9,10] poultry [11].

Because the problem of antimicrobial resistance became a global problem, in 2003 WHO, together with the Food and Agriculture Organization of the United Nations (FAO) and the World Organization for Animal Health (OIE), began work on creating a List of Critically Important Antimicrobials for Human Medicine (WHO CIA List) [12]. Tacconelli et al. in 2018, pointed out that global research and development strategies should also include antibiotics active against more common community bacteria, such as *Salmonella* spp., *Campylobacter* spp. and *H. pylori*, which are resistant to antibiotics [13]. Therefore, the scope of the new edition of the WHO CIA List, published in 2019, is limited to antibacterial drugs of which most are also used in veterinary medicine. It is very important to use critically important antimicrobials the most prudently in human and veterinary medicine. With accordance monitoring of antimicrobial resistance in food and food-producing bacteria, as defined in Commission Implementing Decision 2013/652/EU, *Salmonella* antibiotics resistance, isolated from food and food-producing animals, should be targeted at broilers, fattening pigs, calves less than 1 year old, and their meat (CID 2013/652/EU).

The aim of our research is to determine the antibiotic resistance of *Salmonella* spp. isolated from raw meat products from beef, pork, and poultry production plants.

2. Results

Of the 170 meat samples tested, no *Salmonella* spp. were found in beef samples; but, three *Citrobacter braakii* were isolated from them. Only one of the pork samples was positive for *Salmonella* spp. and three *Citrobacter braakii* were isolated from them. Details of any identification difficulties during the isolation of *Salmonella* spp. from meat samples tested were presented by Pławińska-Czarnak in 2021 [14]. From the poultry samples, 38 were positive for *Salmonella* spp. All *Salmonella* strains of the isolated species belong to *Salmonella enterica* subsp. *enterica* and represented seven serotypes which shown in Table 1.

The most common serovars from all positive samples were: *S.* Enteritidis (58.97%); *S.* Derby (12.82%) and *S.* Newport (12.82%), which were less frequently isolated; *S.* Infantis (5.13%); *S.* Kentucky (5.13%); *S.* Indiana (2.56%); and *S.* Mbandaka (2.56%) (the details of the results are presented in Table 1).

Table 1. The *Salmonella enterica subsp. enterica* variously identified serovars isolated from meat samples of pork and poultry.

Sample of Meat	Salmonella enterica spp. enterica	Antigenic Formula	Number of Isolated Strains
pork	Enteritidis	1,9,12:g,m (without phase II)	1
poultry			22
poultry	Derby	1,4,12:f,g:-(without phase II)	5
poultry	Newport	6,8,20:e,h:1,2	5
poultry	Infantis	6,7:r:1,5	2
poultry	Kentucky	8,20:i:z$_6$	2
poultry	Indiana	4,12:z:1,7	1
poultry	Mbandaka	6,7:z$_{10}$:e,n,z$_{15}$	1
Total	Salmonella spp.		n = 39

Annotation: Antigenic formula according to White-Kauffmann-Le Minor scheme somatic; somatic antigen O (1,9,12 group O9, 1,4,12; 4,12 group O4, 6,8,20; 8,20 group O8, 6,7 group O8, flagellar antigen H phase I and II.

2.1. Antibiotic Susceptibility

Antibiotic susceptibility testing conducted on the 39 *Salmonella* strains shows that only one strain (*S. enteritidis*) has resistance to two classes of antibiotics (CPH-GEN-STR) whereas 38 strains (64%) were resistant to one or more of the tested antibiotics. However, no resistance against imipenem or colistin was detected. Surprisingly, we detected that 100% of *Salmonella* strains were phenotypically resistant to streptomycin and gentamycin. *Salmonella* strains had intermediate resistance to: amoxicillin (5.13%, *S. Kentucky*, *S. Newport*), cephalexin (30.77%, *S. Infantis, S. enteritidis*), ceftiofur (2.56%, *S. Infantis*), neomycin (7.96%, *S. Newport*), enrofloxacin (23.08%, *S. Infantis, S. Mbandaka, S. Newport, S. enteritidis*), norfloxacin (15.8%, *S. derby, S. Indiana, S. Enteritidis*), doxycycline and oxytetracycline (5.13%, *S. Derby, S. Enteritidis*), florfenicol (56.41%, *S. Mbandaka, S. Kentucky, S. Newport, S. Enteritidis*), and trimethoprim-sulfamethoxazole (2.26%, *S. Derby*). In total, 35.9% (14/39) of the strains were resistant to ampicillin, 38.46% (15/39) to amoxicillin, and 7.69% (3/39) to amoxicillin and clavulanic acid. In the case of cephalosporins 46.15% (18/39) of the strains were resistant to cephalexin, 38.46% (14/39) to cefalotin, 97.43% (38/39) to cefapirin, 17.95% (7/39) to cefoperazone, 23.08% (9/39) to ceftiofur, and 12.82% (5/39) to cefquinome. In the case of aminoglycosides, 10.25% (4/39) were resistant to neomycin. In the case of fluoroquinolones, 28.2% (11/39) were resistant to enrofloxacin, 82.05% (32/39) to flumequine, 33.33% (13/39) to marbofloxacin, and 10.25% (4/39) to norfloxacin. A total of 25.64% (10/39) were resistant to tetracyclines, 38.46% (14/39) to florfenicol, 56.41% (22/39) to lincomycin/spectinomycin, and 7.69% (3/39) to trimethoprim/sulfamethoxazole.

2.2. Prevalence of Multiple Drug Resistance

In our study, most of *S. Enteritidis* showed an MAR index lower than 0.3, whereas one (*S. Newport*) showed an MAR index above 0.5. We observed a high prevalence of multiple antibiotic resistance amongst the isolates where 53.84% of the isolates were MDR strains, with resistance from three to six different classes of antibiotics.

2.3. Antimicrobial Resistance Profile

All *Salmonella* strains of the isolated species belongs to *Salmonella enterica subsp. enterica* and represented seven serotypes (Derby, Indiana, Infantis, Mbandaka, Kentucky, Newport, and Enteritidis). All isolated *Salmonella* were sensitive to imipenem (IMP) and colistin (COL)/polymixin B (PB).

A total of 53.84% *Salmonella* spp. strains isolated from meat were classified as MDR strains that were resistant to the six antibiotic classes: penicillins, cephalosporins, aminoglycosides, fluorochinolones, sulfonamides, and tetracyclines. *S. Newport* (sample 1) presented the most extensive resistance profiles to 17 antibiotics (AMP-AMX-AMX/CL-CFX-CFT-CPH-GEN-NEO-STR-ENR-UB-MRB-NOR-DOX-OXY-TET-LIN/SP), belonging to 5 classes of antibiotics (β-lactams, aminoglycoside, fluorochinolones, tetracyclines and lincosamides with spectinomycin. In one of S. Derby (AMP-AMX-CFX-CFT-CPH-CFP-CFTI-CFQ-GEN-STR-ENR-UB-MRB-FLR-LIN/SP-TR/SMX) and S. Newport (AMP-AMX-AMX/CL-CFX-CFT-CPH-GEN-STR-ENR-UB-MRB-NOR-DOX-OXY-TET-LIN/SP), extensive resistance profiles to 16 antibiotics were present. In *S. indiana* (AMX-AMX/CL-CTX-CPH-CFTI-GEN-NEO-STR-DOX-OXY-TET-FLR-LIN/SP-TR/SMX), extensive resistance profiles to 14 antibiotics were present.

The classes to which it presented the highest resistance were β-lactams (AMP, AMX) and beta-lactam/beta-lactamase inhibitor combination (AMX/CL), I generation cephalosporin (CFX-CFT-CPH), III generation cephalosporin (CFTI, CFP), aminoglycosides (GEN-NEO-STR), fluorochinolones (ENR-UB-MRB-NOR), and tetracyclines (DOX-OXY-TET). The most diverse serotype in terms of antimicrobial resistance turned out to be S. Enteritidis, in which 13 patterns of resistance were observed. Serovar S. Mbandaka showed complete resistance to 9 antibiotics (AMP-AMX-CFX-CFT-CPH-GEN-STR-UB-LIN/SP), and S. Infantis showed resistance to 10 antibiotics to varying degrees. The least resistant strain of S. Enteritidis was strain from pork meat resistant to 3 antibacterial substances (CPH-GEN-STR), and the most resistance to S. Enteritidis was strain 11 from poultry meat (AMP-CFX-CFT-CPH-CFTI-GEN-STR-UB-MRB-FLR-LIN/SP).

For the particular serotypes of *Salmonella enterica* spp. *enterica*, all individual patterns of resistance to multiple antibiotics are presented in Table 2.

The isolates were subjected to antibiotic susceptibility tests against 33 antibiotics belonging to ten different classes using the MIC method Merlin MICRONAUT (MERLIN Diagnostika GmbH, Niemcy) and AST-GN96 CARD and VITEK2 system (Biomerieux, Marcy-l'Étoile, France). The AST card is essentially a miniaturised and abbreviated version of the doubling dilution technique for MICs determined by the microdilution [15]. The multiple antibiotics resistance index (MAR) was performed for isolates showing resistance to more than two antibiotics and is presented in the Table 2 [16].

Table 2. Multiple Antibiotic Resistance Index and phenotype pattern of *Salmonella enterica* spp. *enterica* all identified serovars isolates from meat samples of pork and poultry.

Salmonella Strains	Sample Source	Antibiotics Resistance Profiles	MAR Index
Salmonella Derby (BO4)	10 poultry	AMP-CFX-CFT-CPH-CFP-CFTI-CFQ-GEN-STR-ENR-UB-MRB-FLR-LIN/SP	0.42
	22 poultry	AMX-CPH-GEN-STR-LIN/SP-TR/SMX	0.18
	36 poultry	AMP-CFX-CFT-CPH-CFP-CFTI-CFQ-GEN-STR-ENR-UB-MRB-FLR-LIN/SP	0.42
	45 poultry	AMP-CFX-CFT-CPH-CFP-CFTI-CFQ-GEN-STR-ENR-UB-MRB-FLR-LIN/SP	0.42
	46 poultry	AMP-AMX-CFX-CFT-CPH-CFP-CFTI-CFQ-GEN-STR-ENR-UB-MRB-FLR-LIN/SP-TR/SMX	0.48
	47 poultry	AMP-AMX-CFX-CFT-CPH-CFP-CFTI-CFQ-GEN-STR-ENR-UB-MRB-FLR	0.42
Salmonella Indiana (BO4)	61 poultry	AMX-AMX/CL-CTX-CPH-CFTI-GEN-NEO-STR-DOX-OXY-TET-FLR-LIN/SP-TR/SMX	0.42
Salmonella Infantis (CO7)	3 poultry	AMX-CPH-GEN-STR-UB-DOX-OXY-TET-FLR-LIN/SP	0.30
Salmonella Infantis (CO7)	38 poultry	CPH-CFTI-GEN-STR-DOX-OXY-TET-FLR-LIN/SP	0.30
Salmonella Mbandaka (CO7)	9 poultry	AMP-AMX-CFX-CFT-CPH-GEN-STR-UB-LIN/SP	0.27
Salmonella Kentucky (CO8)	24 poultry	AMP-AMX-CFX-CFT-CPH-CFP-GEN-STR-ENR-UB-MRB-DOX-OXY-TET	0.42
	27 poultry	AMP-AMX-CFX-CFT-CPH-CFP-GEN-STR-ENR-UB-MRB-DOX-OXY-TET	0.42
Salmonella Newport (CO8)	1 poultry	AMP-AMX-AMX/CL-CFX-CFT-CPH-GEN-NEO-STR-ENR-UB-MRB-NOR-DOX-OXY-TET-LIN/SP	0.51
	6 poultry	AMP-AMX-AMX/CL-CFX-CFT-CPH-GEN-STR-ENR-UB-MRB-NOR-DOX-OXY-TET-LIN/SP	0.48
	8 poultry	AMP-CFX-CFT-CPH-GEN-STR-UB-MRB-DOX-OXY-TET-FLR	0.36
	12 poultry	AMP-CFX-CFT-CPH-GEN-STR-ENR-UB-MRB-DOX-OXY-TET-FLR	0.39
	13 poultry	AMP-AMX-CFX-CFT-CPH-GEN-STR-ENR-UB-MRB-DOX-OXY-TET-FLR	0.42

Table 2. Cont.

Salmonella Strains	Sample Source	Antibiotics Resistance Profiles	MAR Index
	2 pork	CPH-GEN-STR	0.09
	4 poultry	AMX-CPH-GEN-STR-UB-FLR-LIN/SP	0.21
	5 poultry	AMX-CPH-GEN-STR-UB-NOR-LIN/SP	0.21
	7 poultry	GEN-STR-UB-LIN/SP	0.12
	11 poultry	AMP-CFX-CFT-CPH-CFTI-GEN-STR-UB-MRB-FLR-LIN/SP	0.33
	30 poultry	CPH-GEN-STR-UB	0.12
	31 poultry	CPH-GEN-STR-UB	0.12
	32 poultry	CPH-GEN-STR-LIN/SP	0.12
	33 poultry	CPH-GEN-STR-LIN/SP	0.12
	34 poultry	CPH-GEN-STR-UB-NOR-LIN/SP	0.18
	35 poultry	CPH-GEN-STR-UB	0.12
Salmonella Enteritidis (DO9)	37 poultry	CPH-GEN-STR-UB-LIN/SP	0.15
	39 poultry	CPH-GEN-STR-UB	0.12
	40 poultry	CPH-GEN-STR-UB-LIN/SP	0.15
	41 poultry	CPH-GEN-STR-LIN/SP	0.12
	42 poultry	CPH-GEN-STR-UB-LIN/SP	0.15
	43 poultry	AMX-CPH-GEN-STR-UB-LIN/SP	0.18
	44 poultry	CPH-GEN-STR	0.09
	48 poultry	AMX-CFX-CFT-CPH-CFTI-GEN-STR-UB-FLR	0.27
	49 poultry	CPH-GEN-STR-UB	0.12
	64 poultry	CFX-CPH-GEN-NEO-STR-UB	0.18
	68 poultry	CFX-CPH-GEN-NEO-STR-UB	0.18

Letter abbreviations correspond to the individual antibiotics according to list: ampicilln (AMP), amoxicillin (AMX), amoxicillin and clavulanic acid (AMX/CL), cephalexin (CFX), cefalotin (CFT), cefapirin (CPH), cefoperazone (CFP), ceftiofur (CFTI), cefquinome (CFQ), imipenem (IPM), gentamicin (GEN), neomycin (NEO), streptomycin (STR), enrofloxacin (ENR), flumequine (UB), marbofloxacin (MRB), norfloxacin (NOR), docycycline (DOX), oxytetracycline (OXY), tetracycline (TET), florfenicol (FLR), lincomycin/spectinomycin (LIN/SP), trimethoprim-sulfamethoxazole (TR/SMX).

2.4. Genotypic Resistance

The gene bla_{CMY-2} that confers resistance to cefoperazone/ceftiofur was detected in 41.02%, and bla_{SHV} in 35.9%. of strains. However, some *Salmonella* spp. strains did not exhibit phenotypic resistance to III generation cephalosporins. In addition, 30.77% of the strains demonstrated the presence of the genes bla_{PSE-1} and 48.72% bla_{TEM} that conferred resistance to ampicillin. Most of ampicillin-resistant strains (85.71%) contained bla_{PSE-1} and bla_{TEM}, and 14.28% harboured only bla_{TEM} gene. The gene *aadB* was detected in eight strains, mainly in *S*. Derby. However, all *Salmonella* spp. strains were phenotypically resistant to gentamicin. The genes *aadA*, *strA*/*strB* that confers resistance to streptomycin was detected in all strains. All of neomycin resistant strains carried *aphA1* and *aphA2* genes. The *tetA* and *tetB* genes were detected in all strains resistant to doxycycline and oxytetracycline. Sulphonamide-resistant strains contained at least one *sul* (1, 2, 3) and *adfR* gene, of which the *sul2* and *adfR1* were the most frequently detected genes. The gene *floR*, that confers resistance to florfenicol, was detected in all strains resistant to florfenicol.

Distribution of the various resistance genes and the prevalence of the corresponding serovars are shown in Table 3.

Table 3. Distribution of resistance genes in relation to antimicrobial resistance patterns.

Salmonella Strains	Sample	Phenotypic Antimicrobial Resistance Profile	Genotypic Antimicrobial Resistance Profile
	10	AMP-CFX-CFT-CPH-CFP-CFTI-CFQ-GEN-STR-ENR-UB-MRB-FLR-LIN/SP	bla_{CMY-2}, bla_{PSE-1}, bla_{TEM}, aadA, strA/strB, floR
	22	AMX-CPH-GEN-STR-LIN/SP-TR/SMX	dfrA1, sul1, sul2, aadA, strA/strB, aadB
	36	AMP-CFX-CFT-CPH-CFP-CFTI-CFQ-GEN-STR-ENR-UB-MRB-FLR-LIN/SP	bla_{CMY-2}, bla_{PSE-1}, bla_{SHV}, bla_{TEM}, aadA, strA/strB, aadB, floR
Salmonella Derby (BO4)	45	AMP-CFX-CFT-CPH-CFP-CFTI-CFQ-GEN-STR-ENR-UB-MRB-FLR-LIN/SP	bla_{CMY-2}, bla_{PSE-1}, bla_{TEM}, dfrA1, dfrA12, sul2, sul3, aadA, strA/strB, aadB, floR
	46	AMP-AMX-CFX-CFT-CPH-CFP-CFTI-CFQ-GEN-STR-ENR-UB-MRB-FLR-LIN/SP-TR/SMX	bla_{CMY-2}, bla_{PSE-1}, bla_{TEM}, dfrA1, dfrA12, sul2, sul3, aadA, strA/strB, aadB, floR
	47	AMP-AMX-CFX-CFT-CPH-CFP-CFTI-CFQ-GEN-STR-ENR-UB-MRB-FLR	bla_{CMY-2}, bla_{PSE-1}, bla_{TEM}, aadA, strA/strB, floR

Table 3. Cont.

Salmonella Strains	Sample	Phenotypic Antimicrobial Resistance Profile	Genotypic Antimicrobial Resistance Profile
Salmonella Indiana (BO4)	61	AMX-AMX/CL-CTX-CPH-CFTI-GEN-NEO-STR-DOX-OXY-TET-FLR-LIN/SP-TR/SMX	bla_{CMY-2}, bla_{TEM}, $dfrA1$, $sul1$, $sul2$, $aadA$, $strA/strB$, $aadB$, $aphA1$, $aphA2$, $tetA$, $tetB$, $floR$
Salmonella Infantis (CO7)	3	AMX-CPH-GEN-STR-UB-DOX-OXY-TET-FLR-LIN/SP	bla_{SHV}, $aadA$, $strA/strB$, $tetA$, $tetB$, $floR$
	38	CPH-CFTI-GEN-STR-UB-DOX-OXY-TET-FLR-LIN/SP	bla_{CMY-2}, $aadA$, $strA/strB$, $tetA$, $tetB$, $floR$
Salmonella Mbandaka (CO7)	9	AMP-AMX-CFX-CFT-CPH-GEN-STR-UB-LIN/SP	bla_{PSE-1}, bla_{TEM}, $aadA$, $strA/strB$
Salmonella Kentucky (CO8)	24	AMP-AMX-CFX-CFT-CPH-CFP-GEN-STR-ENR-UB-MRB-DOX-OXY-TET	bla_{CMY-2}, bla_{PSE-1}, bla_{TEM}, $aadA$, $strA/strB$, $aadB$, $tetA$, $tetB$
	27	AMP-AMX-CFX-CFT-CPH-CFP-GEN-STR-ENR-UB-MRB-DOX-OXY-TET	bla_{CMY-2}, bla_{PSE-1}, bla_{TEM}, $aadA$, $strA/strB$, $tetA$, $tetB$
Salmonella Newport (CO8)	1	AMP-AMX-AMX/CL-CFX-CFT-CPH-GEN-NEO-STR-ENR-UB-MRB-NOR-DOX-OXY-TET-LIN/SP	bla_{CMY-2}, bla_{TEM}, $aadA$, $strA/strB$, $aadB$, $aphA1$, $aphA2$, $tetA$, $tetB$
	6	AMP-AMX-AMX/CL-CFX-CFT-CPH-GEN-STR-ENR-UB-MRB-NOR-DOX-OXY-TET-LIN/SP	bla_{CMY-2}, bla_{TEM}, $aadA$, $strA/strB$, $tetA$, $tetB$
	8	AMP-CFX-CFT-CPH-GEN-STR-UB-MRB-DOX-OXY-TET-FLR	bla_{PSE-1}, bla_{TEM}, $aadA$, $strA/strB$, $tetA$, $tetB$, $floR$
	12	AMP-CFX-CFT-CPH-GEN-STR-ENR-UB-MRB-DOX-OXY-TET-FLR	bla_{PSE-1}, bla_{TEM}, $aadA$, $strA/strB$, $tetA$, $tetB$, $floR$
	13	AMP-AMX-CFX-CFT-CPH-GEN-STR-ENR-UB-MRB-DOX-OXY-TET-FLR	bla_{PSE-1}, bla_{TEM}, $aadA$, $strA/strB$, $aadB$, $tetA$, $tetB$, $floR$
Salmonella Enteritidis (DO9)	2	CPH-GEN-STR	$aadA$, $strA/strB$
	4	AMX-CPH-GEN-STR-UB-FLR-LIN/SP	bla_{CMY-2}, $aadA$, $strA/strB$, $floR$
	5	AMX-CPH-GEN-STR-UB-NOR-LIN/SP	bla_{SHV}, $aadA$, $strA/strB$
	7	GEN-STR-UB-LIN/SP	$aadA$, $strA/strB$
	11	AMP-CFX-CFT-CPH-CFTI-GEN-STR-UB-MRB-FLR-LIN/SP	bla_{CMY-2}, bla_{PSE-1}, bla_{TEM}, $aadA$, $strA/strB$, $floR$
	30	CPH-GEN-STR-UB	bla_{SHV}, $aadA$, $strA/strB$
	31	CPH-GEN-STR-LIN/SP	bla_{SHV}, $aadA$, $strA/strB$
	32	CPH-GEN-STR-LIN/SP	bla_{SHV}, $aadA$, $strA/strB$
	33	CPH-GEN-STR-UB-NOR-LIN/SP	bla_{SHV}, $aadA$, $strA/strB$
	34	CPH-GEN-STR-UB	bla_{CMY-2}, $aadA$, $strA/strB$
	35	CPH-GEN-STR-UB-LIN/SP	bla_{SHV}, $aadA$, $strA/strB$
	37	CPH-GEN-STR-UB	bla_{SHV}, $aadA$, $strA/strB$
	39	CPH-GEN-STR-UB	bla_{SHV}, $aadA$, $strA/strB$
	40	CPH-GEN-STR-UB-LIN/SP	bla_{TEM}, $aadA$, $strA/strB$
	41	CPH-GEN-STR-LIN/SP	bla_{TEM}, $aadA$, $strA/strB$
	42	CPH-GEN-STR-UB-LIN/SP	bla_{SHV}, $aadA$, $strA/strB$
	43	AMX-CPH-GEN-STR-UB-LIN/SP	bla_{SHV}, $aadA$, $strA/strB$
	44	CPH-GEN-STR	bla_{CMY-2}, $aadA$, $strA/strB$
	48	AMX-CFX-CFT-CPH-CFTI-GEN-STR-UB-FLR	bla_{CMY-2}, $aadA$, $strA/strB$, $floR$
	49	CPH-GEN-STR-UB	bla_{SHV}, $aadA$, $strA/strB$
	64	CFX-CPH-GEN-NEO-STR-UB	bla_{TEM}, $aadA$, $strA/strB$, $aphA1$, $aphA2$
	68	CFX-CPH-GEN-NEO-STR-UB	bla_{TEM}, $aadA$, $strA/strB$, $aphA1$, $aphA2$

Letter abbreviations correspond to the individual antibiotics according to list: ampicilln (AMP), amoxicillin (AMX), amoxicillin and clavulanic acid (AMX/CL), cephalexin (CFX), cefalotin (CFT), cefapirin (CPH), cefoperazone (CFP), ceftiofur (CFTI), cefquinome (CFQ), imipenem (IPM), gentamicin (GEN), neomycin (NEO), streptomycin (STR), enrofloxacin (ENR), flumequine (UB), marbofloxacin (MRB), norfloxacin (NOR), docycycline (DOX), oxytetracycline (OXY), tetracycline (TET), florfenicol (FLR), lincomycin/spectinomycin (LIN/SP), trimethoprim-sulfamethoxazole (TR/SMX).

3. Materials and Methods

3.1. Sampling

A total number of 190 raw meat samples (60 beef, 60 pork, and 70 poultry) were obtained from three sources within the meat industry, such as cuttings of beef, pork and poultry carcasses in central Poland. All samples were obtained from carcass parts of animals recognised as healthy: the tissues and organs of which were classified by the veterinary inspection as fit for human consumption. All samples were considered a single sample, weighing at least 200 g for each type of meat. The meat samples were collected randomly, using an aseptic technique and packed into sterile bags, which were labeled. All samples were transported to the laboratory in refrigerated containers at a temperature 4 °C and processed within five hours.

3.2. Salmonella spp. Isolation and Identification

Salmonella spp. from all samples were isolated in accordance with PN-EN ISO 6579-1:2017-04 Microbiology of the food chain—Horizontal method for the detection, enumeration and serotyping of Salmonella—Part 1: Detection of Salmonella spp. (ISO 6579-1:2017). Samples were pre-enriched: for pork and beef samples, the 10 g of each sample was mixed with 90 mL Buffered Pepton Water (GRASO, Gdansk, Poland), and the 25 g of each poultry meat sample was mixed with 225 mL BPW with a temperature of 25 °C (±3 °C) in a sterile stomacher bag (Whirl-Pak, Nasco, Madison, WI, USA), and crushed for 2 min. After that, they were incubated at 37 °C for 18 h. Selective proliferation of Salmonella spp. was carried out using the MSRV agar (Modified semi-solid Rappaport-Vassiliadis—MSRV agar, GRASO, Poland) with 0.1 mL of the pre-enriched culture as three equally spaced spots on the surface of the MSRV agar were incubated at 41.5 °C for 24 h and 1 mL of the culture obtained was put to a tube containing 10 mL of Muller-Kauffmann tetrathionate-novobiocin (MKTTn) broth (GRASO, Gdansk, Poland) and incubated at 37 °C for 24 h. From the positive growth obtained on the MSRV agar, it was chosen as the furthest point of opaque growth from the inoculation points, and picked up a 1 µL loop and was inoculated on two selective agars: XLD (Xylose Lysine Deoxycholate agar, GRASO, Gdansk, Poland) and BGA (Brilliant Green agar, OXOID, Hampshire, UK). From the liquid culture obtained in the MKTTn, broth was picked up of a 10 µL loop and spread on XLD agar and BGA agar to obtain well-isolated colonies. All selective agars were incubated at 37 °C for 24 h (±3 h). Salmonella-suspect colonies were transferred to Nutrient agar (GRASO, Gdansk, Poland) to obtain the pure culture for further testing.

3.2.1. DNA Preparation and Presumptive Salmonella Confirmation

The Real-time PCR method, and an amplification based on detection gene specific for Salmonella, was used to confirm presumptive identification. DNA for real-time PCR was extracted from bacterial cells, using commercial Kylt® DNA Extraction-Mix II (Anicon, Emstek, Germany). For the detection of Salmonella spp. commercial Kylt® Salmonella spp. (Anicon, Germany) was used, and for the simultaneous detection of Salmonella Enteritidis, the Typhimurium commercial Spp-Se-St PCR (BioChek, Reeuwijk, The Netherland) kit was used. The Real Time PCR method to detect Salmonella was performed according to the manufacturer's instructions with using Applied Biosystems 7500 Fast Real-Time PCR System (Thermo, Waltham, MA, USA).

3.2.2. Biochemical Strain Identification

For identification of the strains, two commercially available biochemical tests were used according to the manufacturer's instructions: Api20E (BioMérieux, Marcy-l'Étoile, France) and the VITEK® 2 GN cards (Biomerieux, Marcy-l'Étoile, France).

3.2.3. Serological Testing

Serotyping was performed according to the White-Kauffmann-Le Minor scheme. Serological testing was carried out by slide agglutination with commercial H poly antisera to verify the genus of *Salmonella enterica* (IBSS Biomed, Lublin, Poland), O group antisera to determine the O group, (IBSS Biomed, Poland), and H phase and H factor antisera to determine the H phase and H factor (IBSS Biomed, Lublin, Poland, Bio-Rad, Chercules, CA, USA), as described in Pławińska-Czarnak [17].

3.3. Antimicrobial Sensitivity Testing

Each *Salmonella* strain was first subcultured as described previously. From an 18–24 h culture, a DensiCHEK Plus (Biomerieux, Marcy-l'Étoile, France) instrument was used to perform a suspension with a 0.5 McFarland range. Then, 145 µL of this inoculum was transferred to another VITEK® tube containing 3 mL 0.45% saline. The card was automatically filled by a vacuum device and automatically sealed. It was manually inserted in the VITEK2 Compact reader-incubator module, and every card was automatically subjected to a kinetic fluorescence measurement every 15 min. This is an automated test methodology based on the MIC technique reported by MacLowry and Marsh [18], and Gerlach [19]. A loop of the suspension was also inoculated onto blood agar (GRASO, Poland) for the purity check.

Antimicrobial susceptibility was assessed by determining the MIC values using a 96 well MICRONAUT Special Plates with antimicrobials: β-lactams/aminopenicillin (amoxicillin—AMX, amoxicillin and clavulanic acid—AMX/CL), β-lactams/I generation cephalosporins (cephalexin—CFX, cephapirin—CPH), β-lactams/III generation cephalosporins (ceftiofur—CFTI), β-lactams/IV generation cephalosporins (cefquinome—CFQ), β-lactams/penicillin cloxacillin—CLO, penicillin G—PG, nafcillin—NAF), aminoglycoside (gentamicin—GEN, neomycin—NEO, streptomycin—STR), polymyxins (colistin—COL), fluorochinolones (enrofloxacin—ENR, norfloxacin—NOR), tetracyclines (doxycycline—DOX, oxytetracycline—OXY), macrolides erythromycin—ERY, tylosin—TYL, florfenicol—FLR), lincosamides (lincomycin—LIN, lincomycin/spectinomycin—LIN/SP), trimethoprim-sulfamethoxazole—TR/SMX, tiamulin—TIA, tylvalosin—TYLV (MERLIN Diagnostika GmbH, Bremen, Niemcy). Simultaneously, antimicrobial susceptibility was assessed by determining the MIC values using a VITEK® 2 System and AST-GN96 cards for Gram-negative bacteria (BioMérieux). The AST card is essentially a miniaturised and abbreviated version of the doubling dilution technique for MICs determined by the microdilution method [c].

The MERLIN antibiotics concentration (µg/mL) is as follows: amoxicillin—0.25, 2, 4, 8, 16; amoxicillin and clavulanic acid—4/2, 8/4, 16/8; cephalexin—8, 16; cephapirin—8, ceftiofur—2; cefquinome—2, 4; cloxacillin—2; penicillin 0.0625, 0.125, 2, 8; nafcillin—2; gentamicin—4, 8; neomycin—8; streptomycin—8; colistin—2; enrofloxacin—0.5, 2; norfloxacin—1, 2; doxycycline—2, 4, 8; oxytetracycline—2, 4, 8; erythromycin—0.25; 0.5, tylosin—TYL; florfenicol—2, 4; lincomycin—2, 8; lincomycin/specinicin—8, 32; trimethoprim-sulfamethoxazole—2/38; tiamulin—16; and tylvalosin—2, 4.

With using AST-GN96 susceptibility for β-lactams/aminopenicillin (ampicillin—AMP, amoxicillin and clavulanic acid—AMX/CL), β-lactams/I generation cephalosporins (cefalexin -CFX), β-lactams/III generation cephalosporins (cefalotin—CFT, cefoperazone CFP), β-lactams/III generation cephalosporins (ceftiofur—CFTI), β-lactams/IV generation cephalosporins (cefquinome—CFQ), carbapenems (imipenem—IPM), polymyxin (polymixin B -PB), aminoglycoside (gentamicin—GEN, neomycin—NEO), fluorochinolones (enrofloxacin—ENR), flumequine—UB), marbofloxacin—MRB), tetracycline -TET, florfenicol—FLR, and trimethoprim/sulfamethoxazole (TR/SMX), were assessed.

The AST-GN96 antibiotics concentration (µg/mL) is as follows: ampicillin—4, 8, 32; amoxicillin and clavulanic acid—4/2, 16/8, 32/16; cephalexin—8, 16, 32; efalotin—2, 8, 32; cefoperazone 4, 8, 32; cefquinome—0.5, 1.5, 4; imipenem 1, 2, 6, 12; polymixin B 0.25, 1, 4, 16; gentamicin—4, 16, 32; neomycin—8, 16, 64; enrofloxacin—0.25, 1, 4; flumequine—2, 4, 8; marbofloxacin—1, 2; tetracycline—2, 4, 8; florfenicol—1, 4, 8; trimethoprim/sulfamethoxazole—1/19, 4/76, 16/304.

The MICs were interpreted according to Clinical and Laboratory Standards Institute (CLSI) and FDA breakpoints (CLSI M100-ED28, 2018). The AST card is essentially a miniaturised and abbreviated version of the doubling dilution technique for MICs determined by the microdilution method.

3.4. Determination of Antibiotics Resistance Profile of Salmonella spp. Isolates

In order to calculate multiple antibiotics resistance, we used the formula according to the Akinola 2019, MAR index [16]:

$$\text{MAR} = \frac{\text{Number of resistance to antibiotics}}{\text{Total number of antibiotics tested}}$$

Detection of Antimicrobial Resistance Genes by PCR

Mueller–Hinton agar was used to culture the bacterial isolates overnight at 35 °C. Bacterial DNA isolation was performed using a standard bacterial DNA isolation Kylt® DNA Extraction-Mix II (Anicon, Emstek, Germany). Eighteen resistance genes (*aadA*, *strA/strB*, *aphA1*, *aphA2*, *aadB*, *tetA*, *tetB*, *sul1*, *sul2*, *sul3*, *dfrA1*, *dfrA10*, *dfrA12*, *floR*, bla_{TEM}, bla_{SHV}, bla_{CMY-2}, bla_{PSE-1} and bla_{CTX-M}) were analysed by conventional PCR, using specific primer pairs in multiplex or a single PCR reaction. The primer sequences predicted PCR product sizes and references shown in Table 4.

Table 4. Description of primer sets, annealing temperature and product size for the molecular gene identification [20–22].

Multiplex PCR or Single PCR	Gene/Antibiotic	Primer Sequences 5′-3′	Annealing Temperature	Product Size (bp)
Multiplex 1	*aadA* streptomycin	F-GTG GAT GGC GGC CTG AAG CC R-AAT GCC CAG TCG GCA GCG	63 °C	525 bp
Multiplex 1	*strA/strB* streptomycin	F-ATG GTG GAC CCT AAA ACT CT R-CGT CTA GGA TCG AGA CAA AG	63 °C	893 bp
Multiplex 2	*aphA1* neomycin	F-ATG GGC TCG CGA TAA TGT C R-CTC ACC GAG GCA GTT CCA T	55 °C	634 bp
Multiplex 2	*aphA2* neomycin	F-GAT TGA ACA AGA TGG ATT GC R-CCA TGA TGG ATA CTT TCT CG	55 °C	347 bp
Multiplex 2	*aadB* gentamicin	F-GAG GAG TTG GAC TATGGA TT R-CTT CAT CGG CAT AGT AAA AG	55 °C	208 bp
Multiplex 3	*tetA* tetracycline	F-GGC GGT CTT CTT CAT CAT GC R-CGG CAG GCA GAG CAA GTA GA	63 °C	502 bp
Multiplex 3	*tetB* tetracycline	F-CGC CCA GTG CTG TTG TTG TC R-CGC GTT GAG AAG CTG AGG TG	63 °C	173 bp
Multiplex 4	*sul1* sulfamethoxazole	F-CGG CGT GGG CTA CCT GAA CG R-GCC GAT CGC GTG AAG TTC CG	66 °C	433 bp
Multiplex 4	*sul2* sulfamethoxazole	F-CGG CAT CGT CAA CAT AAC CT R-TGT GCG GAT GAA GTC AGC TC	66 °C	721 bp
Single PCR	*sul3* sulfamethoxazole	F-GGGAGCCGCTTCCAGTAAT R-TCCGTGACACTGCAATCATTA	60 °C	500 bp
Single PCR	*dfrA1* trimethoprim	F-CAATGGCTGTTGGTTGGAC R-CCGGCTCGATGTCTATTGT	62 °C	253 bp
Single PCR	*dfrA10* trimethoprim	F-TCAAGGCAAATTACCTTGGC R-ATCTATTGGATCACCTACCC	59 °C	433 bp
Single PCR	*dfrA12* trimethoprim	F-TTCGCAGACTCACTGAGGG R-CGGTTGAGACAAGCTCGAAT	63 °C	330 bp
Single PCR	*floR* florfenicol	F-CACGTTGAGCCTCTATATGG R-ATGCAGAAGTAGAACGCGAC	61 °C	888 bp
5	bla_{TEM} ampicillin	F-TTAACTGGCGAACTACTTAC R-GTCTATTTCGTTCATCCATA	55 °C	247 bp
5	bla_{SHV} ceftiofur	F-AGGATTGACTGCCTTTTTG R-ATTTGCTGATTTCGCTCG	55 °C	393 bp
5	bla_{CMY-2} ceftiofur	F-GACAGCCTCTTTCTCCACA R-TGGACACGAAGGCTACGTA	55 °C	1000 bp
Single PCR	bla_{PSE-1} ampicillin	F-GCAAGTAGGGCAGGCAATCA R-GAGCTAGATAGATGCTCACAA	60 °C	461 bp
Single PCR	bla_{CTX-M}	F-CGCTTTGCGATGTGCAG R-ACCGCGATATCGTTGGT	60 °C	585 bp

3.5. Statistical Assessment

Statistical testing was performed with Statistica software, version 13.1. Descriptive statistics were computed to determine the proportions of isolates resistant to different antimicrobial agents. Chi square tests were adopted for the determination of statistical significance of differences between the proportions.

4. Discussion

Our data show that poultry meat is a relevant source of *Salmonella*, and the prevalent serovar was Enteritidis (56.41%). We estimate the antibiotic susceptibility profiles of *Salmonella* strains, and we found a high rate of strains showing at least one phenotypic resistance. In our study, sensitivity to 25 antibiotics were assessed. Penicillins (cloxacillin, penicillin G, nafcillin), macrolides (erythromycin, tylvalosin), lincomycin, tiamulin, and tylvalosin were excluded from analysis, due to a natural lack of activity against *Salmonella*.

The results of the antibiotic resistance indicate that the *Salmonella* spp. strains isolated from meat can be categorized as resistant to MDR: that is, bacteria exhibiting resistance to one or more antibiotics from three or more classes of antibiotics. These bacteria are resistant to β-lactams, aminoglycosides, cephalosporins, fluorochinolones, sulfonamides, and tetracyclines. Resistance to third generation cephalosporins exhibited by the strains isolated from meats represents a concern, because these antibiotics are used for salmonellosis treatment in human, thus rendering the transmission of resistant bacteria a public health problem. All strains isolated from meat were resistant to gentamycin, which is one of the major antibiotics used in the treatment of urinary infections in humans, and were resistant to streptomycin used to treat tuberculosis and *Burkholderia* infection. Although streptomycin is an aminoglycoside and not used for *Salmonella* treatment, streptomycin resistance has been widely used as an epidemiological marker. Resistance to streptomycin is analogous to the phenotypic characteristics observed in multi-drug resistance to ampicillin, chloramphenicol, streptomycin, sulfonamides, and tetracyclines [23,24]. Regarding the resistance to ampicillin (35.89%), previous studies from different countries report highest resistance rates [25].

Moreover, *Salmonella* Derby from meat shows resistance to cefequinome, fourth generation cephalosporins, and antibiotics used in the treatment of mastitis and bovine pneumonia. In *Salmonella* Derby and Indiana (both in the BO4 group), we found resistance against sulphonamides, a class of antibiotics used in severe *Salmonella* infections. We also observed resistance to third generation cephalosporins (cefoperazone and ceftiofur) in four *Salmonella* Derby strains isolated from poultry meat. In addition, a high percentage of strains (Indiana, Infantis, Kentucky, and Newport) showed resistance to tetracyclines (24.64%), despite the fact that, in 2006, the European Union, imposed a ban on the non-therapeutic use of antibiotics important to humans, such as tetracyclines, in animal treatment. A total of 53.84% of tested strains showed an MDR profile with resistance to one or more antibiotics from three or more classes of antibiotics. On the other hand, all the *Salmonella* spp. strains were susceptible to imipenem, which is similar to the result reported previously [26]. Carbapenems are the final choice of antibiotics used in the treatment of salmonellosis when the bacteria exhibit resistance to antibiotics, such as ciprofloxacin and third generation cephalosporins.

These data are alarming for consumers because of the real possibility of an infection with an MDR strain in food, but also because these strains showed resistance to antibiotic classes crucial in human medicine, such as beta-lactamases.

Finally, because these antibiotic phenotypes can be conferred by several ARGs, the detection of resistance genes was performed in order to confirm phenotypic pattern.

In *Salmonella*, the main mechanism of resistance to β-lactams is the acquisition *bla* gene encodes beta-lactamase hydrolytic enzymes, which inactivate the antibiotic [27]. Extended-spectrum beta-lactamases (ESBLs), which inactivates first-, second-, and third-generation cephalosporins and penicillins, and are encoded multi-variant bla_{TEM}, bla_{SHV} and bla_{CTX-M} genes [28]. The bla_{CTX-M} genes encode for the extended-spectrum of β-lactamases (ESBLs) were not present in analysed strains. These types of β-lactamases are active against cephalosporins and monobactams (but not carbapenems), and are currently of great epidemiological and clinical interest. The bla_{SHV} gene was found to be the most prevalent gene amongst our isolates, mainly in *S. enteritidis*. The bla_{SHV} gene is associated with *Enterobacteriaceae* in causing nosocomial infections, but also in isolates from different sources (human, animal, and environment). The gene bla_{CMY-2} encodes an extended-spectrum beta-lactamase that is responsible for hydrolyzing the β-lactam ring that was detected in 35.89% of strains. However, some *Salmonella* spp. strains did not expose phenotypic resistance to this antibiotic. This gene confers resistance to ampicillin, ceftiofur, cefoperazone and is associated with mobile elements, thus increasing the probability of transmission between bacteria [29]. In our study, 28.21% of the strains demonstrate the presence of the genes $blaPSE-1$ and bla_{TEM} that encode β-lactamases that confer resistance to ampicilin. In a study conducted in Colombia, 69.4% of the strains isolated from broiler farms had both genes; thus, a frequency was higher than that found in the present study [30]. Five *S. derby*, one *S. enteritidis*, and all *S. Kentucky* that were phenotypically resistant to ampicillin and third generation cephalosporins, showed the presence of the genes bla_{PSE-1}, bla_{TEM}, bla_{CMY-2}, but not and bla_{CTX-M}. The streptomycin resistance gene *aadA* and *strA/strB* were detected in all of the strains. Interestingly, White et al. [31] showed that *Salmonella* strains isolated from meat that had the *aadA* genes but were susceptible to streptomycin, probably due to gene silencing. The gene *sul2* encodes DHPS (dihydropteroate synthase) was found in 7.69% of the strains (*S. derby* and *S. indiana*). In a previous study, the gene *sul1* is reported to be the most prevalent (57.1%) [24], whereas in the present study, it was found in only 5.13% of the strains. Trimethoprim resistance is mediated by the expression of the enzyme DHFR (dihydrofolate reductase) and is encoded by the *dfrA1* gene that was detected in 7.69% of the strains. In general, the strains that were resistant to trimethoprim-sulfamethoxazole showed the *sul* (*sul1*, *sul2* or *sul3*) and *dfrA* (*dfrA1*, *dfrA12*) resistance genes, mainly in *S. Derby*. However, all strains were resistant to this antibiotic. This resistance may be mediated by other resistance genes, which are not assessed in this study. In *S. derby*, *S. indiana*, *S. newport*, and in two *S. Enteritidis*, the *floR* gene was detected. This gene encodes an efflux pump that confers resistance to amphenicols, which has been reported in the genomic island of *Salmonella* (SGI1) [32].

Our data are very alarming, since all of our strains came from food samples, mainly poultry meat for human consumption. Thermal processing of these products may reduce the risk of foodborne disease, but ARGs can be transferred to the gut microbiota and transfer resistance to other bacteria [33]. Therefore, our data are in line with recommendations, which confirm how important it is in the monitoring and control of antibiotic resistance to assess the presence or absence of ARGs in foodborne strains, especially in a One Health approach that recognises the circularity of human, animal, and environmental health.

5. Conclusions

The *Salmonella* spp. strains exhibited resistance to multiple antibiotics, as well as multiple genes associated with them. A high resistance rate to multiple antibiotics combined with multiple ARGs in isolates from raw meat, as revealed in this study, suggests that the situation is alarming in where irrational use of antibiotics is combined with inadequate surveillance and facilities to detect MDR. Continued monitoring of antimicrobial resistance in *Salmonella* strain collection along the food chain is required so that comparisons of antimicrobial resistance from the different origins can be effectively performed.

Author Contributions: Conceptualization, J.P.-C. and M.K.-Ś.; methodology, J.P.-C., K.W. and M.K.-Ś.; validation, J.P.-C., K.W., M.K.-Ś. and J.B.; formal analysis, J.P.-C., K.W., M.K.-Ś., T.N. and Z.S.; investigation, J.P.-C., P.K. and K.A.; resources, J.P.-C.; data curation, J.P.-C., K.W. and M.K.-Ś.; writing—original draft preparation, J.P.-C., K.W., M.K.-Ś., T.N., Z.S. and J.B.; writing—review and editing, J.P.-C., K.W., M.K.-Ś., K.A., Z.S. and P.K.; visualization, J.P.-C., K.W. and M.K.-Ś.; supervision, J.P.-C. and K.A.; project administration, J.P.-C.; funding acquisition, K.A. and P.K. All authors have read and agreed to the published version of the manuscript.

Funding: This research received no external funding.

Institutional Review Board Statement: Not applicable.

Informed Consent Statement: Not applicable.

Data Availability Statement: The data presented in this study are available on request from the corresponding author. The data are not publicly available due to their containing information that could compromise the image of the meat processing plants.

Acknowledgments: Special thanks to Jolanta Przybylska for help with the laboratory work and Maria Górka for help with editing the text.

Conflicts of Interest: The authors declare no conflict of interest. The funders had no role in the design of the study; in the collection, analyses, or interpretation of data; in the writing of the manuscript, or in the decision to publish the results.

References

1. European Food Safety Authority; European Centre for Disease Prevention and Control. The European Union One Health 2020 Zoonoses Report. *EFSA J.* **2021**, *19*, e06971. [CrossRef]
2. Issenhuth-Jeanjean, S.; Roggentin, P.; Mikoleit, M.; de Pinna, E.; Nair, S.; Fields, P.I.; Issenhuth-jeanjean, S.; Roggentin, P.; Mikoleit, M.; Guibourdenche, M.; et al. Supplement 2008–2010 (no. 48) to the White–Kauffmann–Le Minor scheme. *Res. Microbiol.* **2014**, *165*, 526–530. [CrossRef]
3. Gutema, F.D.; Agga, G.E.; Abdi, R.D.; De Zutter, L.; Duchateau, L.; Gabriël, S. Prevalence and serotype diversity of *Salmonella* in apparently healthy cattle: Systematic review and meta-analysis of published studies, 2000–2017. *Front. Vet. Sci.* **2019**, *6*, 102. [CrossRef]
4. European Food Safety Authority; European Centre for Disease Prevention and Control. The European Union Summary Report on Antimicrobial Resistance in zoonotic and indicator bacteria from humans, animals and food in 2018/2019. *EFSA J.* **2022**, *20*, e07209. [CrossRef]
5. Kong-Ngoen, T.; Santajit, S.; Tunyong, W.; Pumirat, P.; Sookrung, N.; Chaicumpa, W.; Indrawattana, N. Antimicrobial Resistance and Virulence of Non-Typhoidal *Salmonella* from Retail Foods Marketed in Bangkok, Thailand. *Foods* **2022**, *11*, 661. [CrossRef]
6. Threlfall, E.J.; Rowe, B.; Ward, L.R. A comparison of multiple drug resistance in *Salmonellas* from humans and food animals in England and Wales, 1981 and 1990. *Epidemiol. Infect.* **1993**, *111*, 189–198. [CrossRef]
7. Barza, M. Potential mechanisms of increased disease in humans from antimicrobial resistance in food animals. *Clin. Infect. Dis.* **2002**, *34*, 123–125. [CrossRef]
8. Lai, J.; Wu, C.; Wu, C.; Qi, J.; Wang, Y.; Wang, H.; Liu, Y.; Shen, J. Serotype distribution and antibiotic resistance of *Salmonella* in food-producing animals in Shandong province of China, 2009 and 2012. *Int. J. Food Microbiol.* **2014**, *180*, 30–38. [CrossRef]
9. Barilli, E.; Bacci, C.; Villa, Z.S.; Merialdi, G.; D'Incau, M.; Brindani, F.; Vismarra, A. Antimicrobial resistance, biofilm synthesis and virulence genes in *Salmonella* isolated from pigs bred on intensive farms. *Ital. J. Food Saf.* **2018**, *7*, 131–137. [CrossRef]
10. Campos, J.; Mourão, J.; Peixe, L.; Antunes, P. Non-typhoidal *Salmonella* in the pig production chain: A comprehensive analysis of its impact on human health. *Pathogens* **2019**, *8*, 19. [CrossRef]
11. Yang, X.; Wu, Q.; Zhang, J.; Huang, J.; Chen, L.; Wu, S.; Zeng, H.; Wang, J.; Chen, M.; Wu, H.; et al. Prevalence, bacterial load, and antimicrobial resistance of *Salmonella* serovars isolated from retail meat and meat products in China. *Front. Microbiol.* **2019**, *10*, 2121. [CrossRef]
12. WHO. *WHO List of Critically Important Antimicrobials (CIA)*; World Health Organization: Geneva, Switzerland, 2019; ISBN 978-924-151-552-8.
13. Tacconelli, E.; Carrara, E.; Savoldi, A.; Harbarth, S.; Mendelson, M.; Monnet, D.L.; Pulcini, C.; Kahlmeter, G.; Kluytmans, J.; Carmeli, Y.; et al. Discovery, research, and development of new antibiotics: The WHO priority list of antibiotic-resistant bacteria and tuberculosis. *Lancet Infect. Dis.* **2018**, *18*, 318–327. [CrossRef]
14. Pławińska-Czarnak, J.; Wódz, K.; Kizerwetter-świda, M.; Nowak, T.; Bogdan, J.; Kwieciński, P.; Kwieciński, A.; Anusz, K. *Citrobacter braakii* yield false-positive identification as *Salmonella*, a note of caution. *Foods* **2021**, *10*, 2177. [CrossRef]
15. Ramtahal, M.A.; Somboro, A.M.; Amoako, D.G.; Abia, A.L.K.; Perrett, K.; Bester, L.A.; Essack, S.Y. Molecular Epidemiology of *Salmonella enterica* in Poultry in South Africa Using the Farm-to-Fork Approach. *Int. J. Microbiol.* **2022**, *2022*, 5121273. [CrossRef]
16. Akinola, S.A.; Mwanza, M.; Ateba, C.N. Occurrence, genetic diversities and antibiotic resistance profiles of *Salmonella* serovars isolated from chickens. *Infect. Drug Resist.* **2019**, *12*, 3327–3342. [CrossRef]
17. Pławińska-Czarnak, J.; Wódz, K.; Piechowicz, L.; Tokarska-Pietrzak, E.; Bełkot, Z.; Bogdan, J.; Wiśniewski, J.; Kwieciński, P.; Kwieciński, A.; Anusz, K. Wild Duck (*Anas platyrhynchos*) as a Source of Antibiotic-Resistant *Salmonella enterica* subsp. diarizonae O58—The First Report in Poland. *Antibiotics* **2022**, *11*, 530. [CrossRef]
18. MacLowry, J.D.; Marsh, H.H. Semi-automatic microtechnique for serial dilution antibiotic sensitivity testing in the clinical laboratory. *J. Lab. Clin. Med.* **1968**, *72*, 685–687.

19. Gerlach, E. Microdilution 1: A Comparative Study. In *Current Techniques for Antibiotic Susceptibility Testing*; Charles C. Thomas: Springfield, IL, USA, 1974; pp. 63–76.
20. Kozak, G.K.; Boerlin, P.; Janecko, N.; Reid-Smith, R.J.; Jardine, C. Antimicrobial resistance in *Escherichia coli* isolates from Swine and wild small mammals in the proximity of swine farms and in natural environments in Ontario, Canada. *Appl. Environ. Microbiol.* **2009**, *75*, 559–566. [CrossRef]
21. Chuanchuen, R.; Padungtod, P. Antimicrobial resistance genes in *Salmonella* enterica isolates from poultry and swine in Thailand. *J. Vet. Med. Sci.* **2009**, *71*, 1349–1355. [CrossRef]
22. Koleri, J.; Petkar, H.M.; Husain, A.A.M.; Almaslamani, M.A.; Omrani, A.S. *Moraxella osloensis* bacteremia, a case series and review of the literature. *IDCases* **2022**, *27*, e01450. [CrossRef]
23. Doran, G.; NiChulain, M.; DeLappe, N.; O'Hare, C.; Corbett-Feeney, G.; Cormican, M. Interpreting streptomycin susceptibility test results for *Salmonella enterica* serovar Typhimurium. *Int. J. Antimicrob. Agents* **2006**, *27*, 538–540. [CrossRef] [PubMed]
24. Mengistu, G.; Dejenu, G.; Tesema, C.; Arega, B.; Awoke, T.; Alemu, K.; Moges, F. Epidemiology of streptomycin resistant *Salmonella* from humans and animals in Ethiopia: A systematic review and meta-analysis. *PLoS ONE* **2020**, *15*, e0244057. [CrossRef] [PubMed]
25. Nair, D.V.T.; Venkitanarayanan, K.; Johny, A.K. Antibiotic-resistant *Salmonella* in the food supply and the potential role of antibiotic alternatives for control. *Foods* **2018**, *7*, 167. [CrossRef]
26. Ali Shah, S.A.; Nadeem, M.; Syed, S.A.; Fatima Abidi, S.T.; Khan, N.; Bano, N. Antimicrobial Sensitivity Pattern of *Salmonella* Typhi: Emergence of Resistant Strains. *Cureus* **2020**, *12*, 10–14. [CrossRef]
27. Iredell, J.; Brown, J.; Tagg, K. Antibiotic resistance in Enterobacteriaceae: Mechanisms and clinical implications. *BMJ* **2016**, *352*, h6420. [CrossRef]
28. Philippon, A.; Slama, P.; Dény, P.; Labia, R. A structure-based classification of class A β-Lactamases, a broadly diverse family of enzymes. *Clin. Microbiol. Rev.* **2016**, *29*, 29–57. [CrossRef]
29. Oladeinde, A.; Cook, K.; Lakin, S.M.; Woyda, R.; Abdo, Z.; Looft, T.; Herrington, K.; Zock, G.; Lawrence, J.P.; Thomas, J.C.; et al. Horizontal gene transfer and acquired antibiotic resistance in *Salmonella enterica* serovar heidelberg following in vitro incubation in broiler ceca. *Appl. Environ. Microbiol.* **2019**, *85*, e01903-19. [CrossRef]
30. Herrera-Sánchez, M.P.; Rodríguez-Hernández, R.; Rondón-Barragán, I.S. Molecular characterization of antimicrobial resistance and enterobacterial repetitive intergenic consensus-PCR as a molecular typing tool for *Salmonella* spp. isolated from poultry and humans. *Vet. World* **2020**, *13*, 1771–1779. [CrossRef]
31. White, P.A.; Iver, C.J.M.C.; Rawlinson, W.D. Integrons and Gene Cassettes in the Enterobacteriaceae. *Antimicrob. Agents Chemother.* **2001**, *45*, 2658–2661. [CrossRef]
32. Doublet, B.; Boyd, D.; Mulvey, M.R.; Cloeckaert, A. The *Salmonella* genomic island 1 is an integrative mobilizable element. *Mol. Microbiol.* **2005**, *55*, 1911–1924. [CrossRef]
33. Groussin, M.; Poyet, M.; Sistiaga, A.; Kearney, S.M.; Moniz, K.; Noel, M.; Hooker, J.; Gibbons, S.M.; Segurel, L.; Froment, A.; et al. Elevated rates of horizontal gene transfer in the industrialized human microbiome. *Cell* **2021**, *184*, 2053–2067.e18. [CrossRef] [PubMed]

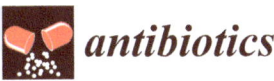

Article

ESBL-Producing *Escherichia coli* Carrying CTX-M Genes Circulating among Livestock, Dogs, and Wild Mammals in Small-Scale Farms of Central Chile

Julio A. Benavides [1,2,3,*], Marília Salgado-Caxito [3,4], Andrés Opazo-Capurro [3,5], Paulina González Muñoz [3,5,6], Ana Piñeiro [7], Macarena Otto Medina [1], Lina Rivas [3,8], Jose Munita [3,8] and Javier Millán [1,9,10]

1. Departamento de Ecología y Biodiversidad, Facultad de Ciencias de la Vida, Universidad Andrés Bello, Santiago 8320000, Chile; mottomed@gmail.com (M.O.M.); syngamustrachea@hotmail.com (J.M.)
2. Centro de Investigación para la Sustentabilidad, Facultad de Ciencias de la Vida, Universidad Andrés Bello, Santiago 8320000, Chile
3. Millennium Initiative for Collaborative Research on Bacterial Resistance (MICROB-R), Santiago 7550000, Chile; mariliasalgadovet@gmail.com (M.S.-C.); andopazo@udec.cl (A.O.-C.); paulinagonzalez@udec.cl (P.G.M.); linarivas@udd.cl (L.R.); munita.jm@gmail.com (J.M.)
4. School of Veterinary Medicine, Pontificia Universidad Católica de Chile, Santiago 7820244, Chile
5. Departamento de Microbiología, Facultad de Ciencias Biológicas, Universidad de Concepción, Concepción 4070386, Chile
6. Departamento de Ciencias Biológicas y Químicas, Facultad de Medicina y Ciencia, Universidad San Sebastián, Concepción 4030000, Chile
7. Escuela de Medicina Veterinaria, Facultad de Ciencias de la Vida, Universidad Andrés Bello, Santiago 8320000, Chile; anapimo@yahoo.es
8. Genomics and Resistance Microbes (GeRM) Lab, Facultad de Medicina CAS—UDD, Instituto de Ciencias e Innovación en Medicina (ICIM), Santiago 7550000, Chile
9. Instituto Agroalimentario de Aragón-IA2, Universidad de Zaragoza-CITA, Miguel Servet 177, 50013 Zaragoza, Spain
10. Fundación ARAID, Avda. de Ranillas, 50018 Zaragoza, Spain
* Correspondence: benavidesjulio@yahoo.fr

Abstract: Antibiotic-resistant bacteria of critical importance for global health such as extended-spectrum beta-lactamases-producing (ESBL)-*Escherichia coli* have been detected in livestock, dogs, and wildlife worldwide. However, the dynamics of ESBL-*E. coli* between these animals remains poorly understood, particularly in small-scale farms of low and middle-income countries where contact between species can be frequent. We compared the prevalence of fecal carriage of ESBL-*E. coli* among 332 livestock (207 cows, 15 pigs, 60 horses, 40 sheep, 6 goats, 4 chickens), 82 dogs, and wildlife including 131 European rabbits, 30 rodents, and 12 Andean foxes sharing territory in peri-urban localities of central Chile. The prevalence was lower in livestock (3.0%) and wildlife (0.5%) compared to dogs (24%). Among 47 ESBL-*E. coli* isolates recovered, CTX-M-group 1 was the main ESBL genotype identified, followed by CTX-M-groups 2, 9, 8, and 25. ERIC-PCR showed no cluster of *E. coli* clones by either host species nor locality. To our knowledge, this is the first report of ESBL-*E. coli* among sheep, cattle, dogs, and rodents of Chile, confirming their fecal carriage among domestic and wild animals in small-scale farms. The high prevalence of ESBL-*E. coli* in dogs encourages further investigation on their role as potential reservoirs of this bacteria in agricultural settings.

Keywords: antimicrobial resistance; bla_{CTX-M}; Chile; domestic animals; *E. coli*; extended-spectrum beta-lactamases; wildlife

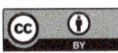

1. Introduction

The current increase of antimicrobial resistance (AMR) is considered a main global threat to human and animal health [1,2]. AMR is responsible for thousands of human fatalities annually [3] and large economic losses that could reduce global GDP in 1–4% by 2050 [2,4]. The intense use of antibiotics in livestock production and humans is the main cause of the emergence and rapid spread of AMR [2,5]. In the last decade, the global growth of livestock has been associated with an increase in antibiotics use [2]. For example, 70% of antibiotics used in human medicine are consumed by animal production in the USA [6,7]. Extended-spectrum beta-lactamase-producing *Escherichia coli* (ESBL-*E. coli*) represent one of the highest burdens of AMR to public health and have globally spread in both hospital settings and the community [8]. ESBL-*E. coli* are commonly isolated from domestic animals such as cattle and dogs, but also wild animals [9–12]. Similar to humans, the misuse of third-generation cephalosporins in livestock generated a selective pressure resulting in the emergence and spread of ESBL-*E. coli* in this sector [9,13]. In contrast, the presence of ESBL-*E. coli* in wildlife is assumed to result from contamination in human-dominated environments [10,12,14].

The circulation of ESBL-*E. coli* across different animal populations requires an integrated One Health approach to better understand, predict, and prevent their dissemination [15]. However, most studies on ESBL-*E. coli* have focused on either one population (e.g., domestic or wild animals) or a large spatial scale (e.g., across cities or countries) [16–19]. For example, ESBL-*E. coli* have been detected worldwide in several livestock settings [13,20–22]. Likewise, ESBL-producing *Enterobacterales* have been found in at least 80 wildlife species since 2006 including rodents, bats, foxes, and wild birds [23–26]. Livestock or human proximity are often suggested as drivers of ESBL-*E. coli* in wildlife but, to our knowledge, no study has proven transmission from humans to wild animals [10,14,23]. Dogs living on farms could also contribute to the spread of ESBL-*E. coli* among agricultural settings because contact with livestock has been associated with an increased probability of ESBL-*E. coli* fecal carriage in dogs [27–30]. However, the circulation of ESBL-*E. coli* at the livestock and wildlife interface is still poorly understood [12,31,32].

Few studies on the circulation of ESBL-*E. coli* at the livestock and wildlife interface have been conducted in low- and middle-income countries (LMICs) [10,33–36]. Paradoxically, the consequences of AMR can be exacerbated in these countries by a higher number of bacterial infections and limited access to health facilities providing the appropriate antibiotic treatment [37,38]. Surveillance of AMR in livestock has been recommended by the World Health Organization (WHO), the Food and Agriculture Organization of the United Nations (FAO), and the World Organisation for Animal Health (OIE), but remains limited in LMICs [1,2,33]. Surveillance of AMR in wildlife and dogs is also mostly inexistent in LMICs. In this study, we use a One Health approach to compare the prevalence of ESBL-*E. coli* fecal carriage among livestock, dogs, and wild mammals located in small-scale agricultural settings of central Chile.

Chile, considered a high income economy but with an agricultural production more similar to LMICs, launched the 'National plan to combat antimicrobial resistance' in 2017, but no national surveillance has been implemented yet in the agricultural sector. ESBL-*E. coli* have not been detected in Chilean cattle herds [39,40], but have been isolated in feces from dogs [41], owls in rehabilitation centers [42], wild Andean condors (*Vultur gryphus*) [43] and gulls (*Leucophaeus pipixcan*) [36]. To our knowledge, no study has investigated the ESBL-*E. coli* fecal carriage of livestock nor simultaneously focused on dogs and wild mammals living closely to livestock. Central Chile hosts a large diversity of endemic terrestrial mammals including foxes and rodents [44,45] but also invasive species such as the European rabbit (*Oryctolagus cuniculus*) that has colonized most of the country [46–48]. Rodents and rabbits are commonly found living on farms and interacting with dogs and livestock [49,50]. Similarly, 85% of the territory of the Andean fox (*Lycalopex culpaeus*) overlaps with human-dominated habitat in central Chile [51]. This creates the potential for fecal-oral and environmental bacterial transmission between livestock and wild animals, which remains largely unknown. Previous studies focusing on foxes in the central region have identified the presence of bla_{CTX-M} genes, but the bacteria carrying the gene was unknown [52]. The aims of this study were (i) to estimate and compare the prevalence of ESBL-*E. coli* fecal carriage between livestock, dogs, and wild mammals living in the same agricultural setting of central Chile, (ii) to detect the presence of the most common ESBL genes including bla_{CTX-M}, bla_{TEM}, and bla_{SHV}, and (iii) use high resolution molecular typing to assess potential ESBL-*E. coli* transmission within farms or between different species.

2. Materials and Methods

2.1. Sample Collection

Fresh fecal samples were collected between March 2019 and September 2019 from livestock, dogs, and wildlife in and around 13 farming localities located in the municipalities of Colina (33.1045° S, 70.6159° W) and Lampa (33.2827° S, 70.8793° W) of the Chacabuco province in the Metropolitan Region of central Chile, in the peri-urban area of the Santiago Capital City (Figure 1). A farming locality was either a single private farm or an area where livestock from different owners grazed together and received the same health treatments. The province of Chacabuco includes mainly small- to medium-scale farmers, with an estimated livestock population of 10,662 cattle (mean: 38 animals/farm), 45,821 pigs (587/farm), 5490 goats (59/farm), 4441 sheep (42/farm), and 2897 horses (4/farm) [53]. Farms were randomly selected from a list provided by the Municipality's agrarian unit, accounting for areas overlapping with the known territory of wildlife as previously described [52]. Our sampling focused mainly on cattle because they had the highest potential of overlapping with wild mammals since they often free-ranged within wildlife habitat during our study period.

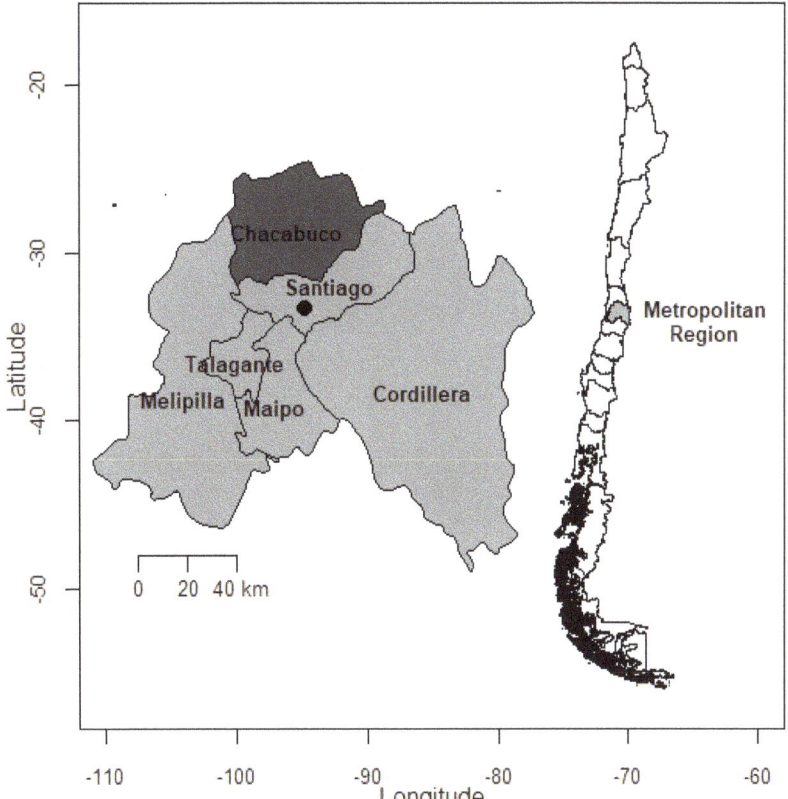

Figure 1. Study area. The inset figure shows the Chacabuco province within the Metropolitan region where farms and wildlife were sampled. Exact farm locations are not given to maintain our confidentiality agreement with farmers. Maps were obtained from the GADM (http://www.gadm.org//, accessed on 15 April 2021) database using the *getData* function from the *raster* package of R.

We focused on sampling the most common wild mammals encountered in those farms including several species of endemic and invasive rodents, the invasive European wild rabbit and the Andean fox, who predates these herbivore species [54,55]. These species were previously determined by discussions with farmers and the municipality's agrarian unit during preliminary visits to the farms. Peri-urban and wild rodents were live captured, sampled, and released using Sherman traps. Fifty traps were placed in and around each sampled farm for at least 4 consecutive days and checked for captured rodents daily. Rectal swabs were collected from alive individuals immobilized, using gloves and protective equipment. Rodents were identified at the genus or species level based on morphological characteristics. Fresh fecal samples from European rabbits were collected early in the morning by identifying rabbit dens in areas where farmers commonly observed rabbits. To avoid sampling the same individual twice, we only collected fresh sample feces from the same den if they were more than 4 m apart, and only sampled each den once. Fresh fecal samples from foxes were collected by walking known paths where foxes were previously captured in the area [56]. Fresh samples from foxes were identified and differentiated from dog feces by their distinct 'fruit' seeds and morphology contained on the sample. To avoid sampling the same individual twice, we only collected a fresh sample in localities that were more than 5 km apart, considering 5 km^2 as the average home range size of foxes in this area [52]. Dogs were sampled by directly taking rectal swabs or waiting until the dog defecated, depending on whether the owner considered that the dog could be aggressive or not during sampling. For all samples taken from the ground, we only collected the portion that was not in contact with the ground to avoid bacterial contamination from the soil. This study was approved by the Ethical Committee of the Universidad Andrés Bello (permit number: 018/2018). The capture and sampling of rodents were also approved by the Servicio Agricola Ganadero (permit number: 2118/2019).

2.2. Sample Size and Prevalence Estimation

The required sample size needed to estimate the prevalence of ESBL-*E. coli* in livestock (defined as the number of animals harboring at least one isolate of ESBL-*E. coli* over the total number of sampled animals) was calculated with the program Epi Info 7.2.2.6^{TM} [57]. To our knowledge, no previous study has estimated the prevalence of fecal carriage of ESBL-*E. coli* among livestock in Chile. Thus, we assumed an expected prevalence of ESBL-*E. coli* of 30%, similar to a study conducted around the Lima capital in Peru with similar farm characteristics [12]. Based on this expected prevalence, a margin of acceptable error of 5% and a confidence interval of 95%, the minimum number of livestock to be sampled in the region was 323.

Based on previous studies on wildlife and dogs, we assumed an expected prevalence of 5% to estimate our sample size. In fact, 5% prevalence of ESLB-*E. coli* was found in wild rodents in China [34,58], no bacteria were found in a previous study conducted in European wild rabbit in Portugal [59], 4% prevalence was found in wild foxes of Portugal [60], and 8% was found in the only study conducted on dogs in Chile [41]. Based on an expected ESBL-*E. coli* prevalence of 5%, a margin of acceptable error of 5% and a confidence interval of 95%, the minimum number of animals to be sampled was 73. We aimed to collect 73 samples per wildlife group (e.g., foxes, rabbits, and rodents). However, giving the intrinsic lower density of foxes compared to small mammals and logistic constraints for finding foxes, we expected a much lower sample size for this species.

2.3. Microbiology Analyses

Fresh fecal samples were collected using Stuart Transport Medium (Deltalab®) and cultured within 3 days of sampling. Swabs were screened for cefotaxime non-susceptible *E. coli* by direct incubation in standard atmospheric conditions (100 kPa) at 37 °C for 24 h in a MacConkey medium containing 2 µg/mL of cefotaxime sodium salt (Sigma-Aldrich, St. Louis, MO, USA) [61]. Up to 3 isolates with different morphotypes compatible with *E. coli* per sample/plate were purified and then stored at −80 °C for further analyses. Bacterial species were confirmed by matrix-assisted laser desorption ionization-time of flight (MALDI-TOF) mass spectrometry (BioMérieux, Marcy l'Etoile, France) at the Genomics and Resistant Microbes (GeRM) Group of the Millennium Initiative for Collaborative Research on Bacterial Resistance (MICROB-R).

Cefotaxime non-susceptible *E. coli* isolates indicating ESBL were tested for antimicrobial susceptibility to 8 antibiotics from 6 classes including chloramphenicol (phenicol), ciprofloxacin (quinolone), sulfamethoxazole (sulfonamide), amikacin (aminoglycoside), tobramycin (aminoglycoside), ertapenem (carbapenem), tetracycline, and gentamicin (aminoglycoside). Multidrug resistance (MDR) was defined as resistance to at least 1 agent of 3 or more antibiotic classes [62]. The *E. coli* ATCC25922 strain was used for quality control and clinical breakpoints were in accordance with CLSI M100:28ED recommendations [61].

Extended-spectrum beta-lactamase production was confirmed in all cefotaxime non-susceptible *E. coli* isolates by the double-disk synergy test [30] on Müller Hinton agar (Difco, BD, Sparks, MD, USA) with and without the AmpC inhibitor phenylboronic acid (Sigma-Aldrich). Briefly, disks of ceftriaxone (30 µg), ceftazidime (30 µg), cefepime (30 µg), and aztreonam (30 µg) were used along with a disk of amoxicillin with clavulanic acid (30 µg) placed in the center of the plate at approximately 20 mm. Inhibition zones (ghost zones) observed around any of the cephalosporin disks towards the disk containing the clavulanic acid after 18–20 h of incubation at 37 °C aerobically were considered as a positive result to produce ESBL.

The presence of the most common ESBL-encoding genes in *E. coli* isolates including bla_{CTX-M}, bla_{TEM}, and bla_{SHV}, was tested by a previously described multiplex PCR [63]. DNA samples from reference bla_{CTX-M}, bla_{TEM}, and bla_{SHV} strains stored at the Universidad de Concepción's Laboratory of Research in Antimicrobial Agents were used as positive PCR controls. The specific group of each CTX-M alleles (CTX-M groups 1, 2, 8, 9, and 25) were detected by multiplex-PCR as described previously [64]. In order to explore the phylogenetic relationships between ESBL-*E. coli* isolates within and between host species or localities, isolates were fingerprinted by ERIC-PCR according to Bilung et al. [65].

2.4. Statistical Analyses

The prevalence of ESBL-*E. coli* was reported and 95% confidence intervals were calculated using the *binom.confint* function (Agresti-Coull method) in the *binom* package in R 3.6.1 [66]. Significant differences in prevalence between populations were tested using the Fisher's exact test in R, since the limited number of observations prevented the use of a Chi-Squared test. We constructed a dendrogram based on the ERIC-PCR electrophoretic patterns using the BioNumerics software v8.0 (Applied Maths, Belgium) and R [65,66]. An UMPGA dendrogram was built based on scaled densitometry curves from the ERIC-PCR obtained from BioNumeric using the *hclust* function of the *dendextended* R package.

3. Results

ESBL-*E. coli* fecal carriage was detected in chickens, cattle, pigs, sheep, goats, dogs, and one wild rodent (*Octodon degus*). The prevalence of ESBL-*E. coli* fecal carriage was significantly higher among dogs (24% [CI: 16–35%]; 20 out of 82) compared to livestock (3% [CI: 2–6%]; 10 out of 324, Fisher's exact test, Odds Ratio (OR) = 10.0, $p < 0.0001$) and wildlife (0.5% [CI: 0–3%]; 1 out of 186, Fisher's exact test, OR = 58.8, $p < 0.0001$) (Figure 2). The prevalence of ESBL-*E. coli* in livestock was also significantly higher than the prevalence in wildlife (Fisher's exact test, OR = 25.4, $p < 0.0001$). At least 1 animal carrying ESBL-*E. coli* was detected in 7 out of the 13 (54%) farm localities sampled. In all 3 farms where livestock carried ESBL-*E. coli* and dogs were sampled, at least 1 dog also carried ESBL-*E. coli*. Likewise, the wild rodent carrying ESBL-*E. coli* was detected in a farm where one cow also carried ESBL-*E. coli*.

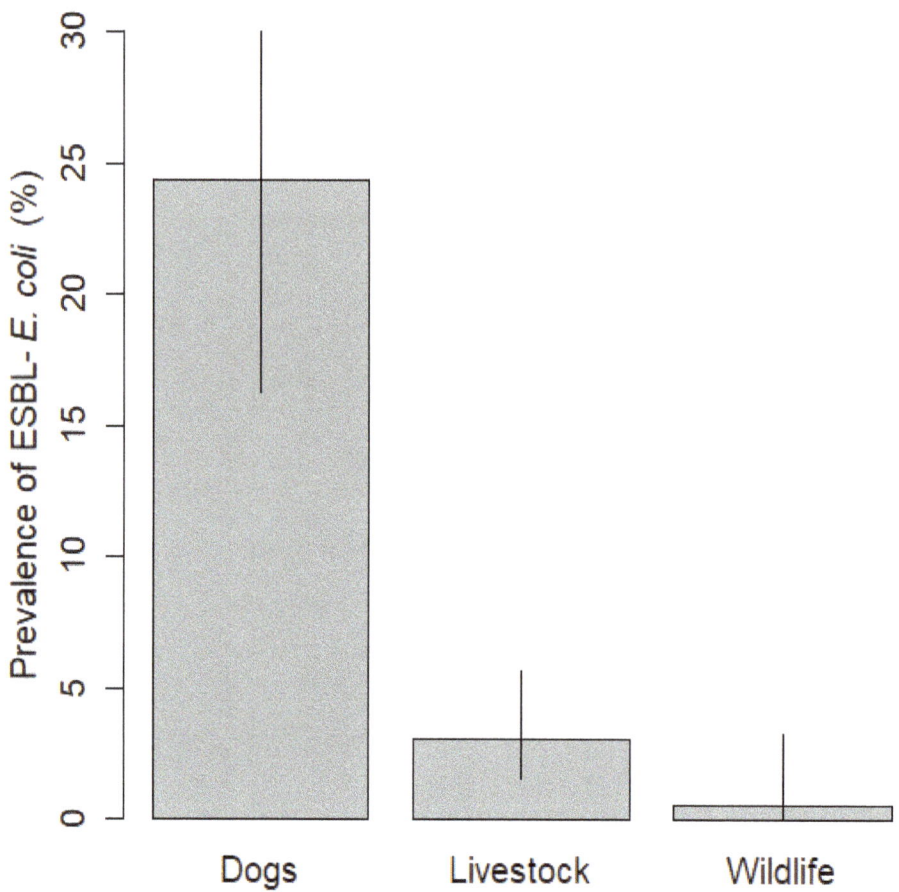

Figure 2. Prevalence of ESBL-*E. coli* per species in small-scale farms of central Chile; 95% confidence intervals were estimated using the *binom.confint* function (Agresti-Coull method) in the *binom* package in R.

A total of 47 ESBL-*E. coli* isolates (confirmed by the double-disk synergy test) from 33 animals were analyzed. Fourteen ESBL-*E. coli* isolates were obtained from 10 livestock, 32 isolates from dogs and 1 isolate from a mouse. ESBL-*E. coli* isolates from livestock were resistant to a median (mean) of 1 (2.6) (range: 0–6) out of 8 antibiotics tested, while ESBL-*E. coli* isolates from dogs were resistant to a median (mean) of 1 antibiotic (1.9) (range: 0–6) (Figure 3A). Overall, 21% of ESBL-*E. coli* isolates from livestock and 31% from dogs were susceptible to all antibiotics, 36% of ESBL-*E. coli* isolates from livestock and 21% from dogs were resistant to one antibiotic, and 43% of ESBL-*E. coli* isolates from livestock and 48% from dogs were resistant to two or more antibiotics. Additionally, 43% of ESBL-*E. coli* isolates from livestock, 47% from dogs and an isolate from one rodent were multidrug resistant (MDR). The ESBL-*E. coli* isolated from a rodent sample was resistant to chloramphenicol, sulfamethoxazole, and ciprofloxacin. More than 20% of ESBL isolates were resistant to ciprofloxacin, chloramphenicol, sulfamethoxazole, and tetracycline in both dogs and livestock. In contrast, no resistance was observed against ertapenem. Among ESBL isolates, the prevalence of resistance to each antibiotic was highly correlated between livestock and dogs (Spearman's test, Rho = 0.90, $p < 0.0001$), but livestock had a slightly higher prevalence than dogs for most antibiotics (Figure 3B).

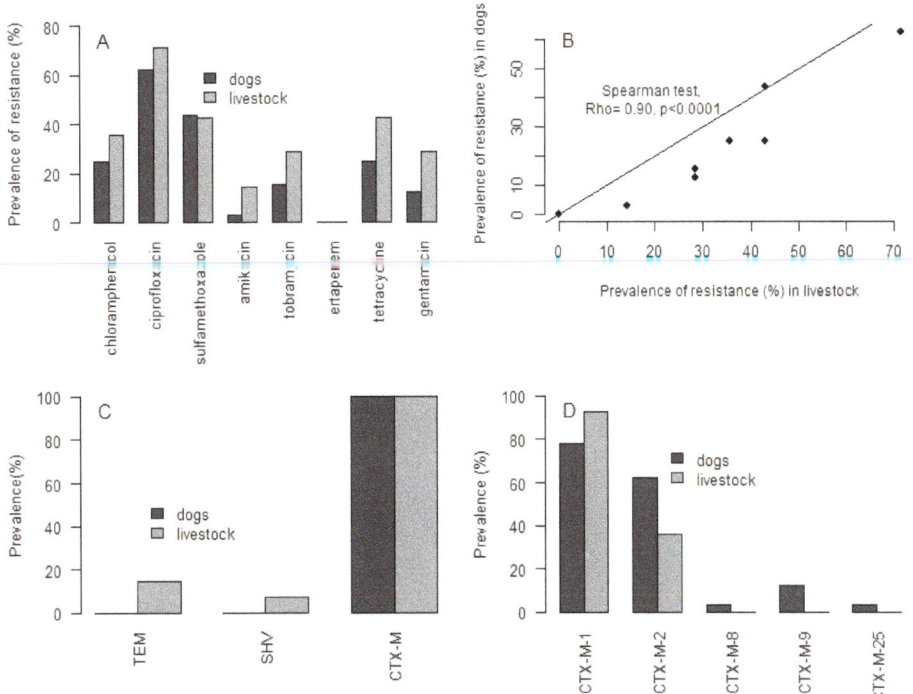

Figure 3. (**A**) Prevalence of resistance to other antibiotic families among ESBL-*E. coli* isolates in dogs and livestock; (**B**) Correlation of the prevalence of resistance to each antibiotic between livestock and dogs; (**C**) Prevalence of bla_{TEM}, bla_{SHV}, and bla_{CTX-M} in ESBL-*E. coli* isolated from livestock and dogs; (**D**) Prevalence of CTX-M groups identified in ESBL-*E. coli* isolates from livestock and dogs.

ESBL-*E. coli* isolates from dogs were only encoded by the CTX-M genotype while all isolates from livestock carried CTX-M (100%), followed by TEM (14%), and SHV (7%) genotypes (Figure 3C). Among the most common CTX-M groups searched, 93% of ESBL-*E. coli* from livestock carried $bla_{CTX-M-group\ 1}$ and 36% carried $bla_{CTX-M-group\ 2}$ genes (Figure 3D). Isolates from dogs carried a more diverse pool of CTX-M genotypes with 78% carrying CTX-M from group 1, followed by group 2 (63%), group 9 (12.5%), group 8 (3%, one isolate), and group 25 (3%). The ESBL-*E. coli* isolate found on a wild mouse carried CTX-M from group 1.

The dendrogram analysis of the ERIC-PCR results showed a high diversity of ESBL-*E. coli* clones within species and farm localities. No visual clustering by species nor farm localities was observed (Figure 4). However, ESBL-*E. coli* isolates from a cow and a dog from the same farm locality clustered together.

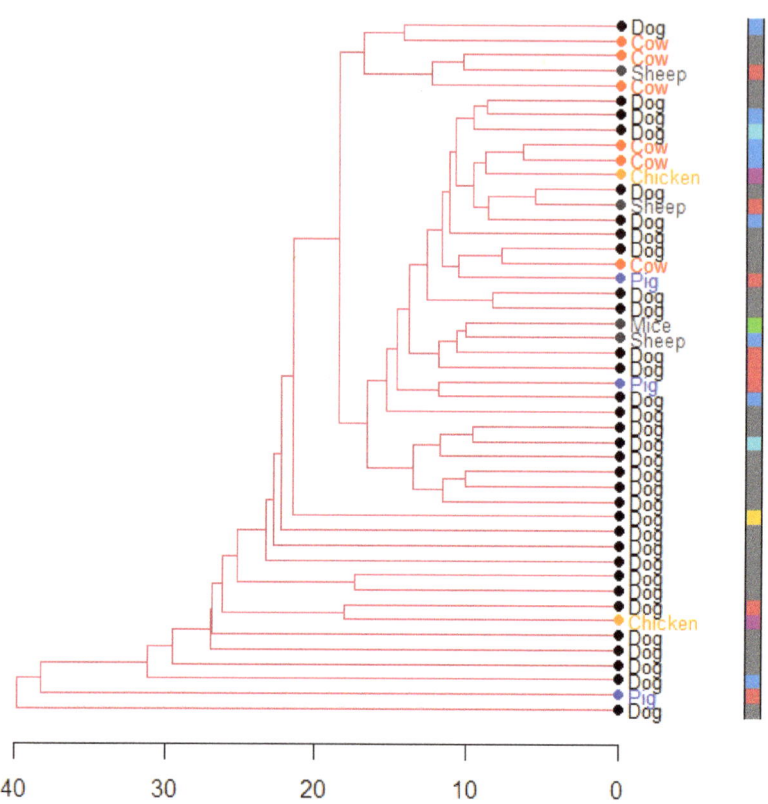

Figure 4. Dendrogram produced by the analysis of the ERIC-PCR of ESBL-*E. coli* isolates from livestock and dogs using the UMPGA method in R. The colored column on the right side represents different farm localities where isolates were recovered.

4. Discussion

The spread of AMR at the interface between domestic animals and wildlife remains poorly understood, particularly in low-income rural areas without specific barriers to limit the interaction between domestic and wild animals. In this study, we simultaneously estimated the prevalence of ESBL-*E. coli* fecal carriage among livestock, dogs, and wild mammals among small-scale agricultural localities of central Chile. The prevalence of ESBL-*E. coli* fecal carriage was lower in livestock (3%) and wildlife (less than 1%) compared to dogs (24%), suggesting that dogs can be an important carrier of these bacteria in agricultural settings. Dogs carried ESBL-*E. coli* in the three farms where ESBL-*E. coli* were detected in livestock, highlighting the potential sharing of these bacteria between dogs and livestock. Among ESBL-*E. coli* isolates, five CTX-M groups including groups 1, 2, 8, 9, and 25 were detected, with most isolates carrying CTX-M group 1. Molecular typing of ESBL-*E. coli* by ERIC-PCR showed no cluster of isolates by neither species nor locality, suggesting a wide range of ESBL-*E. coli* strains circulating on agricultural settings and highlighting the potential for cross-species transmission of either bacteria or antibiotic resistance genes.

ESBL-*E. coli* have been detected across livestock in South America, with prevalence in cattle ranging from 18% in Brazil to 48% in Peru [12,67]. In this study, we detected ESBL-*E. coli* fecal carriage in cattle, swine, sheep, and chicken, showing the widespread dissemination of these bacteria in agricultural settings. This is the first report of ESBL-*E. coli* in cattle in Chile, although their prevalence was low (3%) compared to a similar study in

Peru estimating a prevalence of 48% among small-scale farmers in the Lima region [12]. The observed prevalence in Chile is similar to farms in high-income countries such as France or Denmark, where the restriction of third-generation cephalosporins has been associated with a reduction in ESBL-*E. coli* [68,69]. The high prevalence of resistance to ciprofloxacin (over 60%) found in ESBL-*E. coli* isolated from domestic animals in this study is consistent with the high level of plasmid-mediated quinolone resistant found in 74% of ESBL-*E. coli* isolated from Chilean hospitals [70] and a high prevalence of resistance to ciprofloxacin (84%) in ESBL-*E. coli* recovered from intensive care units of Southern Chile [71]. The presence of ESBL-*E. coli* could result from low but existing selective pressure by the use of third generation cephalosporins in these farms, which requires further investigation. In a similar agricultural setting of Peru, the low use of cephalosporins [72] was associated to a high prevalence of ESBL-*E. coli* in livestock (50%) [12], suggesting that factors other than antibiotic use can influence AMR. For example, farm hygiene, herd size, contact with humans or other husbandry conditions such as storage of slurry in a pit have been associated with the presence of ESBL-*E. coli* in livestock [13,20,21].

The low prevalence of ESBL-*E. coli* in wildlife (less than 1%) is similar to other studies focusing on ESBL-*E. coli* among wildlife in Latin America and other LMICs [12,73]. For example, a previous study estimated a 4% prevalence of ESBL-*E. coli* among vampire bats (*Desmodus rotundus*) in Peru using a similar methodology for screening [12]. Previous studies conducted in Chile and Latin America have detected the presence of ESBL-*E. coli* on wild birds including gulls [36], Andean condors [43], and three species of owls [42]. Likewise, *bla*$_{CTX-M}$ genes have been previously detected using qPCR methods from feces in Andean foxes [52] and the guiña (*Leopardus guigna*) [74], although the bacteria species carrying the genes, and whether it was expressed or not, remains unknown. To our knowledge, this is the first study to report *E. coli* carrying CTX-M group 1 on wild mammals in Chile. The origin of ESBL-*E. coli* found in a rodent remains to be clarified. Given the presence of similar *bla*$_{CTX-M}$ genes among a nearby farm and a wide variety of ESBL-*E. coli* strains circulating, one potential explanation is the transmission of *bla*$_{CTX-M}$ from domestic animals, although other potential contamination sources (e.g., humans, water contamination) cannot be discarded.

The high prevalence of ESBL-*E. coli* found in dogs (24%) highlights their role as either passive 'receivers' or reservoirs of ESBL-*E. coli* in agricultural settings. Although there are only a limited number of studies estimating the prevalence of ESBL-*E. coli* among dogs, previous studies have shown a prevalence in Latin American dogs ranging from 9–30%, and a global prevalence of 7% [30,75–79]. The detection of ESBL-*E. coli* in dogs has been associated with previous antibiotic treatment, but also close contact with livestock, implying the potential transmission of these bacteria between livestock and dogs [29,30,80]. The latest is also suggested by our study, as the three farms where we detected ESBL-*E. coli* in livestock also had a dog carrying ESBL-*E. coli*. Molecular typing by ERIC-PCR showed no cluster of ESBL-*E. coli* by host species, while isolates sampled from a cow and a dog at the same farm clustered together. These results suggest that bacterial strains or ESBL genes such as *bla*$_{CTX-M}$ could be exchanged between host populations. Overall, the circulation of ESBL-*E. coli* among dogs highlights the potential public health risk for domestic animals but also for dog owners, given the potential spillover of bacteria from dogs to humans [28,29,81]. Moreover, the higher prevalence observed in dogs compared to livestock suggests that ESBL-*E. coli* could be spreading from dogs to livestock, and not necessarily in the other direction, as most previous studies have assumed.

Our study constitutes one of the first One Health approaches to simultaneously address the circulation of ESBL-*E. coli* among livestock, dogs, and wildlife in a rural setting. However, several future research can complement our findings and provide further insight into the selection and spread of AMR among these compartments. First, the limited sample size of foxes prevented a more accurate estimation of ESBL-*E. coli* prevalence in this species. Thus, we could not conclude whether predators or preys are more likely to carry ESBL-*E. coli* in this setting. Secondly, the low selective pressure for ESBL-*E. coli* should be confirmed by studies on antibiotic use among farmers in these agricultural settings [72], which are currently lacking in Chile. Although the use of antibiotics in Chilean terrestrial livestock remains unknown, the national health authority (Servicio Agricola Ganadero) advises the use of fluroquinolones and cephalosporins as a last resource antibiotic in livestock, following a susceptibility test [82]. Antibiotic residues of tetracyclines, beta-lactams, aminoglycosides, and macrolides have been found in eggs from backyard poultry production [83]. Thirdly, although the ERIC-PCR technique used has a high resolution and allows us to differentiate among *E. coli* strains from the same locality and host species [65], several other molecular techniques can improve our understanding of the transmission dynamics of resistance genes and *E. coli*. For example, future work could determine the pathogenic potential of these strains using whole genome sequencing, or whether bla_{CTX-M} genes are carried by specific mobile elements such as plasmids. Finally, future research should identify associated factors to ESBL-*E. coli* fecal carriage in each animal population (e.g., individual characteristics of dogs and cattle).

Author Contributions: Conceptualization, J.A.B.; Data curation, J.A.B.; Formal analysis, J.A.B. and A.O.-C.; Funding acquisition, J.A.B.; Investigation, J.A.B., M.S.-C. and A.O.-C.; Methodology, J.A.B., M.S.-C., A.O.-C., P.G.M., A.P., M.O.M., L.R., J.M. (Jose Munita) and J.M. (Javier Millán); Project administration, J.A.B.; Resources, J.A.B.; Software, J.A.B.; Supervision, J.A.B.; Validation, J.A.B.; Visualization, J.A.B.; Writing—original draft, J.A.B.; Writing—review and editing, J.A.B., M.S.-C. and J.M. (Javier Millán). All authors have read and agreed to the published version of the manuscript.

Funding: This work was funded by the National Agency for Research and Development (ANID) FONDECYT Iniciación 11181017, awarded to J.A.B. Jose M. Munita was supported by Comisión Nacional de Investigación Científica y Tecnológica (CONICYT) (grant number: FONDECYT 1171805) and the ANID Millennium Science Initiative, MICROB-R, NCN17_081, Government of Chile.

Institutional Review Board Statement: This study was approved by the Ethical Committee of the Universidad Andrés Bello (permit number: 018/2018). Capture and sampling of rodents were also approved by Servicio Agricola Ganadero (permit number: 2118/2019).

Informed Consent Statement: Informed consent was obtained from all farmers for the inclusion of their dogs and/or livestock.

Data Availability Statement: The data presented in this study are available within this article.

Acknowledgments: We thank all farmers involved in this study for their cooperation and help with livestock and dog sampling. We also thank the personnel of the Municipalidad de Colina (particularly Carlos Telleria y Maximiliano Larrain) for their great help contacting farmers and helping us accessing farms. We thank all the staff members of @themonkey_lab for their assistance in the laboratory. We thank Gabriel Carrasco for participating in the collection of rodents.

Conflicts of Interest: The authors declare no conflict of interest.

References

1. World Health Organization. *2019 Antibacterial Agents in Clinical Development: An Analysis of the Antibacterial Clinical Development Pipeline*; WHO: Geneva, Switzerland, 2019; Available online: https://www.who.int/medicines/areas/rational_use/antibacterial_agents_clinical_development/en/ (accessed on 28 December 2020).
2. Wall, B.A.; Mateus, A.; Marshall, L.; Pfeiffer, D.; Lubroth, J.; Ormel, H.J.; Otto, P.; Patriarchi, A.; Food and Agriculture Organization of the United Nations. *Drivers, Dynamics and Epidemiology of Antimicrobial Resistance in Animal Production*; Food and Agriculture Organization (FAO): Rome, Italy, 2016; ISBN 978-92-5-109441-9.
3. IACG. No Time to Wait: Securing the Future from Drug-Resistant Infections. Available online: http://www.who.int/antimicrobial-resistance/interagency-coordination-group/final-report/en/ (accessed on 23 July 2020).
4. World Bank. *Drug-Resistant Infections: A Threat to Our Economic Future*; World Bank: Washington, DC, USA, 2017.
5. *Antimicrobial Resistance: Global Report on Surveillance*; World Health Organization: Geneva, Switzerland, 2014; ISBN 978-92-4-156474-8.
6. O'Neill, J. The Review on Antimicrobial Resistance—Tackling Drug-Resistant Infections Globally: Final Report and Recommendations. Available online: https://amr-review.org/ (accessed on 29 July 2020).
7. Van Boeckel, T.P.; Brower, C.C.; Gilbert, M.; Grenfell, B.T.; Levin, S.A.S.; Robinson, T.P.; Teillant, A.; Laxminarayan, R.R. Global trends in antimicrobial use in food animals. *Proc. Natl. Acad. Sci. USA* **2015**, *112*, 5649–5654. [CrossRef]

8. Doi, Y.; Iovleva, A.; Bonomo, R.A. The ecology of extended-spectrum β-lactamases (ESBLs) in the developed world. *J. Travel Med.* **2017**, *24*, S44–S51. [CrossRef]
9. Smet, A.; Martel, A.; Persoons, D.; Dewulf, J.; Heyndrickx, M.; Herman, L.; Haesebrouck, F.; Butaye, P. Broad-spectrum β-lactamases among Enterobacteriaceaeof animal origin: Molecular aspects, mobility and impact on public health. *FEMS Microbiol. Rev.* **2010**, *34*, 295–316. [CrossRef]
10. Eguenther, S.; Eewers, C.; Wieler, L.H. Extended-Spectrum Beta-Lactamases Producing *E. coli* in Wildlife, yet Another Form of Environmental Pollution? *Front. Microbiol.* **2011**, *2*, 246. [CrossRef]
11. Loayza, F.; Graham, J.P.; Trueba, G. Factors Obscuring the Role of *E. coli* from Domestic Animals in the Global Antimicrobial Resistance Crisis: An Evidence-Based Review. *Int. J. Environ. Res. Public Health* **2020**, *17*, 3061. [CrossRef]
12. Benavides, J.A.; Shiva, C.; Virhuez, M.; Tello, C.; Appelgren, A.; Vendrell, J.; Solassol, J.; Godreuil, S.; Streicker, D.G. Extended-spectrum beta-lactamase-producing *Escherichia coli* in common vampire bats Desmodus rotundus and livestock in Peru. *Zoonoses Public Health* **2018**, *65*, 454–458. [CrossRef]
13. Snow, L.; Warner, R.; Cheney, T.; Wearing, H.; Stokes, M.; Harris, K.; Teale, C.; Coldham, N. Risk factors associated with extended spectrum beta-lactamase *Escherichia coli* (CTX-M) on dairy farms in North West England and North Wales. *Prev. Vet. Med.* **2012**, *106*, 225–234. [CrossRef]
14. Atterby, C.; Börjesson, S.; Ny, S.; Järhult, J.D.; Byfors, S.; Bonnedahl, J. ESBL-producing *Escherichia coli* in Swedish gulls—A case of environmental pollution from humans? *PLoS ONE* **2017**, *12*, e0190380. [CrossRef]
15. Jamborova, I.; Johnston, B.D.; Papousek, I.; Kachlikova, K.; Micenkova, L.; Clabots, C.; Skalova, A.; Chudejova, K.; Dolejska, M.; Literak, I.; et al. Extensive Genetic Commonality among Wildlife, Wastewater, Community, and Nosocomial Isolates of *Escherichia coli* Sequence Type 131 (H30R1 and H30Rx Subclones) That Carry blaCTX-M-27 or blaCTX-M-15. *Antimicrob. Agents Chemother.* **2018**, *62*, 00519-18. [CrossRef]
16. Joosten, P.; Ceccarelli, D.; Odent, E.; Sarrazin, S.; Graveland, H.; Van Gompel, L.; Battisti, A.; Caprioli, A.; Franco, A.; Wagenaar, J.A.; et al. Antimicrobial Usage and Resistance in Companion Animals: A Cross-Sectional Study in Three European Countries. *Antibiotics* **2020**, *9*, 87. [CrossRef]
17. Van Boeckel, T.P.; Pires, J.; Silvester, R.; Zhao, C.; Song, J.; Criscuolo, N.G.; Gilbert, M.; Bonhoeffer, S.; Laxminarayan, R. Global trends in antimicrobial resistance in animals in low- and middle-income countries. *Science* **2019**, *365*, eaaw1944. [CrossRef]
18. Chantziaras, I.; Boyen, F.; Callens, B.; Dewulf, J. Correlation between veterinary antimicrobial use and antimicrobial resistance in food-producing animals: A report on seven countries. *J. Antimicrob. Chemother.* **2014**, *69*, 827–834. [CrossRef]
19. de Jong, A.; Thomas, V.; Klein, U.; Marion, H.; Moyaert, H.; Simjee, S.; Vallé, M. Pan-European resistance monitoring programmes encompassing food-borne bacteria and target pathogens of food-producing and companion animals. *Int. J. Antimicrob. Agents* **2013**, *41*, 403–409. [CrossRef]
20. Hille, K.; Felski, M.; Ruddat, I.; Woydt, J.; Schmid, A.; Friese, A.; Fischer, J.; Sharp, H.; Valentin, L.; Michael, G.B.; et al. Association of farm-related factors with characteristics profiles of extended-spectrum β-lactamase-/plasmid-mediated AmpC β-lactamase-producing *Escherichia coli* isolates from German livestock farms. *Vet. Microbiol.* **2018**, *223*, 93–99. [CrossRef]
21. Gay, N.; LeClaire, A.; Laval, M.; Miltgen, G.; Jégo, M.; Stéphane, R.; Jaubert, J.; Belmonte, O.; Cardinale, E. Risk Factors of Extended-Spectrum β-Lactamase Producing Enterobacteriaceae Occurrence in Farms in Reunion, Madagascar and Mayotte Islands, 2016–2017. *Vet. Sci.* **2018**, *5*, 22. [CrossRef]
22. Dahms, C.; Hübner, N.-O.; Kossow, A.; Mellmann, A.; Dittmann, K.; Kramer, A. Occurrence of ESBL-Producing *Escherichia coli* in Livestock and Farm Workers in Mecklenburg-Western Pomerania, Germany. *PLoS ONE* **2015**, *10*, e0143326. [CrossRef]
23. Wang, J.; Ma, Z.B.; Zeng, Z.L.; Yang, X.W.; Huang, Y.; Liu, J.H. The role of wildlife (wild birds) in the global transmission of antimicrobial resistance genes. *Zool. Res.* **2017**, *38*, 55. [CrossRef]
24. Poeta, P.; Radhouani, H.; Pinto, L.; Martinho, A.; Rego, V.; Rodrigues, R.; Gonçalves, A.; Rodrigues, J.; Estepa, V.; Torres, C.; et al. Wild boars as reservoirs of extended-spectrum beta-lactamase (ESBL) producing *Escherichia coli* of different phylogenetic groups. *J. Basic Microbiol.* **2009**, *49*, 584–588. [CrossRef]
25. Alonso, C.; González-Barrio, D.; Tenorio, C.; Ruiz-Fons, F.; Torres, C. Antimicrobial resistance in faecal *Escherichia coli* isolates from farmed red deer and wild small mammals. Detection of a multiresistant *E. coli* producing extended-spectrum beta-lactamase. *Comp. Immunol. Microbiol. Infect. Dis.* **2016**, *45*, 34–39. [CrossRef]
26. Alonso, C.A.; Alcalá, L.; Simón, C.; Torres, C. Novel sequence types of extended-spectrum and acquired AmpC beta-lactamase producing *Escherichia coli* and *Escherichia* clade V isolated from wild mammals. *FEMS Microbiol. Ecol.* **2017**, *93*, fiy066. [CrossRef]
27. Seni, J.; Falgenhauer, L.; Simeo, N.; Mirambo, M.M.; Imirzalioglu, C.; Matee, M.; Rweyemamu, M.; Chakraborty, T.; Mshana, S.E. Multiple ESBL-Producing *Escherichia coli* Sequence Types Carrying Quinolone and Aminoglycoside Resistance Genes Circulating in Companion and Domestic Farm Animals in Mwanza, Tanzania, Harbor Commonly Occurring Plasmids. *Front. Microbiol.* **2016**, *7*, 142. [CrossRef] [PubMed]
28. Dupouy, V.; Abdelli, M.; Moyano, G.; Arpaillange, N.; Bibbal, D.; Cadiergues, M.-C.; Lopez-Pulin, D.; Sayah-Jeanne, S.; De Gunzburg, J.; Saint-Lu, N.; et al. Prevalence of Beta-Lactam and Quinolone/Fluoroquinolone Resistance in Enterobacteriaceae From Dogs in France and Spain—Characterization of ESBL/pAmpC Isolates, Genes, and Conjugative Plasmids. *Front. Vet. Sci.* **2019**, *6*, 279. [CrossRef]

29. Bunt, G.V.D.; Fluit, A.C.; Spaninks, M.P.; Timmerman, A.J.; Geurts, Y.; Kant, A.; Scharringa, J.; Mevius, D.; Wagenaar, J.A.; Bonten, M.J.M.; et al. Faecal carriage, risk factors, acquisition and persistence of ESBL-producing Enterobacteriaceae in dogs and cats and co-carriage with humans belonging to the same household. *J. Antimicrob. Chemother.* **2020**, *75*, 342–350. [CrossRef] [PubMed]
30. Salgado-Caxito, M.; Benavides, J.A.; Munita, J.M.; Rivas, L.; García, P.; Listoni, F.J.; Moreno-Switt, A.I.; Paes, A.C. Risk factors associated with faecal carriage of extended-spectrum cephalosporin-resistant Escherichia coli among dogs in Southeast Brazil. *Prev. Vet. Med.* **2021**, *190*, 105316. [CrossRef]
31. Barth, S.A.; Blome, S.; Cornelis, D.; Pietschmann, J.; Laval, M.; Maestrini, O.; Geue, L.; Charrier, F.; Etter, E.; Menge, C.; et al. Faecal*Escherichia coli*as biological indicator of spatial interaction between domestic pigs and wild boar (Sus scrofa) in Corsica. *Transbound. Emerg. Dis.* **2018**, *65*, 746–757. [CrossRef] [PubMed]
32. Mercat, M.; Clermont, O.; Massot, M.; Ruppe, E.; De Garine-Wichatitsky, M.; Miguel, E.; Fox, H.V.; Cornelis, D.; Andremont, A.; Denamur, E.; et al. Escherichia coli Population Structure and Antibiotic Resistance at a Buffalo/Cattle Interface in Southern Africa. *Appl. Environ. Microbiol.* **2015**, *82*, 1459–1467. [CrossRef]
33. Founou, L.L.; Founou, R.C.; Essack, S.Y. Antibiotic Resistance in the Food Chain: A Developing Country-Perspective. *Front. Microbiol.* **2016**, *7*, 1881. [CrossRef]
34. Ho, P.L.; Chow, K.H.; Lai, E.L.; Lo, W.U.; Yeung, M.K.; Chan, J.; Chan, P.Y.; Yuen, K.Y. Extensive dissemination of CTX-M-producing Escherichia coli with multidrug resistance to 'critically important' antibiotics among food animals in Hong Kong, 2008–2010. *J. Antimicrob. Chemother.* **2011**, *66*, 765–768. [CrossRef]
35. Hasan, B.; Laurell, K.; Rakib, M.M.; Ahlstedt, E.; Hernandez, J.; Caceres, M.; Järhult, J.D. Fecal Carriage of Extended-Spectrum β-Lactamases in Healthy Humans, Poultry, and Wild Birds in León, Nicaragua—A Shared Pool of blaCTX-M Genes and Possible Interspecies Clonal Spread of Extended-Spectrum β-Lactamases-Producing *Escherichia coli*. *Microb. Drug Resist.* **2016**, *22*, 682–687. [CrossRef]
36. Hernandez, J.; Johansson, A.; Stedt, J.; Bengtsson, S.; Porczak, A.; Granholm, S.; González-Acuña, D.; Olsen, B.; Bonnedahl, J.; Drobni, M. Characterization and Comparison of Extended-Spectrum β-Lactamase (ESBL) Resistance Genotypes and Population Structure of *Escherichia coli* Isolated from Franklin's Gulls (*Leucophaeus pipixcan*) and Humans in Chile. *PLoS ONE* **2013**, *8*, e76150. [CrossRef]
37. Nweneka, C.V.; Tapha-Sosseh, N.; Sosa, A. Curbing the menace of antimicrobial resistance in developing countries. *Harm Reduct. J.* **2009**, *6*, 31. [CrossRef] [PubMed]
38. Ahmad, M.; Khan, A.U. Global economic impact of antibiotic resistance: A review. *J. Glob. Antimicrob. Resist.* **2019**, *19*, 313–316. [CrossRef] [PubMed]
39. González, C.M.A. Susceptibilidad Microbiana: Un Test Rápido Para el Análisis de Resistencia Bacteriana en Cepas Aisladas de Mastitis Clínica. Bachelor's Thesis, Universidad de Chile, Santiago, Chile, 2006.
40. Ewers, C.; Bethe, A.; Semmler, T.; Guenther, S.; Wieler, L. Extended-spectrum β-lactamase-producing and AmpC-producing Escherichia coli from livestock and companion animals, and their putative impact on public health: A global perspective. *Clin. Microbiol. Infect.* **2012**, *18*, 646–655. [CrossRef]
41. Moreno, A.; Bello, H.; Guggiana, D.; Domínguez, M.; González, G. Extended-spectrum β-lactamases belonging to CTX-M group produced by Escherichia coli strains isolated from companion animals treated with enrofloxacin. *Vet. Microbiol.* **2008**, *129*, 203–208. [CrossRef]
42. Fuentes-Castillo, D.; Farfán-López, M.; Esposito, F.; Moura, Q.; Fernandes, M.R.; Lopes, R.; Cardoso, B.; Muñoz, M.E.; Cerdeira, L.; Najle, I.; et al. Wild owls colonized by international clones of extended-spectrum β-lactamase (CTX-M)-producing Escherichia coli and Salmonella Infantis in the Southern Cone of America. *Sci. Total Environ.* **2019**, *674*, 554–562. [CrossRef]
43. Fuentes-Castillo, D.; Esposito, F.; Cardoso, B.; Dalazen, G.; Moura, Q.; Fuga, B.; Fontana, H.; Cerdeira, L.; Dropa, M.; Rottmann, J.; et al. Genomic data reveal international lineages of critical priority*Escherichia coli*harbouring wide resistome in Andean condors (*Vultur gryphus* Linnaeus, 1758). *Mol. Ecol.* **2020**, *29*, 1919–1935. [CrossRef]
44. Simonetti, J.A. Diversity and Conservation of Terrestrial Vertebrates in Mediterranean Chile. *Rev. Chil. Hist. Nat.* **1999**, *72*, 493–500.
45. Cofre, H.; A Marquet, P. Conservation status, rarity, and geographic priorities for conservation of Chilean mammals: An assessment. *Biol. Conserv.* **1999**, *88*, 53–68. [CrossRef]
46. Iriarte, J.A.; Lobos, G.A.; Jaksic, F.M. Invasive vertebrate species in Chile and their control and monitoring by governmental agencies. *Rev. Chil. Hist. Nat.* **2005**, *78*, 143–151. [CrossRef]
47. Silva, C.; Saavedra, B. Knowing for controlling: Ecological effects of invasive vertebrates in Tierra del Fuego. *Rev. Chil. Hist. Nat.* **2008**, *81*, 123–136. [CrossRef]
48. Sanguinetti, J.; Kitzberger, T. Factors controlling seed predation by rodents and non-native Sus scrofa in Araucaria araucana forests: Potential effects on seedling establishment. *Biol. Invasions* **2010**, *12*, 689–706. [CrossRef]
49. Castro, S.; Bozinovic, F.; Jaksic, F. Ecological efficiency and legitimacy in seed dispersal of an endemic shrub (Lithrea caustica) by the European rabbit (*Oryctolagus cuniculus*) in central Chile. *J. Arid. Environ.* **2008**, *72*, 1164–1173. [CrossRef]
50. Muñoz-Zanzi, C.; Mason, M.; Encina, C.; Gonzalez, M.; Berg, S. Household Characteristics Associated with Rodent Presence and Leptospira Infection in Rural and Urban Communities from Southern Chile. *Am. J. Trop. Med. Hyg.* **2014**, *90*, 497–506. [CrossRef]
51. Salvatori, V.; Vaglio-Laurin, G.; Meserve, P.L.; Boitani, L.; Campanella, A. Spatial Organization, Activity, and Social Interactions of Culpeo Foxes (*Pseudalopex culpaeus*) in North-Central Chile. *J. Mammal.* **1999**, *80*, 980–985. [CrossRef]

52. Cevidanes, A.; Esperón, F.; Di Cataldo, S.; Neves, E.; Sallaberry-Pincheira, N.; Millán, J. Antimicrobial resistance genes in Andean foxes inhabiting anthropized landscapes in central Chile. *Sci. Total Environ.* **2020**, *724*, 138247. [CrossRef]
53. INE. Instituto Nacional de Estadísticas—Censo Agropecuario. Available online: http://www.ine.cl/estadisticas/economia/agricultura-agroindustria-y-pesca/censos-agropecuarios (accessed on 24 March 2021).
54. Milstead, W.B.; Meserve, P.L.; Campanella, A.; Previtali, M.A.; Kelt, D.A.; Gutiérrez, J.R. Spatial Ecology of Small Mammals in North-central Chile: Role of Precipitation and Refuges. *J. Mammal.* **2007**, *88*, 1532–1538. [CrossRef]
55. Jaksic, F.M.; Soriguer, R.C. Predation Upon the European Rabbit (*Oryctolagus cuniculus*) in Mediterranean Habitats of Chile and Spain: A Comparative Analysis. *J. Anim. Ecol.* **1981**, *50*, 269. [CrossRef]
56. Cevidanes, A.; Ulloa-Contreras, C.; Di Cataldo, S.; Latrofa, M.S.; Gonzalez-Acuña, D.; Otranto, D.; Millán, J. Marked host association and molecular evidence of limited transmission of ticks and fleas between sympatric wild foxes and rural dogs. *Med. Vet. Entomol.* **2021**. [CrossRef]
57. CDC. Downloads | Support | Epi InfoTM | CDC. Available online: https://www.cdc.gov/epiinfo/support/downloads.html (accessed on 18 June 2020).
58. Ho, P.-L.; Liu, M.C.-J.; Lo, W.-U.; Lai, E.L.-Y.; Lau, T.C.-K.; Law, O.-K.; Chow, K.-H. Prevalence and characterization of hybrid blaCTX-M among Escherichia coli isolates from livestock and other animals. *Diagn. Microbiol. Infect. Dis.* **2015**, *82*, 148–153. [CrossRef]
59. Silva, N.; Igrejas, G.; Figueiredo, N.; Gonçalves, A.; Radhouani, H.; Rodrigues, J.; Poeta, P. Molecular characterization of antimicrobial resistance in enterococci and Escherichia coli isolates from European wild rabbit (*Oryctolagus cuniculus*). *Sci. Total Environ.* **2010**, *408*, 4871–4876. [CrossRef]
60. Radhouani, H.; Igrejas, G.; Gonçalves, A.; Estepa, V.; Sargo, R.; Torres, C.; Poeta, P. Molecular characterization of extended-spectrum-beta-lactamase-producing Escherichia coli isolates from red foxes in Portugal. *Arch. Microbiol.* **2012**, *195*, 141–144. [CrossRef]
61. CLSI. *Performance Standards for Antimicrobial Susceptibility Testing*, 28th ed.; CLSI Supplement M100; Clinical and Laboratory Standards Institute: Wayne, PA, USA, 2018; ISBN 978-1-56238-838-6.
62. Magiorakos, A.-P.; Srinivasan, A.; Carey, R.B.; Carmeli, Y.; Falagas, M.E.; Giske, C.G.; Harbarth, S.; Hindler, J.F.; Kahlmeter, G.; Olsson-Liljequist, B.; et al. Multidrug-resistant, extensively drug-resistant and pandrug-resistant bacteria: An international expert proposal for interim standard definitions for acquired resistance. *Clin. Microbiol. Infect.* **2012**, *18*, 268–281. [CrossRef]
63. Dallenne, C.; Da Costa, A.; Decré, D.; Favier, C.; Arlet, G. Development of a set of multiplex PCR assays for the detection of genes encoding important β-lactamases in Enterobacteriaceae. *J. Antimicrob. Chemother.* **2010**, *65*, 490–495. [CrossRef]
64. Woodford, N.; Fagan, E.J.; Ellington, M.J. Multiplex PCR for rapid detection of genes encoding CTX-M extended-spectrum β-lactamases. *J. Antimicrob. Chemother.* **2005**, *57*, 154–155. [CrossRef] [PubMed]
65. Bilung, L.M.; Pui, C.F.; Su'Ut, L.; Apun, K. Evaluation of BOX-PCR and ERIC-PCR as Molecular Typing Tools for PathogenicLeptospira. *Dis. Markers* **2018**, *2018*, 1–9. [CrossRef] [PubMed]
66. Brasil. Decreto—Lei n° 227, de 28 de Fevereiro de 1967. Dá nova Redação ao Decreto-Lei n° 1.985, de 29 de Janeiro de 1940 (Código de Minas) Brasília. 1967. Available online: http://www.planalto.gov.br/ccivil_03/Decreto-Lei/Del0227.htm (accessed on 19 October 2020).
67. Palmeira, J.D.; Haenni, M.; Metayer, V.; Madec, J.-Y.; Ferreira, H.M.N. Epidemic spread of IncI1/pST113 plasmid carrying the Extended-Spectrum Beta-Lactamase (ESBL) blaCTX-M-8 gene in Escherichia coli of Brazilian cattle. *Vet. Microbiol.* **2020**, *243*, 108629. [CrossRef] [PubMed]
68. Résapath, B. *Réseau D'épidémiosurveillance de L'antibiorésistance des Bactéries Pathogènes Animales*; Ploufragan-Plouzané-Niort: Lyon, France, 2020; p. 155.
69. Levy, S. Reduced Antibiotic Use in Livestock: How Denmark TackledResistance. *Environ. Health Perspect.* **2014**, *122*, A160-5. [CrossRef]
70. Elgorriaga-Islas, E.; Guggiana-Nilo, P.; Domínguez-Yévenes, M.; González-Rocha, G.; Mella-Montecinos, S.; Labarca-Labarca, J.; García-Cañete, P.; Bello-Toledo, H. Prevalencia del determinante de resistencia plasmídica a quinolonas aac(6')-Ib-cr en cepas de Escherichia coli y Klebsiella pneumoniae productoras de BLEE aisladas en diez hospitales de Chile. *Enferm. Infecc. Microbiol. Clín.* **2012**, *30*, 466–468. [CrossRef]
71. Pavez, M.; Troncoso, C.; Osses, I.; Salazar, R.; Illesca, V.; Reydet, P.; Rodríguez, C.; Chahin, C.; Concha, C.; Barrientos, L. High prevalence of CTX-M-1 group in ESBL-producing enterobacteriaceae infection in intensive care units in southern Chile. *Braz. J. Infect. Dis.* **2019**, *23*, 102–110. [CrossRef]
72. Benavides, J.A.; Streicker, D.G.; Gonzales, M.S.; Rojas-Paniagua, E.; Shiva, C. Knowledge and use of antibiotics among low-income small-scale farmers of Peru. *Prev. Vet. Med.* **2021**, *189*, 105287. [CrossRef]
73. Albrechtova, K.; Papousek, I.; De Nys, H.M.; Pauly, M.; Anoh, E.; Mossoun, A.; Dolejska, M.; Masarikova, M.; Metzger, S.; Couacy-Hymann, E.; et al. Low Rates of Antimicrobial-Resistant Enterobacteriaceae in Wildlife in Taï National Park, Côte d'Ivoire, Surrounded by Villages with High Prevalence of Multiresistant ESBL-Producing Escherichia coli in People and Domestic Animals. *PLoS ONE* **2014**, *9*, e113548. [CrossRef]
74. Sacristán, I.; Esperón, F.; Acuña, F.; Aguilar, E.; García, S.; López, M.J.; Cevidanes, A.; Neves, E.; Cabello, J.; Hidalgo-Hermoso, E.; et al. Antibiotic resistance genes as landscape anthropization indicators: Using a wild felid as sentinel in Chile. *Sci. Total Environ.* **2020**, *703*, 134900. [CrossRef]

75. Ortega-Paredes, D.; Haro, M.; Leoro-Garzón, P.; Barba, P.; Loaiza, K.; Mora, F.; Fors, M.; Vinueza-Burgos, C.; Fernández-Moreira, E. Multidrug-resistant Escherichia coli isolated from canine faeces in a public park in Quito, Ecuador. *J. Glob. Antimicrob. Resist.* **2019**, *18*, 263–268. [CrossRef] [PubMed]
76. Melo, L.C.; Oresco, C.; Leigue, L.; Netto, H.M.; Melville, P.A.; Benites, N.R.; Saras, E.; Haenni, M.; Lincopan, N.; Madec, J.-Y. Prevalence and molecular features of ESBL/pAmpC-producing Enterobacteriaceae in healthy and diseased companion animals in Brazil. *Vet. Microbiol.* **2018**, *221*, 59–66. [CrossRef] [PubMed]
77. Carvalho, A.; Barbosa, A.; Arais, L.; Ribeiro, P.; Carneiro, V.; Cerqueira, A. Resistance patterns, ESBL genes, and genetic relatedness of Escherichia coli from dogs and owners. *Braz. J. Microbiol.* **2016**, *47*, 150–158. [CrossRef] [PubMed]
78. Rocha-Gracia, R.; Cortés-Cortés, G.; Lozano-Zarain, P.; Bello, F.; Martínez-Laguna, Y.; Torres, C. Faecal Escherichia coli isolates from healthy dogs harbour CTX-M-15 and CMY-2 β-lactamases. *Vet. J.* **2015**, *203*, 315–319. [CrossRef] [PubMed]
79. Salgado-Caxito, M.; Benavides, J.A.; Adell, A.D.; Paes, A.C.; Moreno-Switt, A.I. Global prevalence and molecular characterization of extended-spectrum β-lactamase producing- in dogs and cats—A scoping review and meta-analysis. *One Health* **2021**, *100236*, 100236. [CrossRef] [PubMed]
80. Wedley, A.L.; Dawson, S.; Maddox, T.W.; Coyne, K.P.; Pinchbeck, G.L.; Clegg, P.; Nuttall, T.; Kirchner, M.; Williams, N.J. Carriage of antimicrobial resistant Escherichia coli in dogs: Prevalence, associated risk factors and molecular characteristics. *Vet. Microbiol.* **2017**, *199*, 23–30. [CrossRef]
81. Ljungquist, O.; Ljungquist, D.; Myrenås, M.; Rydén, C.; Finn, M.; Bengtsson, B. Evidence of household transfer of ESBL-/pAmpC-producing Enterobacteriaceae between humans and dogs—A pilot study. *Infect. Ecol. Epidemiol.* **2016**, *6*, 31514. [CrossRef] [PubMed]
82. *Sag Resolución Exenta No: 4579/2018*; Servicio Agricola Ganadero: Santiago, Chile, 2018.
83. Cornejo, J.; Pokrant, E.; Figueroa, F.; Riquelme, R.; Galdames, P.; Di Pillo, F.; Jimenez-Bluhm, P.; Hamilton-West, C. Assessing Antibiotic Residues in Poultry Eggs from Backyard Production Systems in Chile, First Approach to a Non-Addressed Issue in Farm Animals. *Animals* **2020**, *10*, 1056. [CrossRef]

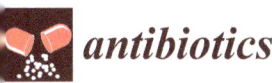

Article

Poultry and Wild Birds as a Reservoir of CMY-2 Producing *Escherichia coli*: The First Large-Scale Study in Greece

Zoi Athanasakopoulou [1], Katerina Tsilipounidaki [2], Marina Sofia [1], Dimitris C. Chatzopoulos [1], Alexios Giannakopoulos [1], Ioannis Karakousis [3], Vassilios Giannakis [3], Vassiliki Spyrou [4], Antonia Touloudi [1], Maria Satra [5], Dimitrios Galamatis [6], Vassilis Diamantopoulos [7], Spyridoula Mpellou [8], Efthymia Petinaki [2] and Charalambos Billinis [1,5,*]

1. Faculty of Veterinary Science, University of Thessaly, 43100 Karditsa, Greece; zathanas@uth.gr (Z.A.); msofia@uth.gr (M.S.); dchatzopoulos@uth.gr (D.C.C.); algiannak@uth.gr (A.G.); atoul@uth.gr (A.T.)
2. Faculty of Medicine, University of Thessaly, 41500 Larissa, Greece; tsilipou@uth.gr (K.T.); petinaki@uth.gr (E.P.)
3. Elanco Hellas S.A.C.I., 15231 Athens, Greece; jkarakousis@elanco.com (I.K.); vgiannakis@elanco.gr (V.G.)
4. Faculty of Animal Science, University of Thessaly, 41110 Larissa, Greece; vasilikispyrou@uth.gr
5. Faculty of Public and Integrated Health, University of Thessaly, 43100 Karditsa, Greece; msatra@uth.gr
6. Hellenic Agricultural Organization DIMITRA (ELGO DIMITRA), 57001 Thessaloniki, Greece; galamatis@elog.gr
7. Directorate of Public Health, Prefecture of Peloponnese, 22132 Tripoli, Greece; diamantopoulos@ppel.gov.gr
8. Bioefarmoges Eleftheriou LP-Integrated Mosquito Control, 19007 Marathon, Greece; smpellou@bioefarmoges.com
* Correspondence: billinis@uth.gr

Abstract: Resistance mediated by β-lactamases is a globally spread menace. The aim of the present study was to determine the occurrence of *Escherichia coli* producing plasmid-encoded AmpC β-lactamases (pAmpC) in animals. Fecal samples from chickens (n = 159), cattle (n = 104), pigs (n = 214), and various wild bird species (n = 168), collected from different Greek regions during 2018–2020, were screened for the presence of pAmpC-encoding genes. Thirteen *E. coli* displaying resistance to third-generation cephalosporins and a positive AmpC confirmation test were detected. bla_{CMY-2} was the sole pAmpC gene identified in 12 chickens' and 1 wild bird (Eurasian magpie) isolates and was in all cases linked to an upstream IS*Ecp1*-like element. The isolates were classified into five different sequence types: ST131, ST117, ST155, ST429, and ST1415. Four chickens' stains were assigned to ST131, while five chickens' strains and the one from the Eurasian magpie belonged to ST117. Seven pAmpC isolates co-harbored genes conferring resistance to tetracyclines (*tetM*, *tetB*, *tetC*, *tetD*), 3 carried sulfonamide resistance genes (*sul*I and *sul*II), and 10 displayed mutations in the quinolone resistance-determining regions of *gyrA* (S83L+D87N) and *parC* (S80I+E84V). This report provides evidence of pAmpC dissemination, describing for the first time the presence of CMY-2 in chickens and wild birds from Greece.

Keywords: *Escherichia coli*; AmpC β-lactamases; antimicrobial resistance; CMY-2 type; IS*Ecp1*; chickens; wild birds; livestock; Greece

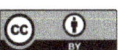

1. Introduction

Antimicrobial resistance (AMR) is a globally emergent, constantly evolving threat affecting humans, animals, and the environment, thus today constituting one of the greatest One Health challenges. Bacterial resistance to cephalosporins is mainly mediated by the production of extended-spectrum β-lactamases (ESBL) and AmpC β-lactamases. AmpC enzymes confer resistance to β-lactams, with the exception of fourth-generation cephalosporins and carbapenems, and subsequently render this essential class of antibiotics ineffective [1,2]. The presence of an AmpC combined with loss of outer membrane porins can, notably, further mediate resistance to carbapenems [2,3]. Hence, although plasmid-encoded AmpC enzymes (pAmpC) are less prevalent than ESBL in most parts of the world, they may lead to resistance of a broader spectrum, while additionally being harder to detect [2].

The most common pAmpC β-lactamase reported in *Escherichia coli* (*E. coli*) isolates of both human and animal origin globally is CMY-2 [4]. The zoonotic potential of this resistance determinant is illustrated by the detection of bla_{CMY-2} on related plasmids and *E. coli* clones in various hosts [5–7]. Insertion sequences, such as IS*Ecp1*, are known to play an important role in the mobilization and thus, the spread of this gene [8,9]. Among animals, poultry have been described as the most frequent bla_{CMY-2} carrier that can also act as an important infection source for humans, especially through meat and meat products [10,11]. On the contrary, cattle and pigs are less frequently detected to harbor this gene [12]. Alarmingly, the worldwide spread of pAmpC has additionally been evidenced in wildlife and the environment [13,14]. Wild birds play an important role as vectors of AMR and have been suggested as sentinels of circulating resistance genes within a certain geographic region [15,16]. Omnivorous, synanthropic birds are more likely to carry and disseminate resistant strains due to their vicinity to human activities and their feeding habits [17]. Despite the well documented role of animals as reservoirs and spreaders of pAmpC, their ability to directly transmit resistant bacteria to humans remains debatable [10,18].

AMR constitutes a serious threat for Greek public health. According to the surveillance report of the European Centre for Disease Prevention and Control (ECDC), Greece is classified among the countries confronting AMR the most [19], while native consumption of anti-infectives for systematic use is the highest in Europe [20]. pAmpC variants of the CMY family seem to circulate among human isolates in the country [21], while there is evidence to support that this case applies for companion animal isolates as well [22,23]. In livestock and poultry, the presence of pAmpC strains has also been ascertained [12,24]. However, there is hitherto paucity of knowledge regarding the molecular characteristics of pAmpC strains isolated from farmed and wild animals, as well as their possible relationship to human hosts.

Considering the emergence of AMR and the lack of detailed data in Greece, this study aimed to evaluate the presence of pAmpC-producing *E. coli* from poultry, cattle, pigs, and wild birds, to detect the responsible pAmpC genes and to identify the *E. coli* sequence types (ST). All pAmpC-producing *E. coli* isolates that were phenotypically resistant to antimicrobials other than β-lactams, including tetracyclines, sulfonamides, and quinolones, were further tested for the respective resistance determinants.

2. Results

2.1. Detection of pAmpC Genes in E. coli Isolates

Among the 646 animal samples, 168 were derived from wild bird species, 104 from cattle, 214 from pigs, and the remaining 159 from chickens. A total of 13 *E. coli*, 12 from chickens (12/159, 7.5%) and 1 from a Eurasian magpie (1/168, 0.6%), was found to be resistant to third-generation cephalosporins (3GC) and had a positive pAmpC-confirmation test. Molecular screening for pAmpC encoding genes revealed that all isolates carried the CMY-2 type and no other pAmpC gene type was detected in any isolate.

All strains were positive in the PCR targeting IS*Ecp1* – CMY, and sequencing analysis confirmed that bla_{CMY-2} genes were linked to an upstream IS*Ecp1*-like element.

2.2. Molecular Typing

Molecular typing of the 13 isolates classified them into five different STs. ST117 *E. coli* was recovered from the wild bird as well as from five chickens. Among the remaining seven chicken strains, four were assigned to ST131 and three were identified as either ST155 or ST429 or ST1415.

2.3. Detection of Additional Resistance Genes

According to susceptibility testing, 12 of the 13 CMY-2-positive *E. coli* strains, including the one from the wild bird, exhibited concurrent resistance to at least three classes of antibiotics. ESBL production, by phenotypic testing, was not observed for any strain. Six strains from chickens and the one from a wild bird exhibited resistance to tetracycline (TET^R). Out of the seven tetracycline-resistant strains, six carried *tetM*, while co-occurrence of *tetB*, *tetC*, and *tetD* was observed in the remaining one. Resistance to sulphonamides was expressed in two strains from chickens as well as in the one from the Eurasian magpie, which all harbored both *sul*I and *sul*II genes. Ten strains showed resistance to quinolones and fluoroquinolones (QN/FQN^R) although none carried *qnrA*, *qnrB*, or *qnrS*. Sequencing analysis of the QRDRs of *gyrA* and *parC*, performed on the resistant isolates, revealed that all strains displayed a mutation of serine-83 to leucine and a mutation of aspartic acid-87 to asparagine in *gyrA*. In addition, ST131 strains also had alterations of serine-80 to isoleucine and glutamic acid-84 to valine in the QRDR of *parC*.

The antimicrobial resistance and molecular typing results of the strains are summarized in Table 1.

Table 1. Characteristics of the plasmid-encoded AmpC β-lactamase (pAmpC)-producing *E. coli* isolates.

Isolate	Host	Sequence Type	Resistance Profile		Mutations (gyrA/parC)
			Phenotype	Resistance Determinants	
C46	Chicken	ST429	AMP, AMC, TZP, CEX, CF, CEF, CFIX, CTX, CAZ, CTRX	bla$_{CMY-2}$	-
C70	Chicken	ST131	AMP, AMC, TZP, CEX, CF, CEF, CFIX, CTX, CAZ, CTRX, FLU	bla$_{CMY-2}$	S83L+D87N/S80I+E84V
C79	Chicken	ST131	AMP, AMC, TZP, CEX, CF, CEF, CFIX, CTX, CAZ, CTRX, FLU	bla$_{CMY-2}$	S83L+D87N/S80I+E84V
C83	Chicken	ST117	AMP, AMC, TZP, CEX, CF, CFIX, CAZ, CTRX, FLU, TET, SXT	bla$_{CMY-2}$, tetM, sulI, sulII	S83L+D87N
C88	Chicken	ST117	AMP, AMC, TZP, CEX, CF, CFIX, CAZ, CTRX, FLU, TET	bla$_{CMY-2}$, tetM	S83L+D87N
C103	Chicken	ST117	AMP, AMC, TZP, CEX, CF, CFIX, CAZ, CTRX, FLU, TET	bla$_{CMY-2}$, tetM	S83L+D87N
C117	Chicken	ST117	AMP, AMC, TZP, CEX, CF, CFIX, CAZ, CTRX, FLU, TET	bla$_{CMY-2}$, tetM	S83L+D87N
C119	Chicken	ST117	AMP, AMC, TZP, CEX, CF, CFIX, CAZ, CTRX, FLU, TET, SXT	bla$_{CMY-2}$, tetM, sulI, sulII	S83L+D87N
C136	Chicken	ST131	AMP, AMC, TZP, CEX, CF, CEF, CFIX, CTX, CAZ, CTRX, FLU	bla$_{CMY-2}$	S83L+D87N/S80I+E84V
C138	Chicken	ST1415	AMP, AMC, TZP, CEX, CF, CEF, CFIX, CTX, CAZ, CTRX, TET	bla$_{CMY-2}$, tetB, tetC, tetD	-
C147	Chicken	ST131	AMP, AMC, TZP, CEX, CF, CEF, CFIX, CTX, CAZ, CTRX, FLU	bla$_{CMY-2}$	S83L+D87N/S80I+E84V
C156	Chicken	ST155	AMP, AMC, TZP, CEX, CF, CEF, CFIX, CTX, CAZ, CTRX	bla$_{CMY-2}$	-
WB105	Eurasian magpie (*Pica pica*)	ST117	AMP, AMC, TZP, CEX, CF, CEF, CFIX, CTX, CAZ, CTRX, FLU, TET, SXT	bla$_{CMY-2}$, tetM, sulI, sulII	S83L+D87N

AMP—ampicillin, AMC—amoxicillin/clavulanic acid, TZP—piperacillin/tazobactam, CEX—cefalexin, CF—cefalotin, CEF—ceftiofur, CFIX—cefixime, CTX—cefotaxime, CAZ—ceftazidime, CTRX—ceftriaxone, FLU—flumequine, TET—tetracycline, SXT—trimethoprim/sulfamethoxazole.

3. Discussion

In this study, pAmpC-producing *E. coli* strains were detected in 7.5% of chickens and 0.6% of wild birds, while they were not identified in cattle and pig samples. The higher frequency of pAmpC isolates among poultry, compared to other species, was in accordance with previously published data [10,12]. Their absence in cattle and pigs was expected, considering the European Union Summary Report on Antimicrobial Resistance for the years 2017 and 2018 that described low detection among fattening pigs and zero occurrence in bovine meat from Greece [12].

To the best of our knowledge, this is the first time that CMY-2 type is identified from *E. coli* isolates of farmed chickens in Greece and bla_{CMY-2} was the sole pAmpC gene detected, which is in agreement with previous studies [25–27]. Carriage was relatively low (7.5%), compared to recent reports from neighboring countries such as Turkey [28], Romania [29], and Italy [25]. Our finding may be indicative of CMY-2 type low occurrence in Greek poultry but, given the lack of previous screening studies, further investigations would be helpful to verify the aforementioned low prevalence. Considering the European prohibition of cephalosporins' use in poultry, the emergence of ESBL/pAmpC-producing Enterobacteriaceae may be attributed to the treatment of eggs and/or one-day-old chickens in grandparent and parent flocks, along with the current management practices [30,31]. It has been shown that broilers can maintain pAmpC *E. coli* imported to the flock via one-day-old chicks or breeding animals even in the absence of selective antibiotic pressure [32,33]. This can be reflected in poultry meat, raising concern about the zoonotic capacity of pAmpC isolates.

We additionally detected a pAmpC-producing *E. coli* harbored by a Eurasian magpie (*Pica pica*) and, as far as we know, this is the first identification of CMY-2 type gene in a wild bird species from Greece. CMY-2 prevails among pAmpC *E. coli* isolates of corvids from The Czech Republic, Poland [34], Austria [16], Canada [17], and The USA [35,36], and of aquatic birds from The Netherlands [13], Spain [37], and Florida, USA [38]. We found a relatively low pAmpC carriage (0.6%) and our results are comparable with those of Alcala et al. [37] who reported 1.0% detection in Spain. Although higher pAmpC carriage has been published previously, varying from 3.4% in The Netherlands [13] to 26.9% in Florida [38], the low detection reported in our study could be attributed to the wide variety of the sampled wild bird species. Sampling and testing were performed, for screening purposes, not only in corvids and aquatic birds, but additionally in "low-risk" wild bird species, which are neither migratory nor omnivorous or aquatic-associated. Eurasian magpie is an omnivore and opportunistic scavenger, highly adapted to human environments and one of the most abundant corvids in Europe. Its diet and ecology, frequently interacting with humans and domestic animals, could explain the detection of a pAmpC-producing strain, as previously described for corvid populations [17]. Eurasian magpies are also known to form large communal roosts outside the breeding season, which could contribute to CMY-2 persistence and dissemination by bird-to-bird transmission during winter.

IS*Ecp1* was found in the upstream region of bla_{CMY-2} in all our isolates. Co-existence of IS*Ecp1* with ESBL/pAmpC genes in *E. coli* strains is well documented and has been associated with their efficient capture, expression, and mobilization [39,40]. Being responsible for bla_{CMY-2} transposition to different plasmids, IS*Ecp1* probably has an important role in the dissemination of this beta-lactamase and subsequently the enhancement of its zoonotic potential [41].

MLST analysis demonstrated that the CMY-2-producing *E. coli* isolates of chickens were distributed in five different STs. Four chickens' strains were assigned to ST131, a clone with a worldwide distribution that has contributed to the dissemination of the ubiquitous ESBL variant CTX-M-15, as well as other resistance genes [42,43]. This finding highlights the potential of acquired AmpC enzymes to arise as an important zoonotic issue. Further supporting this claim, we also detected bla_{CMY-2} type in a chicken *E. coli* ST155, a clone commonly reported in poultry but additionally significant for public health [44,45]. On the contrary, ST429 that was detected to express CMY-2, is a predominant avian pathogenic lineage, related only to incidental human infections [46,47]. In Greece, CMY-2-producing *E. coli* ST429 has previously been isolated from a healthy household dog [23], which could imply inter-species circulation of the clone in the country. The CMY-2 type-producing *E. coli* isolated from the Eurasian magpie (*Pica pica*) belonged to ST117, previously reported in corvids both in Europe and in Canada [17,34]. Five chickens' isolates were also assigned to this clinically important multiresistant ST, suggesting possible strain transmission among different animal hosts in the country. Detection of ST117 in poultry and a wild bird raises concern, given its frequent association to hospital-based and community-acquired human infections worldwide [48–50]. Finally, an *E. coli* of chicken origin was classified as ST1415, a rather rare ST that, to our knowledge, has not been previously related to CMY-2.

Tetracycline resistance genes were identified in 6 out of the 12 CMY-2-producing poultry isolates, as well as in the Eurasian magpie isolate. Five chickens' strains carried *tetM*, while *tetB*, *tetC*, and *tetD* were detected in the remaining one. The high frequency of tetracycline resistance among chicken pAmpC-producing isolates probably depicts the widespread use of this antibiotic in poultry husbandry all over the world [51]. Co-occurrence of bla_{CMY-2} and *tet* genes has formerly been reported in *E. coli* isolates from chicken carcasses in South Brazil [41], retail chicken meat in Canada [52], as well as in avian pathogenic *E. coli* from septicemic broilers in Egypt [53]. Additionally, the Eurasian magpie CMY-2 type-positive isolate displayed tetracycline resistance mediated by *tetM* and our finding complies with Sen et al. [35], who detected co-occurrence of *tetM* and bla_{CMY-2} in crow isolates.

Resistance to sulfonamides was detected in three strains, two from chickens and the one from the Eurasian magpie, which all harbored *sul*I and *sul*II sulfonamide resistance genes. In the past, sulfonamides were extensively used in traditional poultry production systems in order to achieve higher population densities and increased production. Over-consumption of this antimicrobial class resulted in the development of high resistance rates, reducing significantly its role in the poultry production nowadays [54,55]. As far as the Eurasian magpie isolate is concerned, resistance against chemically synthesized antibiotic classes such as sulphonamides has been reported in wild fauna, even though these antimicrobials are not expected to be widespread in the environment [56]. Co-occurrence of ESBL/pAmpC and sulfonamide resistance determinants on the same plasmid could probably explain the latter's detection in the wild bird isolate [57].

Quinolone resistance was also reported in CMY-2 *E. coli* strains from nine chickens and the Eurasian magpie. Mutations were responsible for the QN/FQN^R phenotype and all isolates possessed the same amino acid substitution pattern in *gyrA* gene. ST131 *E. coli* possessed the S83L + D87N in *gyrA* combined with S80I + E84V in *parC*. Notably, the same mutations have been found in a collection of ST131 *E. coli* isolated from humans in Central Greece [58]. That study suggested that fluoroquinolone resistance in humans could be related to the use of these antimicrobials in the veterinary practice and the poultry production of the area. Our results verify that this specific substitutional pattern exists in *E. coli* strains of poultry origin. However, no isolate in our study co-harbored bla_{CMY-2} and plasmid mediated quinolone resistance (PMQR) genes, as has previously been described for ESBL/pAmpC-producing *E. coli* of poultry and wild bird origin [13,59,60].

4. Materials and Methods

4.1. Sample Collection

During 2018–2020, a total of 646 non duplicated fecal samples of clinically healthy animals were collected from different regions of Greece. In particular, 159 stool samples were collected from chickens, 104 from cattle, 214 from pigs, and 168 from thirty different wild bird species (Table 2). Samples were obtained by inserting a sterile cotton swab (Transwab® Amies, UK) into the rectum or the cloaca and gently rotating the tip against the mucosa.

Regarding sampling of different wild bird species, Larsen and Australian type traps as well as modified bird catching nets were used, located in a variety of habitats. The sampling site of each wild bird was recorded using handheld Global Positioning System (GPS) units. All wild birds were released immediately following sampling, according to the prerequisites of the Greek Legislation.

Swabs were transported under refrigeration and laboratory analysis was initiated 24–48 h from the samples' collection day.

Table 2. Number of samples per wild bird species included in the study.

Common Name	Scientific Name	Number of Samples
Common blackbird	*Turdus merula*	4
Common buzzard	*Buteo buteo*	5
Common pheasant	*Phasianus colchicus*	7
Common starling	*Sturnus vulgaris*)	9
Common swift	*Apus apus*	1
Common whitethroat	*Sylvia communis*	2
Common wood pigeon	*Columba palumbus*	3
Domestic Muscovy duck	*Cairina moschata domestica*	1
Domestic goose	*Anser cygnoides domesticus*	1
Eurasian collared dove	*Streptopelia decaocto*	2
Eurasian eagle-owl	*Bubo bubo*	3
European goldfinch	*Carduelis carduelis*	6
Eurasian scops owl	*Otus scops*	1
Eurasian tree sparrow	*Passer montanus*	9
Eurasian woodcock	*Scolopax rusticola*	11
Golden pheasant	*Chrysolophus pictus*	2
Great tit	*Parus major*	5
House sparrow	*Passer domesticus*	14
Lesser kestrel	*Falco naumanni*	1
Leaf warbler	*Phylloscopus spp.*	1
Little owl	*Athene noctua*	2
Long-eared owl	*Asio otus*	2
Eurasian Magpie	*Pica pica*	52
Mallard	*Anas platyrhynchos*	3
Redwing	*Turdus iliacus*	1
Rock partridge	*Alectoris graeca*	3
Sardinian warbler	*Sylvia melanocephala*	1
Short-toed snake eagle	*Circaetus gallicus*	1
Song thrush	*Turdus philomelos*	14
Yellow-legged gull	*Larus michahellis*	1

4.2. Isolation, Identification and Antimicrobial Susceptibility Testing of pAmpC-producing E. coli

For the isolation of pAmpC-producing Enterobacterales, swabs were directly streaked on ESBL selective media (CHROMID® ESBL, BioMérieux, Marcy l'Etoile, France) (a medium able to detect both ESBLs and high-level expressed AmpC cephalosporinases) and then the plates were incubated aerobically at 37 °C for 48 h in order to increase sensitivity [61]. Each morphologically different pink colony, corresponding to *E. coli* grown on the plates, was sub-cultured on MacConkey agar. Identification of the isolated bacteria and antimicrobial susceptibility testing were carried out using the automated Vitek-2 system (BioMérieux, Marcy l'Etoile, France), according to the manufacturer's instructions. The antimicrobial agents tested, using the AST-GN96 card, were ampicillin, amoxicillin/clavulanic acid, ticarcillin/clavulanic acid, cefalexin, cefalotin, cefoperazone, ceftiofur, cefquinome, imipenem, gentamicin, neomycin, flumequine, enrofloxacin, marbofloxacin, tetracycline, florfenicol, polymyxin B, and trimethoprim/sulfamethoxazole. Interpretation of the antimicrobial susceptibility testing was performed automatically by the Vitek-2 software (BioMérieux, system version 8.02). Susceptibility to piperacillin/tazobactam, cefixime, cefotaxime, ceftazidime, and ceftriaxone was also tested by Etest, according to EUCAST guidelines [62].

All *E. coli* isolates that were resistant to 3GC were further tested for phenotypic AmpC production using Etest strips containing cefotetan and cefotetan plus cloxacillin (Liofilchem). Isolates that had a ratio cefotetan/cefotetan + cloxacillin ≥8 were selected for molecular detection of AmpC genes and molecular typing. Additionally, these isolates were phenotypically screened for ESBL production using Etest strips containing cefotaxime +/- clavulanic acid and Ceftazidime +/- clavulanic acid (Liofilchem). An MIC ratio ≥8 or the presence of a deformed ellipse were considered indicative of ESBL production.

4.3. DNA Extraction of the AmpC-Producing E.coli

Bacterial DNA was extracted from overnight cultures of the selected isolates using the PureLink™ Genomic DNA Mini Kit (Invitrogen, Darmstadt, Germany), according to the manufacturer's instructions for Gram-negative bacteria.

4.4. Molecular Confirmation of PAmpC Production and Screening of Insertion Sequence

In all isolates, simplex PCRs were performed for amplification of genes for the most common types of plasmid mediated AmpC β-lactamases using the primers described by Pérez-Pérez and Hanson [63] (Table 3). Post-amplification products were visualized on 2% agarose gel electrophoresis. The PCR products were purified and were analyzed by sequencing (3730xl DNA Analyzer, Applied Biosystems).

Table 3. Primer sequences, amplicon sizes, and optimal annealing temperatures of each simplex PCR performed for the amplification of pAmpC and other resistance genes.

Target	Primer Sequence (5'-3')	Amplicon Size (bp)	Annealing Temperature (°C)	Reference
MOX (MOX-1, MOX-2, CMY-1, CMY-8 to CMY-11)	F: GCTGCTCAAGGAGCACAGGAT R:CACATTGACATAGGTGTGGTGC	520	55	[63]
CIT (LAT-1 to LAT-4, CMY-2 to CMY-7, BIL-1)	F: TGGCCAGAACTGACAGGCAAA R: TTTCTCCTGAACGTGGCTGGC	462	55	[63]
DHA (DHA-1, DHA-2)	F: AACTTTCACAGGTGTGCTGGGT R: CCGTACGCATACTGGCTTTGC	405	56	[63]
ACC	F: AACAGCCTCAGCAGCCGGTTA R: TTCGCCGCAATCATCCCTAGC	346	55	[63]
EBC (MIR-1T ACT-1)	F: TCGGTAAAGCCGATGTTGCGG R: CTTCCACTGCGGCTGCCAGTT	302	58	[63]
FOX (FOX-1 to FOX-5b)	F:AACATGGGGTATCAGGGAGATG R: CAAAGCGCGTAACCGGATTGG	190	55	[63]
tetA	F: GCCTTTCCTTTGGGTTCTCT R: TGTCCGACAAGTTGCATGAT	402	55	[64]
tetB	F: CACCACCAGCCAATAAAATT R: TTTATTTAAAACGATGCCCA	319	52	This study
tetC	F: TCACTGGTTAACTCAGCACG R: TCAAGTTCATTCCAACCAAT	319	52	This study
tetD	F: CTCCAATTCCCATAATTTAT R: ATCAAAATAAAGCTAATAAC	379	52	This study
tetM	F: TTATCAACGGTTTATCAGG R: CGTATATATGCAAGACG	398	57	This study
qnrA	F: AGAGGATTTCTCACGCCAGG R: CCAGGCACAGATCTTGAC	580	55	[58]
qnrB	F: GGGTATGGATATTATTGATAAAG R: CTAATCCGGCAGCACTATTA	264	55	[58]

Table 3. Cont.

Target	Primer Sequence (5'-3')	Amplicon Size (bp)	Annealing Temperature (°C)	Reference
qnrS	F: GCAAGTTCATTGAACAGGGT R: TCTAAACCGTCGAGTTCGGC	428	55	[58]
gyrA	F: TTAATGATTGCCGCCGTCGG R: TACACCGGTCAACATTGAGG	648	54	[58]
parC	F: GTGGTGCCGTTAAGCAAA R: AAACCTGTTCAGCGCCGCATT	395	55	[58]
sulI	F: ACG AGA TTG TGC GGT TCT TC R: GGT TTC CGA GAT GGT GAT TG	347	55	[64]
sulII	F: CCG TCT CGC TCG ACA GTT AT R: GTG TGT GCG GAT GAA GTC AG	506	55	[64]
ISEcp1 – CMY	F- AAAAATGATTGAAAGGTGGT R- TTTCTCCTGAACGTGGCTGGC	546	52	[41]

The presence of ISEcp1 insertion element upstream of the bla_{CMY-2} was investigated by PCR, using a forward primer targeting the ISEcp1 element and a reverse primer targeting the bla_{CMY}, as described previously [41] (Table 3).

4.5. Molecular Typing of Isolates

Molecular typing of isolates was based on Multilocus Sequence Typing (MLST) in which amplification of seven gene loci (adk, fumC, gyrB, icd, mdh, purA, recA) was performed by PCR (Table 3). PCR products were purified using PureLink™ PCR Purification Kit (Thermo Fisher Scientific), according to the manufacturer's instructions. Purified products were sequenced (3730xl DNA Analyzer, Applied Biosystems) and analysis of the alleles was conducted using an online available database (https://pubmlst.org/bigsdb?db=pubmlst_ecoli_achtman_seqdef) (accessed date: 5 February 2021).

4.6. Molecular Detection of Additional Resistance Genes

Strains in which the presence of a pAmpC gene was confirmed and were phenotypically resistant to tetracyclines, sulfonamides, and/or quinolones were additionally tested for the respective resistance genes. In detail, genes conferring resistance to tetracycline (tetA, tetB, tetC, tetD, tetM), to sulfonamides (sulI, sulII), and the PMQR determinants (qnrA, qnrB, qnrS) were investigated by PCR. Quinolone-resistant isolates were also screened for mutations in the quinolone resistance-determining regions (QRDRs) of gyrA and parC by PCR and sequencing of the amplicons was performed (3730xl DNA Analyzer, Applied Biosystems) (Table 3).

5. Conclusions

In this study, we investigated, for the first time, the occurrence of pAmpC-producing *E. coli* from various hosts in Greece. Chicken and wild bird strains harbored bla_{CMY-2} type in a low prevalence, while pAmpC were not detected in cattle and pigs. ST117 and ST131 were the predominant circulating CMY-2 *E. coli* clones. Tetracycline, sulfonamide, and quinolone resistance were also identified in the CMY-2 strains, revealing the presence of *tet* genes, *sul* genes, and of mutations in the QRDRs, respectively.

Author Contributions: Conceptualization, Z.A., K.T., V.S., E.P., and C.B.; methodology, Z.A., K.T., M.S. (Marina Sofia), D.C.C., A.G., I.K., V.G., V.S., E.P., and C.B.; validation, Z.A., E.P., and C.B.; formal analysis, Z.A. and K.T.; investigation, Z.A., K.T., M.S. (Marina Sofia), D.C.C., A.T., and M.S. (Maria Satra); resources, A.G., I.K., V.G., D.G., V.D., and S.M.; data curation, Z.A., K.T., M.S., D.C.C., A.T., and M.S. (Maria Satra); writing—original draft preparation, Z.A., K.T., and M.S.; writing—review and editing, Z.A., V.S., E.P., and C.B.; supervision, V.S., E.P., and C.B.; project administration, V.S., E.P., and C.B.; funding acquisition, M.S. (Marina Sofia), D.C.C., A.G., I.K., V.G., V.S., E.P., and C.B. All authors have read and agreed to the published version of the manuscript.

Funding: This work has been co-funded by the European Union and the General Secretariat for Research and Innovation, Ministry of Development & Investments, under the project «Novel technologies for surveillance and characterization of Extended-spectrum β-lactamase and Carbapenemase producing Enterobacteriaceae, in humans and animals (CARBATECH)» T2DGE-0944, of the Bilateral S&T Cooperation Program Greece–Germany 2017. This support is gratefully acknowledged.

Institutional Review Board Statement: All samples were obtained by noninvasive rectal or cloacal swabs and no research on animals, as defined in the EU Ethics for Researchers document (European Commission, 2013, Ethics for Researchers-Facilitating Research Excellence in FP7, Luxembourg: Office for Official Publications of the European Communities, ISBN 978-92-79-28854-8), was carried out for this study. Official permissions for capturing and sampling crows, migratory and epidemic wild birds were provided by the Hellenic Ministry of Environment and Energy (159169/1920/21 7-2017), (181997/1000/10-5-2019). Capturing, handling and sampling wild birds complied with European and national legislation.

Data Availability Statement: Most data for this study are presented within the manuscript. The remaining data are available on request from the corresponding author. The data are not publicly available as they are part of the PhD thesis of the first author, which has not yet been examined, approved and uploaded in the official depository of PhD theses from Greek Universities.

Conflicts of Interest: The authors declare no conflict of interest.

References

1. *Critically Important Antimicrobials for Human Medicine*, 6th ed.; World Health Organization: Geneva, Switzerland, 2019.
2. Jacoby, G.A. AmpC B-Lactamases. *Clin. Microbiol. Rev.* **2009**, *22*, 161–182. [CrossRef]
3. Mammeri, H.; Guillon, H.; Eb, F.; Nordmann, P. Phenotypic and Biochemical Comparison of the Carbapenem-Hydrolyzing Activities of Five Plasmid-Borne AmpC β-Lactamases. *Antimicrob. Agents Chemother.* **2010**, *54*, 4556–4560. [CrossRef]
4. Ewers, C.; Bethe, A.; Semmler, T.; Guenther, S.; Wieler, L. Extended-spectrum β-lactamase-producing and AmpC-producing *Escherichia coli* from livestock and companion animals, and their putative impact on public health: A global perspective. *Clin. Microbiol. Infect.* **2012**, *18*, 646–655. [CrossRef] [PubMed]
5. Pietsch, M.; Irrgang, A.; Roschanski, N.; Michael, G.B.; Hamprecht, A.; Rieber, H.; Käsbohrer, A.; Schwarz, S.; Rösler, U. Whole genome analyses of CMY-2-producing *Escherichia coli* isolates from humans, animals and food in Germany. *BMC Genom.* **2018**, *19*, 601. [CrossRef]
6. Hansen, K.H.; Bortolaia, V.; Nielsen, C.A.; Nielsen, J.B.; Schønning, K.; Agersø, Y.; Guardabassi, L. Host-Specific Patterns of Genetic Diversity among IncI1-Iγ and IncK Plasmids Encoding CMY-2 β-Lactamase in *Escherichia coli* Isolates from Humans, Poultry Meat, Poultry, and Dogs in Denmark. *Appl. Environ. Microbiol.* **2016**, *82*, 4705–4714. [CrossRef]
7. Seiffert, S.N.; Carattoli, A.; Schwendener, S.; Collaud, A.; Endimiani, A.; Perreten, V. Plasmids Carrying blaCMY-2/4 in *Escherichia coli* from Poultry, Poultry Meat, and Humans Belong to a Novel IncK Subgroup Designated IncK2. *Front. Microbiol.* **2017**, *8*, 407. [CrossRef] [PubMed]
8. Toleman, M.A.; Walsh, T.R. Combinatorial events of insertion sequences and ICE in Gram-negative bacteria. *FEMS Microbiol. Rev.* **2011**, *35*, 912–935. [CrossRef]
9. Verdet, C.; Gautier, V.; Chachaty, E.; Ronco, E.; Hidri, N.; Decré, D.; Arlet, G. Genetic Context of Plasmid-Carried blaCMY-2-Like Genes in Enterobacteriaceae. *Antimicrob. Agents Chemother.* **2009**, *53*, 4002–4006. [CrossRef] [PubMed]
10. Madec, J.-Y.; Haenni, M.; Nordmann, P.; Poirel, L. Extended-spectrum β-lactamase/AmpC- and carbapenemase-producing Enterobacteriaceae in animals: A threat for humans? *Clin. Microbiol. Infect.* **2017**, *23*, 826–833. [CrossRef] [PubMed]
11. Berg, E.; Wester, A.; Ahrenfeldt, J.; Mo, S.; Slettemeås, J.; Steinbakk, M.; Samuelsen, Ø.; Grude, N.; Simonsen, G.; Løhr, I.; et al. Norwegian patients and retail chicken meat share cephalosporin-resistant *Escherichia coli* and IncK/bla CMY-2 resistance plasmids. *Clin. Microbiol. Infect.* **2017**, *23*, 407.e9–407.e15. [CrossRef]
12. *The European Union Summary Report on Antimicrobial Resistance in Zoonotic and Indicator Bacteria from Humans, Animals and Food in 2017/2018*; Wiley-Blackwell Publishing Ltd.: Hoboken, NJ, USA, 2020; Volume 18.
13. Veldman, K.; van Tulden, P.; Kant, A.; Testerink, J.; Mevius, D. Characteristics of Cefotaxime-Resistant *Escherichia coli* from Wild Birds in The Netherlands. *Appl. Environ. Microbiol.* **2013**, *79*, 7556–7561. [CrossRef]
14. Zhang, A.; Call, D.R.; Besser, T.E.; Liu, J.; Jones, L.; Wang, H.; Davis, M.A. β-lactam resistance genes in bacteriophage and bacterial DNA from wastewater, river water, and irrigation water in Washington State. *Water Res.* **2019**, *161*, 335–340. [CrossRef]
15. Bonnedahl, J.; Järhult, J.D. Antibiotic resistance in wild birds. *Upsala J. Med. Sci.* **2014**, *119*, 113–116. [CrossRef] [PubMed]
16. Loncaric, I.; Stalder, G.L.; Mehinagic, K.; Rosengarten, R.; Hoelzl, F.; Knauer, F.; Walzer, C. Comparison of ESBL—And AmpC Producing Enterobacteriaceae and Methicillin-Resistant *Staphylococcus aureus* (MRSA) Isolated from Migratory and Resident Population of Rooks (*Corvus frugilegus*) in Austria. *PLoS ONE* **2013**, *8*, e84048. [CrossRef]

17. Jamborova, I.; Janecko, N.; Halova, D.; Sedmik, J.; Mezerova, K.; Papousek, I.; Kutilova, I.; Dolejska, M.; Cizek, A.; Literak, I. Molecular characterization of plasmid-mediated AmpC beta-lactamase- and extended-spectrum beta-lactamase-producing *Escherichia coli* and Klebsiella pneumoniae among corvids (*Corvus brachyrhynchos* and *Corvus corax*) roosting in Canada. *FEMS Microbiol. Ecol.* **2018**, *94*. [CrossRef]
18. Dorado-García, A.; Smid, J.H.; van Pelt, W.; Bonten, M.J.M.; Fluit, A.C.; Bunt, G.V.D.; Wagenaar, J.A.; Hordijk, J.; Dierikx, C.M.; Veldman, K.T.; et al. Molecular relatedness of ESBL/AmpC-producing *Escherichia coli* from humans, animals, food and the environment: A pooled analysis. *J. Antimicrob. Chemother.* **2018**, *73*, 339–347. [CrossRef] [PubMed]
19. Surveillance of Antimicrobial Resistance in Europe 2018. Available online: https://www.ecdc.europa.eu/en/publications-data/surveillance-antimicrobial-resistance-europe-2018 (accessed on 2 November 2020).
20. European Centre for Disease Prevention and Control (ECDC) Rates by Country. Available online: https://www.ecdc.europa.eu/en/antimicrobial-consumption/database/rates-country (accessed on 28 November 2020).
21. Kazmierczak, K.M.; de Jonge, B.L.M.; Stone, G.G.; Sahm, D.F. In vitro activity of ceftazidime/avibactam against isolates of Enterobacteriaceae collected in European countries: INFORM global surveillance 2012–15. *J. Antimicrob. Chemother.* **2018**, *73*, 2782–2788. [CrossRef]
22. Vingopoulou, E.I.; Siarkou, V.I.; Batzias, G.; Kaltsogianni, F.; Sianou, E.; Tzavaras, I.; Koutinas, A.; Saridomichelakis, M.N.; Sofianou, D.; Tzelepi, E.; et al. Emergence and maintenance of multidrug-resistant *Escherichia coli* of canine origin harbouring a blaCMY-2-IncI1/ST65 plasmid and topoisomerase mutations. *J. Antimicrob. Chemother.* **2014**, *69*, 2076–2080. [CrossRef] [PubMed]
23. Liakopoulos, A.; Betts, J.; la Ragione, R.; van Essen-Zandbergen, A.; Ceccarelli, D.; Petinaki, E.; Koutinas, C.K.; Mevius, D.J. Occurrence and characterization of extended-spectrum cephalosporin-resistant Enterobacteriaceae in healthy household dogs in Greece. *J. Med. Microbiol.* **2018**, *67*, 931–935. [CrossRef] [PubMed]
24. Investigation of Antimicrobial Resistance Patterns in Commensal Escherichia coli Isolates from Broilers in Greece. Available online: http://ecvmicro.org/Files/ICECVM_2019_Abstract_Book_ver3.pdf#page=119 (accessed on 11 January 2021).
25. Apostolakos, I.; Mughini-Gras, L.; Fasolato, L.; Piccirillo, A. Assessing the occurrence and transfer dynamics of ESBL/pAmpC-producing *Escherichia coli* across the broiler production pyramid. *PLoS ONE* **2019**, *14*, e0217174. [CrossRef] [PubMed]
26. Maamar, E.; Hammami, S.; Alonso, C.A.; Dakhli, N.; Abbassi, M.S.; Ferjani, S.; Hamzaoui, Z.; Saidani, M.; Torres, C.; Boubaker, I.B.-B. High prevalence of extended-spectrum and plasmidic AmpC beta-lactamase-producing *Escherichia coli* from poultry in Tunisia. *Int. J. Food Microbiol.* **2016**, *231*, 69–75. [CrossRef] [PubMed]
27. Päivärinta, M.; Latvio, S.; Fredriksson-Ahomaa, M.; Heikinheimo, A. Whole genome sequence analysis of antimicrobial resistance genes, multilocus sequence types and plasmid sequences in ESBL/AmpC *Escherichia coli* isolated from broiler caecum and meat. *Int. J. Food Microbiol.* **2020**, *315*, 108361. [CrossRef] [PubMed]
28. Aslantaş, Özkan High occurrence of CMY-2-type beta-lactamase-producing *Escherichia coli* among broiler flocks in Turkey. *Trop. Anim. Heal. Prod.* **2019**, *52*, 1681–1689. [CrossRef]
29. Maciuca, I.E.; Williams, N.J.; Tuchilus, C.; Dorneanu, O.; Guguianu, E.; Carp-Carare, C.; Rimbu, C.; Timofte, D. High Prevalence of *Escherichia coli*-Producing CTX-M-15 Extended-Spectrum Beta-Lactamases in Poultry and Human Clinical Isolates in Romania. *Microb. Drug Resist.* **2015**, *21*, 651–662. [CrossRef] [PubMed]
30. Murphy, D.; Ricci, A.; Auce, Z.; Beechinor, J.G.; Bergendahl, H.; Breathnach, R.; Bureš, J.; da Silva, J.P.D.; Hederová, J.; Hekman, P.; et al. EMA and EFSA Joint Scientific Opinion on measures to reduce the need to use antimicrobial agents in animal husbandry in the European Union, and the resulting impacts on food safety (RONAFA). *EFSA J.* **2017**, *15*, e04666. [CrossRef] [PubMed]
31. Dorado-García, A.; Mevius, D.J.; Jacobs, J.J.H.; van Geijlswijk, I.M.; Mouton, J.W.; Wagenaar, J.A.; Heederik, D.J. Quantitative assessment of antimicrobial resistance in livestock during the course of a nationwide antimicrobial use reduction in the Netherlands. *J. Antimicrob. Chemother.* **2016**, *71*, 3607–3619. [CrossRef]
32. Huijbers, P.M.; Graat, E.A.; van Hoek, A.H.; Veenman, C.; de Jong, M.C.; van Duijkeren, E. Transmission dynamics of extended-spectrum β-lactamase and AmpC β-lactamase-producing *Escherichia coli* in a broiler flock without antibiotic use. *Prev. Veter. Med.* **2016**, *131*, 12–19. [CrossRef]
33. Nilsson, O.; Börjesson, S.; Landén, A.; Bengtsson, B. Vertical transmission of *Escherichia coli* carrying plasmid-mediated AmpC (pAmpC) through the broiler production pyramid. *J. Antimicrob. Chemother.* **2014**, *69*, 1497–1500. [CrossRef]
34. Jamborova, I.; Dolejska, M.; Vojtech, J.; Guenther, S.; Uricariu, R.; Drozdowska, J.; Papousek, I.; Pasekova, K.; Meissner, W.; Hordowski, J.; et al. Plasmid-Mediated Resistance to Cephalosporins and Fluoroquinolones in Various *Escherichia coli* Sequence Types Isolated from Rooks Wintering in Europe. *Appl. Environ. Microbiol.* **2014**, *81*, 648–657. [CrossRef]
35. Sen, K.; Berglund, T.; Soares, M.A.; Taheri, B.; Ma, Y.; Khalil, L.; Fridge, M.; Lu, J.; Turner, R.J. Antibiotic Resistance of E. coli Isolated from a Constructed Wetland Dominated by a Crow Roost, With Emphasis on ESBL and AmpC Containing E. coli. *Front. Microbiol.* **2019**, *10*, 1034. [CrossRef]
36. Jamborova, I.; Dolejska, M.; Zurek, L.; Townsend, A.K.; Clark, A.B.; Ellis, J.C.; Papousek, I.; Cizek, A.; Literak, I. Plasmid-mediated resistance to cephalosporins and quinolones in *Escherichia coli* from American crows in the USA. *Environ. Microbiol.* **2017**, *19*, 2025–2036. [CrossRef]
37. Alcalá, L.; Alonso, C.A.; Simón, C.; González-Esteban, C.; Orós, J.; Rezusta, A.; Ortega, C.; Torres, C. Wild Birds, Frequent Carriers of Extended-Spectrum β-Lactamase (ESBL) Producing *Escherichia coli* of CTX-M and SHV-12 Types. *Microb. Ecol.* **2015**, *72*, 861–869. [CrossRef]

38. Poirel, L.; Potron, A.; de la Cuesta, C.; Cleary, T.; Nordmann, P.; Munoz-Price, L.S. Wild Coastline Birds as Reservoirs of Broad-Spectrum-β-Lactamase-Producing Enterobacteriaceae in Miami Beach, Florida. *Antimicrob. Agents Chemother.* **2012**, *56*, 2756–2758. [CrossRef]
39. Poirel, L.; Decousser, J.-W.; Nordmann, P. Insertion Sequence ISEcp1B Is Involved in Expression and Mobilization of a blaCTX-M β-Lactamase Gene. *Antimicrob. Agents Chemother.* **2003**, *47*, 2938–2945. [CrossRef]
40. Saladin, M.; Cao, V.T.B.; Lambert, T.; Donay, J.-L.; Herrmann, J.-L.; Ould-Hocine, Z.; Verdet, C.; Delisle, F.; Philippon, A.; Arlet, G. Diversity of CTX-M β²-lactamases and their promoter regions from Enterobacteriaceae isolated in three Parisian hospitals. *FEMS Microbiol. Lett.* **2002**, *209*, 161–168. [CrossRef]
41. Koga, V.L.; Maluta, R.P.; Da Silveira, W.D.; Ribeiro, R.A.; Hungria, M.; Vespero, E.C.; Nakazato, G.; Kobayashi, R.K.T. Characterization of CMY-2-type beta-lactamase-producing *Escherichia coli* isolated from chicken carcasses and human infection in a city of South Brazil. *BMC Microbiol.* **2019**, *19*, 1–9. [CrossRef]
42. Nicolas-Chanoine, M.-H.; Blanco, J.; Leflon-Guibout, V.; Demarty, R.; Alonso, M.P.; Caniça, M.M.; Park, Y.-J.; Lavigne, J.-P.; Pitout, J.; Johnson, J.R. Intercontinental emergence of *Escherichia coli* clone O25:H4-ST131 producing CTX-M-15. *J. Antimicrob. Chemother.* **2007**, *61*, 273–281. [CrossRef]
43. Pitout, J.D.; Finn, T.J. The evolutionary puzzle of *Escherichia coli* ST131. *Infect. Genet. Evol.* **2020**, *81*, 104265. [CrossRef] [PubMed]
44. Lazarus, B.; Paterson, D.L.; Mollinger, J.L.; Rogers, B.A. Do Human Extraintestinal *Escherichia coli* Infections Resistant to Expanded-Spectrum Cephalosporins Originate from Food-Producing Animals? A Systematic Review. *Clin. Infect. Dis.* **2015**, *60*, 439–452. [CrossRef] [PubMed]
45. Foster-Nyarko, E.; Alikhan, N.-F.; Ravi, A.; Thomson, N.M.; Jarju, S.; Kwambana-Adams, B.A.; Secka, A.; O'Grady, J.; Antonio, M.; Pallen, M.J. Genomic diversity of *Escherichia coli* isolates from backyard chickens and guinea fowl in the Gambia. *Microb. Genom.* **2021**, *7*, mgen000484. [CrossRef]
46. Papouskova, A.; Masarikova, M.; Valcek, A.; Senk, D.; Cejkova, D.; Jahodarova, E.; Cizek, A. Genomic analysis of *Escherichia coli* strains isolated from diseased chicken in the Czech Republic. *BMC Veter. Res.* **2020**, *16*, 1–10. [CrossRef] [PubMed]
47. Xu, J.; Lin, W.; Chen, Y.; He, F. Genomic and phylogenetic analysis of a community-acquired extended-spectrum β-lactamase-producing *Escherichia coli* ST429 strain recovered from a urinary tract infection. *J. Glob. Antimicrob. Resist.* **2020**, *22*, 656–658. [CrossRef] [PubMed]
48. Maluta, R.P.; Logue, C.M.; Casas, M.R.T.; Meng, T.; Guastalli, E.A.L.; Rojas, T.C.G.; Montelli, A.C.; Sadatsune, T.; Ramos, M.D.C.; Nolan, L.K.; et al. Overlapped Sequence Types (STs) and Serogroups of Avian Pathogenic (APEC) and Human Extra-Intestinal Pathogenic (ExPEC) *Escherichia coli* Isolated in Brazil. *PLoS ONE* **2014**, *9*, e105016. [CrossRef]
49. Hall, M.L.-V.; Dierikx, C.; Stuart, J.C.; Voets, G.; Munckhof, M.V.D.; van Essen-Zandbergen, A.; Platteel, T.; Fluit, A.; van de Sande-Bruinsma, N.; Scharinga, J.; et al. Dutch patients, retail chicken meat and poultry share the same ESBL genes, plasmids and strains. *Clin. Microbiol. Infect.* **2011**, *17*, 873–880. [CrossRef]
50. Manges, A.R.; Harel, J.; Masson, L.; Edens, T.J.; Portt, A.; Reid-Smith, R.J.; Zhanel, G.G.; Kropinski, A.M.; Boerlin, P. Multilocus Sequence Typing and Virulence Gene Profiles Associated with *Escherichia coli* from Human and Animal Sources. *Foodborne Pathog. Dis.* **2015**, *12*, 302–310. [CrossRef]
51. Roth, N.; Käsbohrer, A.; Mayrhofer, S.; Zitz, U.; Hofacre, C.; Domig, K.J. The application of antibiotics in broiler production and the resulting antibiotic resistance in *Escherichia coli*: A global overview. *Poult. Sci.* **2019**, *98*, 1791–1804. [CrossRef]
52. Sheikh, A.A.; Checkley, S.; Avery, B.; Chalmers, G.; Bohaychuk, V.; Boerlin, P.; Reid-Smith, R.; Aslam, M. Antimicrobial Resistance and Resistance Genes in *Escherichia coli* Isolated from Retail Meat Purchased in Alberta, Canada. *Foodborne Pathog. Dis.* **2012**, *9*, 625–631. [CrossRef]
53. Ahmed, A.M.; Shimamoto, T.; Shimamoto, T. Molecular characterization of multidrug-resistant avian pathogenic *Escherichia coli* isolated from septicemic broilers. *Int. J. Med. Microbiol.* **2013**, *303*, 475–483. [CrossRef]
54. Navia, M.A. A Chicken in Every Pot, Thanks to Sulfonamide Drugs. *Science* **2000**, *288*, 2132–2133. [CrossRef] [PubMed]
55. Diarra, M.S.; Silversides, F.G.; Diarrassouba, F.; Pritchard, J.; Masson, L.; Brousseau, R.; Bonnet, C.; Delaquis, P.; Bach, S.; Skura, B.J.; et al. Impact of Feed Supplementation with Antimicrobial Agents on Growth Performance of Broiler Chickens, Clostridium perfringens and Enterococcus Counts, and Antibiotic Resistance Phenotypes and Distribution of Antimicrobial Resistance Determinants in *Escherichia coli* Isolates. *Appl. Environ. Microbiol.* **2007**, *73*, 6566–6576. [CrossRef] [PubMed]
56. Marcelino, V.R.; Wille, M.; Hurt, A.C.; González-Acuña, D.; Klaassen, M.; Schlub, T.E.; Eden, J.-S.; Shi, M.; Iredell, J.R.; Sorrell, T.C.; et al. Meta-transcriptomics reveals a diverse antibiotic resistance gene pool in avian microbiomes. *BMC Biol.* **2019**, *17*, 1–11. [CrossRef]
57. Ecanton, R.; Egonzalez-Alba, J.M.; Egalán, J.C. CTX-M Enzymes: Origin and Diffusion. *Front. Microbiol.* **2012**, *3*, 110. [CrossRef]
58. Mavroidi, A.; Miriagou, V.; Liakopoulos, A.; Tzelepi, E.; Stefos, A.; Dalekos, G.N.; Petinaki, E. Ciprofloxacin-resistant *Escherichia coli* in Central Greece: Mechanisms of resistance and molecular identification. *BMC Infect. Dis.* **2012**, *12*, 371. [CrossRef] [PubMed]
59. Baez, M.; Espinosa, I.; Collaud, A.; Miranda, I.; Montano, D.; Feria, A.; Hernández-Fillor, R.; Obregón, D.; Alfonso, P.; Perreten, V. Genetic Features of Extended-Spectrum β-lactamase-Producing *Escherichia coli* from Poultry in Mayabeque Province, Cuba. *Antibiot.* **2021**, *10*, 107. [CrossRef] [PubMed]
60. Oh, J.-Y.; Kwon, Y.K.; Tamang, M.D.; Jang, H.-K.; Jeong, O.-M.; Lee, H.-S.; Kang, M.-S. Plasmid-Mediated Quinolone Resistance in *Escherichia coli* Isolates from Wild Birds and Chickens in South Korea. *Microb. Drug Resist.* **2016**, *22*, 69–79. [CrossRef] [PubMed]

61. Réglier-Poupet, H.; Naas, T.; Carrer, A.; Cady, A.; Adam, J.-M.; Fortineau, N.; Poyart, C.; Nordmann, P. Performance of chromID ESBL, a chromogenic medium for detection of Enterobacteriaceae producing extended-spectrum β-lactamases. *J. Med. Microbiol.* **2008**, *57*, 310–315. [CrossRef] [PubMed]
62. The European Committee on Antimicrobial Susceptibility Testing. *Breakpoint Tables for Interpretation of MICs and Zone Diameters, Version 10.0*; European Committee on Antimicrobial Susceptibility Testing: Växjö, Sweden, 2020; pp. 1–77.
63. Pérez-Pérez, F.J.; Hanson, N.D. Detection of Plasmid-Mediated AmpC-Lactamase Genes in Clinical Isolates by Using Multiplex PCR. *J. Clin. Microbiol.* **2002**, *40*, 2153–2162. [CrossRef]
64. Li, Q.; Sherwood, J.; Logue, C. Characterization of antimicrobial resistant *Escherichia coli* isolated from processed bison carcasses. *J. Appl. Microbiol.* **2007**, *103*, 2361–2369. [CrossRef]

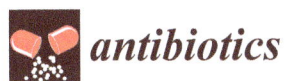

Review

Vancomycin-Resistant Enterococci (VRE) in Nigeria: The First Systematic Review and Meta-Analysis

Yusuf Wada [1,2], Azian Binti Harun [1,3], Chan Yean Yean [1] and Abdul Rahman Zaidah [1,3,*]

1. Department of Medical Microbiology and Parasitology, School of Medical Sciences, Universiti Sains Malaysia, Kubang Kerian 16150, Malaysia; wadayusuf34@gmail.com (Y.W.); azian@usm.my (A.B.H.); yeancyn@yahoo.com (C.Y.Y.)
2. Department of Zoology, Faculty of Life Sciences, Ahmadu Bello University, Zaria 810211, Nigeria
3. Hospital Universiti Sains Malaysia, Universiti Sains Malaysia, Kubang Kerian 16150, Malaysia
* Correspondence: drzaidah@usm.my; Tel.: +60-169227344

Received: 27 July 2020; Accepted: 26 August 2020; Published: 1 September 2020

Abstract: Vancomycin-Resistant Enterococci (VRE) are on the rise worldwide. Here, we report the first prevalence of VRE in Nigeria using systematic review and meta-analysis. International databases MedLib, PubMed, International Scientific Indexing (ISI), Web of Science, Scopus, Google Scholar, and African journals online (AJOL) were searched. Information was extracted by two independent reviewers, and results were reviewed by the third. Two reviewers independently assessed the study quality using the Preferred Reporting Items for Systematic Reviews and Meta-Analysis (PRISMA) checklist. OpenMeta analyst was used. The random effect was used, and publication bias was assessed using a funnel plot. Between-study heterogeneity was assessed, and the sources were analysed using the leave-one-out meta-analysis, subgroup analysis, and meta-regression. Nineteen studies met the eligibility criteria and were added to the final meta-analysis, and the study period was from 2009–2018. Of the 2552 isolates tested, 349 were VRE, and *E. faecalis* was reported the most. The pooled prevalence of VRE in Nigeria was estimated at 25.3% (95% CI; 19.8–30.8%; I^2 = 96.26%; $p < 0.001$). Between-study variability was high (t^2 = 0.011; heterogeneity I^2 = 96.26% with heterogeneity chi-square (Q) = 480.667, degrees of freedom (df) = 18, and $p = 0.001$). The funnel plot showed no publication bias, and the leave-one-out forest plot did not affect the pooled prevalence. The South-East region had a moderate heterogeneity though not significant (I^2 = 51.15%, $p = 0.129$). Meta-regression showed that all the variables listed contributed to the heterogeneity except for the animal isolate source ($p = 0.188$) and studies that were done in 2013 ($p = 0.219$). Adherence to proper and accurate antimicrobial usage, comprehensive testing, and continuous surveillance of VRE are required.

Keywords: *Enterococcus*; vancomycin resistance; systematic review; meta-analysis; Nigeria

1. Introduction

Enterococcus is a Gram-positive and catalase-negative bacterium. It is an important gastrointestinal tract normal flora of most warm-blooded animals and humans [1,2]. However, different species of Gram-positive cocci could be an opportunistic pathogen causing various infectious diseases [3,4]. *Enterococcus* species especially *Enterococcus faecium* and *Enterococcus faecalis* are two common causes of urinary tract infection [5,6], inflammation of the lining of the heart and its valves, intra-abdominal abscesses, wound infections, bacteremia, and sepsis in human [7]. It has been proven that *Enterococcus* is the second leading cause of urinary tract and wound infections and the third leading cause of bacteremia in hospitals [8]. The inherent resistance to several antibiotics and their ability to cause infections has placed enterococci on the pedestal as an important hospital-acquired pathogen [9].

Hospital-acquired infection, especially that caused by Vancomycin-Resistant Enterococci (VRE), has been on the rise regardless of their low pathogenicity and virulence. VRE prevalence in the intensive care unit (ICU) of many hospitals worldwide is high and more so when patients have an underlying health condition such as diabetes mellitus, neutropenia, and impaired renal function [10]. In the treatment of infections caused by *Enterococcus*, vancomycin and sometimes with any other aminoglycoside, is used because of its bactericidal efficacy. These antibiotics are usually used to treat infections caused by methicillin-resistant *Staphylococcus aureus* and other Gram-positive bacteria [11,12]. Vancomycin is used as the last option in the treatment of *Enterococcus* [9] as its resistance to antibiotics is as a result of either an inherent or acquired machinery. Isolates of *E. faecalis* and *E. faecium* exhibit high resistance to vancomycin while the reverse is the case for *E. gallinarum* and *E. flavescens* as they exhibit low resistance [13]. Genetic elements known as *van* genes confer resistance to *Enterococcus* of which *vanA* and *vanB* present mostly in *E. faecium* occur the most and are well-distributed, especially among hospital isolates [13]. There is a disturbing trend following several reports on the resistance of *enterococcus* to linezolid and daptomycin, two potent antibiotics used against VRE infection [14,15] while Melese et al. [16] stated that the persistent increase in nosocomial infection caused by VRE is being reported by several studies.

One of the most important goals of meta-analyses is to provide an accurate and reliable result by increasing the sample size and reducing the width of the 95% CI from the range of the various applicable studies. Several studies are reporting VRE in Nigeria as a result of its role in the livestock industry and the health sector. Nigeria is beginning to generate a lot of revenue from the livestock industry recently as a result of the border closure. This simply means that a lot of farmers would want to sell their product in time and might result in the use of growth promoters such as avoparcin. It is therefore important that this sector is closely guarded given the risk of importation of an infected and tainted product. The knowledge of VRE distribution can be used to develop a policy to curtail the spread of resistant bacteria while addressing the prevention, control, and treatment as it is of public health significance. Such a policy would ensure that healthy livestock products are consumed, and resistant bacteria monitored. It is, however, necessary to obtain the pool prevalence of VRE in Nigeria from different sources using meta-analysis to enable the Nigeria Center for Disease Control (NCDC) to develop a policy and road map for its prevention and elimination. A meta-analysis would help us validate the results of various studies reporting VRE in Nigeria and put forward a measure that is accurate and reliable.

It is based on the above points that this paper was designed to determine the pooled prevalence of VRE using a systematic literature review and meta-analysis in Nigeria.

2. Results

2.1. Search Results and Eligible Studies

Figure 1 shows the search results. A total of 500 studies were found, of which 120 were left after duplicates were removed. Of the 120 studies screened for eligibility, 97 were excluded as they did not meet any of the inclusion criteria. Twenty-three full-text articles were assessed for eligibility with four excluded since vancomycin was not used in their antimicrobial susceptibility test and had insufficient information. A total of 19 full-text studies were used for quantitative analyses.

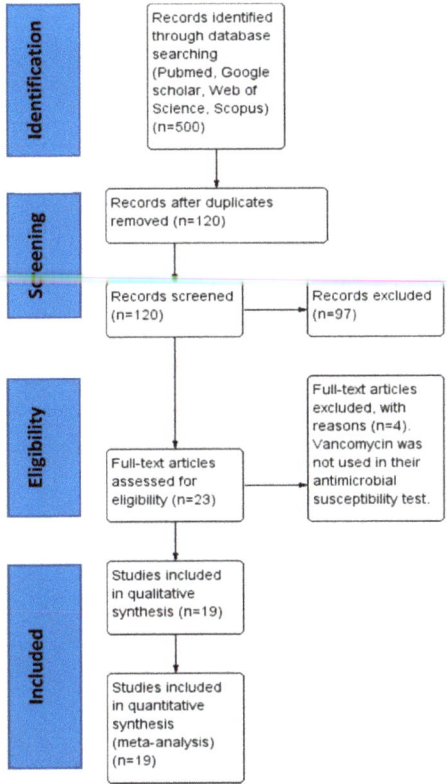

Figure 1. PRISMA flow diagram for the selection of eligible articles included in the study.

2.2. Characteristics of the Eligible Studies

All the 19 studies included in this review were cross sectional by design. Most of the studies were reported from the South-West region (n = 8) [17–24]. Other studies include the North-Central region (n = 3) [25–27], South-East region (n = 3) [28–30], South-South (n = 4) [31–34], and North-West region (n = 1) [35]. No study was reported in the North-East region of the country. Of the 2552 isolates tested, 349 were VRE. The sample size ranges from as low as 7 [17] to as high as 658 [20] and prevalence as high as 88.9% in the South-South region [31] to as low as 1.1% in the North-Central region [27] (Table 1). The highest number of VRE (n = 77) was isolated from environmental sources in the study conducted in the South-West region of Nigeria. The study analysed the highest number of specimens compared to others [20]. Most of the studies utilised the disk diffusion method in their antimicrobial susceptibility testing except for [18] and [27], who utilised agar dilution and VRE chromogenic agar, respectively (Table 1). The majority of the data included in analyses were from clinical studies (n = 8) which involved clinical specimens, and environmental studies (n = 7) with others from animal studies (n = 4) (Table 1). Details of the characteristics of the included studies are summarized in (Table 1) below and a map showing the spatial distribution and number of studies of VRE in Nigeria is shown in Figure 2.

Only 12 studies reported the reported the prevalence of VRE according to species (Table 2). *E. faecalis* was the most reported with a prevalence of 62.98% (148/235) followed by *E. faecium* with a prevalence of 21. 70% (51/235)

Table 1. Characteristics of the selected studies reporting prevalence of Vancomycin-Resistant Enterococci (VRE) in Nigeria.

Author, Publication Year	Study Year	Study Area	Isolate Sources	Sample Size	Number Positive	Prevalence (%)	Detection Method
Olawale et al., 2011 [17]	2009	South-West	Clinical specimens	7	3	42.9	Disc diffusion
Oyedeji et al., 2011 [18]	2010	South-West	Environmental	78	14	18	Agar dilution
Oguntoyinbo & Okueso, 2013 [25]	2012	North-Central	Environmental	95	32	33.7	Disc diffusion
Olawale et al., 2014 [19]	2012	South-West	Environmental	246	10	4.1	Disc diffusion
Anyanwu & Obetta, 2015 [28]	2015	South-East	Animal	75	5	6.7	Disc diffusion
Olawale et al., 2015 [20]	2013	South-West	Environmental	658	77	11.7	Disc diffusion
Ayeni et al., 2016 [21]	2015	South-West	Animal	60	39	65	Disc diffusion
Nsofor et al., 2016 [29]	2016	South-East	Clinical	34	7	20.59	Disc diffusion
Ekuma et al., 2016 [22]	2013	South-West	Clinical	319	13	4.07	E test
Adesida et al., 2017 [23]	2017	South-West	Clinical	65	9	13.85	Disc diffusion
David et al., 2017 [24]	2017	South-West	Clinical	69	27	39.13	Disc diffusion
Enenya et al., 2017 [35]	2014	North-West	Environmental	16	4	25	Disc diffusion
Ndubuisi et al., 2017 [26]	2017	North-Central	Clinical	102	34	33.3	Disc diffusion
Foka et al., 2018 [31]	2018	South-South	Environmental	9	8	88.9	Disc diffusion
Abasiubong et al., 2019 [32]	2018	South-South	Clinical	19	13	68.4	Disc diffusion
Anyanwu et al., 2019 [30]	2018	South-East	Animal	30	7	23.3	Disc diffusion
Igbinosa & Beshiru., 2019 [33]	2018	South-South	Animal	59	22	37.3	Disc diffusion
Igbinosa & Raje, 2019 [34]	2017	South-South	Environmental	64	23	35.9	Disc diffusion
Shettima & Iregbu, 2019 [27]	2015	North-Central	Clinical	545	6	1.1	VRE Chromogenic agar

Table 2. Species distribution of VRE across studies.

Author, Publication Year	E. faecium	E. faecalis	E. gallinarum	E. casseliflavus	E. mundti	E. hirae	E. dispar	Total
Olawale et al., 2011 [17]	1	2	-	-	-	-	-	3
Olawale et al., 2014 [19]	-	10	-	-	-	-	-	10
Olawale et al., 2015 [20]	-	77	-	-	-	-	-	77
Nsofor et al., 2016 [29]	4	3	-	-	-	-	-	7
Ekuma et al., 2016 [22]	3	-	9	1	-	-	-	13
Adesida et al., 2017 [23]	6	3	-	-	-	-	-	9
David et al., 2017 [24]	-	27	-	-	-	-	-	27
Enenya et al., 2017 [35]	2	-	1	1	-	-	-	4
Ndubuisi et al., 2017 [26]	12	10	1	-	9	1	1	34
Igbinosa & Beshiru., 2019 [33]	13	8	1	-	-	-	-	22
Igbinosa & Raje, 2019 [34]	7	8	-	2	-	3	3	23
Shettima & Iregbu, 2019 [27]	3	-	2	1	-	-	-	6
	51 (21.7%)	148 (62.98%)	14 (5.96%)	5 (2.13%)	9 (3.83%)	4 (1.70%)	4 (1.70%)	235

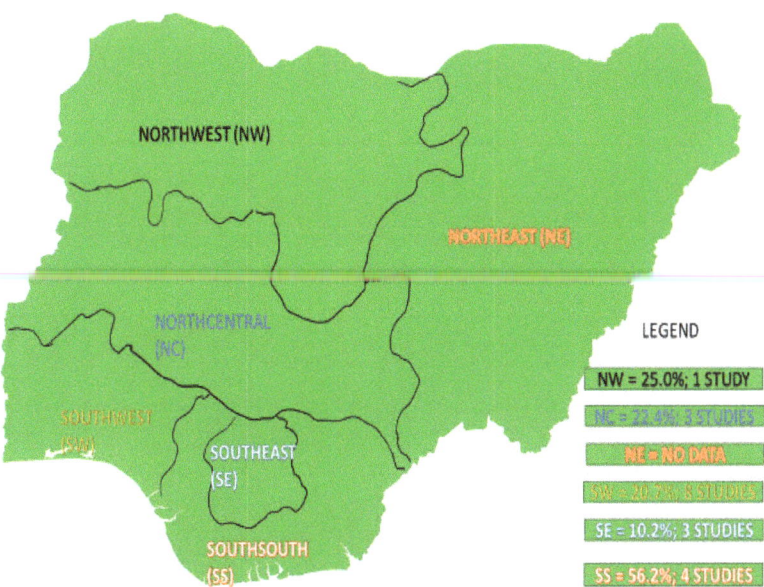

Figure 2. Spatial distribution and number of studies of VRE in Nigeria based on data extracted from eligible studies.

2.3. The Pooled Prevalence of VRE

The pooled prevalence of VRE in Nigeria was estimated at 25.3% (95% CI; 19.8–30.8%; I^2 = 96.26%; $p < 0.001$) (Figure 3). Random-effects meta-analyses were carried out using the total sample size and number of positives (effect size, standard error of effect size) to estimate the prevalence of VRE in Nigeria. Between-study variability was high (t^2 = 0.011; heterogeneity I^2 = 96.26% with heterogeneity chi-square (Q) = 480.667, degrees of freedom (df) = 18, and $p = 0.001$).

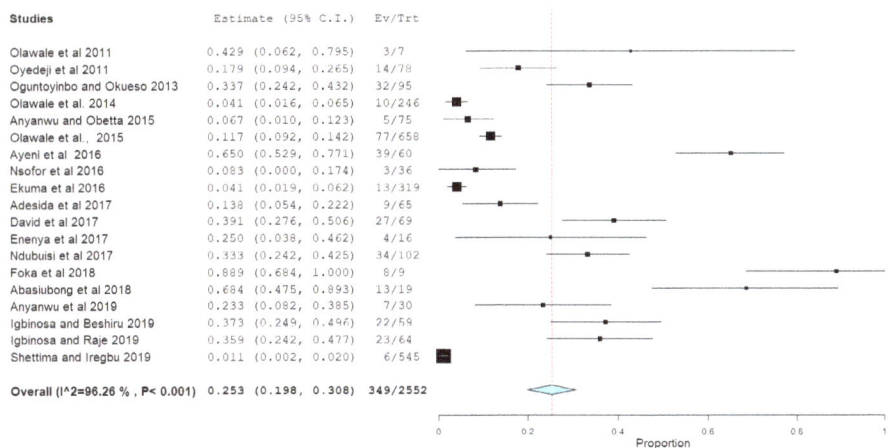

Figure 3. Forest plot showing the pooled prevalence of VRE in Nigeria.

Sensitivity analysis using the leave-one-out forest plot revealed that no single study significantly influenced the heterogeneity and pooled prevalence of VRE (25.3%; 95% CI; 19.8–30.8%; $p < 0.001$) (Figure 4). The presence of publication bias was observed from the drawn asymmetric funnel plot (Figure 5) which indicates no publication bias.

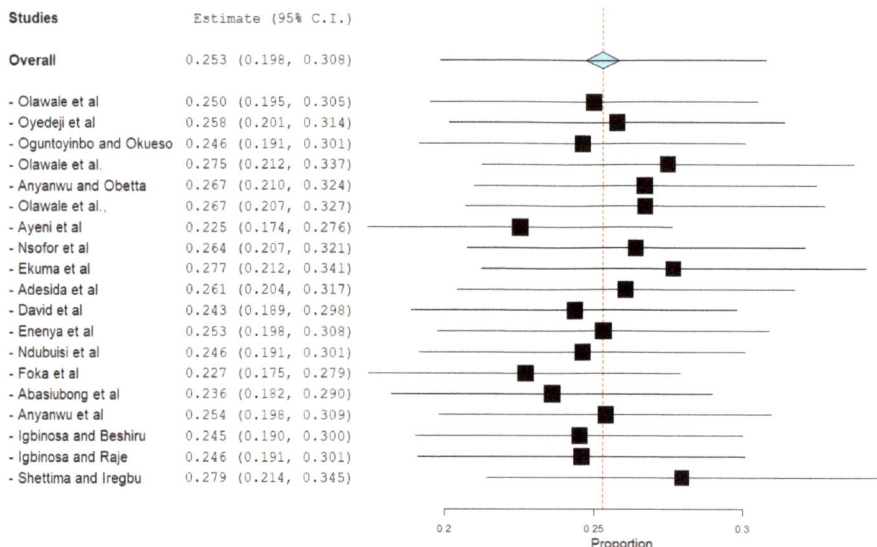

Figure 4. Leave-one-out forest plot of VRE in Nigeria.

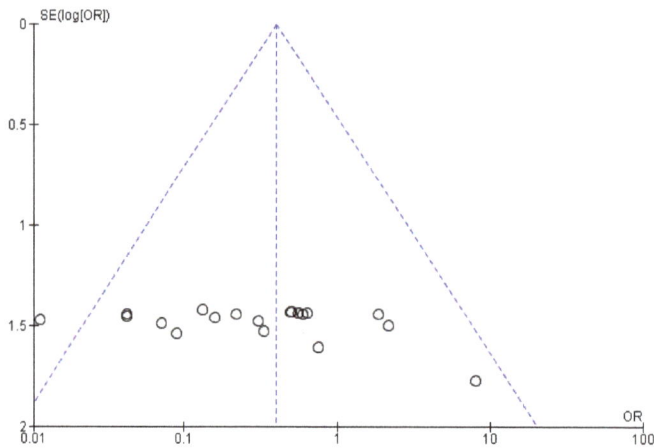

Figure 5. Funnel plot showing no publication bias.

2.4. Subgroup Meta-Analysis

Since this meta-analysis showed substantial heterogeneity, subgroup analysis was done using the study period, study area, isolate sources, and detection method to identify the possible sources of heterogeneity among the studies. The result of subgroup meta-analysis by study region revealed overall large variability in studies reporting the prevalence of VRE (the Higgins I^2 statistic = 96.26% with heterogeneity chi-square (Q) = 480.667, degrees of freedom = 18, and $p < 0.001$). The Southeast region was the only region with moderate heterogeneity, though not significant ($I^2 = 51.15\%$, $p = 0.129$), revealing a probable cause of heterogeneity. The overall statistics are shown in Table 3.

Table 3. Subgroup analysis for comparisons of the prevalence of VRE across study regions.

Study Region	Number of Studies	Prevalence (%)	95% CI	I^2 (%)	Q	Heterogeneity Test	
						DF	p
South-West	8	20.7	13.1–28.2	95.5	155.404	7	<0.001
North-Central	3	22.4	−3.6–48.3	97.81	91.227	2	<0.001
South-East	3	10.2	2.7–17.8	51.15	4.094	2	0.129
North-West	1	25.0	3.8–46.2	NA	-	-	-
South-South	4	56.2	33.5–79.0	88.37	25.802	3	<0.001
Overall	19	25.3	19.8–30.8	96.26	480.667	18	<0.001

Similarly, the result of subgroup meta-analysis by isolate source revealed the highest variability in isolates from clinical ($I^2 = 195.18\%$), followed by the environment ($I^2 = 95.33\%$), and animal sources ($I^2 = 96.37\%$). Isolates from environmental sources had the highest prevalence (27.2%, CI 17.3–13.2%). The overall statistics are shown in Table 4.

Table 4. Subgroup analysis for comparison of prevalence of VRE among isolate sources.

Isolate Source	Number of Studies	Prevalence (%)	95% CI	I^2 (%)	Q	Heterogeneity Test	
						DF	p
Clinical	8	19.9	12.5–27.2	195.18	145.362	7	<0.001
Environmental	7	27.2	17.3–37.2	95.33	128.519	6	<0.001
Animal	4	32.9	5.1–60.7	96.37	82.535	3	<0.001
Overall	19	25.3	19.8–30.8	96.26	480.667	18	<0.001

Further, the result of subgroup meta-analysis by the detection method revealed that 16 of the studies utilised the disc diffusion method in their antimicrobial susceptibility test accounting for a prevalence of 33.8% with a CI of 24.3–43.4% and I^2 of 93.84%. The overall statistics are shown in Table 5.

Table 5. Subgroup analysis for comparison of prevalence of VRE using various detection methods.

Detection Method	Number of Studies	Prevalence (%)	95% CI	I^2 (%)	Q	Heterogeneity Test	
						DF	p
Disc diffusion	15	33.8	24.3–43.4	93.84	227.406	14	<0.001
Disc diffusion	1	4.1	1.6–6.5	-	-	-	-
Agar dilution	1	17.9	9.4–26.5	-	-	-	-
E test	1	1.9	1.9–6.2	-	-	-	-
VRE chromogenic agar	1	1.1	1.1–0.2	-	-	-	-
Overall	19	25.3	19.8–30.8	96.26	480.667	18	<0.001

Finally, the result of subgroup meta-analysis by study period revealed that the years 2017 and 2018 had four studies each, and the study period ranged from 2009 to 2018. The prevalence of VRE ranged from 42.9%, CI 6.2–79.5% in 2009 to 53.6%, CI 26.5–80.7%, indicating an increase in the prevalence of VRE over 10 years. The overall statistics are shown in Table 6.

Table 6. Subgroup analysis for comparison of prevalence of VRE across study periods.

Study Period	Number of Studies	Prevalence (%)	95% CI	I^2 (%)	Q	Heterogeneity Test	
						DF	p
2009	1	42.9	6.2–79.5	-	-	-	-
2010	1	17.9	9.4–26.5	-	-	-	-
2012	2	18.5	−10.4–47.5	97.14	34.954	1	<0.001
2013	2	7.9	4.0–15.3	95.19	20.806	1	<0.001
2014	1	25.0	3.8–46.2	-	-	-	-
2015	3	23.1	0.7–45.5	98.19	110.342	2	<0.001
2016	1	8.3	−0.7–17.4	-	-	-	-
2017	4	30.2	18.0–42.3	82.92	17.560	3	<0.001
2018	4	53.6	26.5–80.7	90.54	31.711	3	<0.001
Overall	19	25.3	19.8–30.8	96.26	480.667	18	<0.001

2.5. Meta-Regression

Meta-regression analysis was done for each variable included in the study individually. The variables included were study region, study year, isolate sources, and detection method. Continuous variables were subjected to assessment to observe a linear relationship with the independent effect size. Variables with p-values < 0.25 were used in the multivariable meta-regression analysis. Independent variables such as study region, study year, isolate sources, and detection method had a reasonably significant value and were retained in the final multivariate analysis. Most of the variables were significantly associated with the prevalence of VRE in the final multivariate meta-regression except for the animal isolate source ($p = 0.188$) and studies done in 2013 ($p = 0.219$). Interestingly, all the variables listed contributed to the heterogeneity observed in this study except for the animal isolate source and studies done in 2013. No result was computed for the study period 2016–2018. The final multivariate meta-regression is shown in Table 7 below.

Table 7. Final multivariable meta-regression model.

Variable	Coefficient	p-Value	95% CI
Study area			
South-West	Reference		
North-Central	0.175	0.005	5.2–29.8
North-West	−1.044	<0.001	−142.1–−66.7
South-East	−0.533	<0.001	−65.9–−40.7
South-South	−0.286	0.003	−47.7–−9.4
Isolates source			
Clinical	Reference		
Animal	0.273	0.188	−13.3–67.9
Environmental	0.865	<0.001	38.4–134.6
Detection method			
Disc diffusion	Reference		
Agar dilution	−1.114	<0.001	−143.7–−79.2
E test	0.371	<0.001	16.7–57.5
VRE chromogenic agar	−0.917	<0.001	−113.9–−69.6
Study period			
2009	Reference		
2010	−1.132	<0.001	−147.8–−78.6
2012	−1.177	<0.001	−148.9–−86.5
2013	−0.093	0.219	−24.1–55.0
2014	−0.230	0.041	−45.1–−0.9
2015	−0.688	<0.001	−87.9–−49.6
Constant	0.429	0.022	6.2–79.5

3. Discussion

To the best of our knowledge, this is the first study to determine the prevalence of VRE in Nigeria using systematic review and meta-analysis. For interventions to be accurately formulated, the prevalence of VRE needs to be known. The NCDC has a program in collaboration with the Federal Ministries of Health, Agriculture and Rural Development and Environment designed to checkmate antimicrobial resistance (AMR) [36]. A National AMR Technical Working Group (AMR-TWG) was inaugurated with members from several sectors such as human and animal health, food animal production, and the environment. The objective of this group is to analyse the situation of AMR in Nigeria and to develop an action plan for its prevention treatment and control. This is a robust plan, but the plan did not list VRE as a priority pathogen given that VRE is one of the most common causes of nosocomial infection worldwide.

The results presented in this report were from the analysis of data obtained through a systematic review of scientific publications on the prevalence of VRE at the country level between the years of 2009–2019, and the literature was heterogeneous. This review did not only take into consideration VRE in clinical settings but also in animals and the environment to get a holistic picture of VRE in Nigeria. The final meta-analysis of the prevalence was done only on 19 articles.

The random effect meta-analysis result showed high variability with Higgin's I^2, which indicates that the variability between studies was not as a result of chance alone. The detection method, study region, study period, and clinical and environmental isolate source were highly significant predictors of the prevalence of VRE, indicating that these variables explain a substantial portion of the variability between studies. However, the animal isolate source and studies done in 2013 retained in the final meta-regression seem statistically insignificant in explaining the study variability.

Although considerable methodological differences between studies existed, these differences were pooled for this review. Therefore, the pooled prevalence of VRE in Nigeria was estimated at 25.3%. This indirectly indicates the potential existence of VRE, not only in health care settings but in in the environment as well as animals in Nigeria, and its likely spread to communities unless properly contained. Our estimate is comparable with reports from Malaysia 25% [37] but higher than those reported in Ethiopia 14.8% [16], Iran 14%, 18.75% [38,39], North America (21%), Asia (24%), Europe (20%) [40], Germany (9.8%) [41], Iran (9.4%) [42], the United Kingdom (9.2%) [43], and Singapore (9.3%) [44]. Our estimate was probably higher because our studies included animal and environmental sources in addition to clinical settings unlike all the studies listed above where they largely centred on clinical settings. This high prevalence could be as a result of various risk factors such as contact with VRE patients, infected animals, surfaces and objects, underlying conditions, serious illness, prior hospitalization, use of catheters, and improper antibiotic usage [45]. Camins et al. [46] stated that health care contacts were the likely source of VRE colonization and infection, and this is plausible in situations where infection control knowledge, attitudes, and practices among healthcare workers, farmworkers, and the general population are poor in third-world countries [47–50] and Nigeria [26]. The antimicrobial susceptibility testing mainly relied on the disc diffusion method and was interpreted according to the Clinical and Laboratory Standard Institute (CLSI) guideline. However, agar dilution and VRE chromogenic agar were also used. Another study in Iran by Shokoohizadeh et al. [51] reported a 48.9% higher prevalence in patients hospitalised than this study estimate. Adams et al. [52] stated that the prevalence of VRE tends to be higher in critically ill and hospitalised patients than n non-hospitalised patients, unlike this present study where isolate sources were diverse. Another probable reason might be the study period as these studies were mostly done in the 1990s and 2000's following the first reports of VRE [53,54], while the oldest study from our analysis was in 2009 and the earliest in 2019 where a ban was already placed on the indiscriminate use of vancomycin [55].

Results obtained from this review indicate that *E. faecalis* is the most reported VRE and this might be because most enterococcal infections are caused by *E. faecalis* [56] and can be treated with aminoglycosides and beta lactams. Because resistance to vancomycin is more regular in homogenous *E. faecalis*, administering of beta lactams should be at the forefront before the use of conventional culture [56]. Arias and Murray [57] and Davis et al. [58] stated that most VRE infections were caused by *E. faecalis*. This has changed as more VRE caused by *E. faecium* are increasingly being reported [59–61] because of their resistance to different group of antibiotics which are mostly expensive [62,63]. In *E. faecalis*, however, there is a marked difference in the occurrence and nature of resistance [64,65] even though *E faecalis* exhibit some level of acquired resistance.

Prevalence of VRE based on study area or region was also estimated. The highest estimated prevalence was in the South-South (56.2%) which is more than twice that estimated in the South-West (20.7%), North-Central (22.4%), South-East (10.2%) and North-West (25.0%). These regional differences could be ascribed to the type of environment and animal samples obtained, study period, the disparity in antibiotic use, detection method, and specimen type. No study or estimate was reported in the North-East of Nigeria. This is probably because this region has been plagued by insecurity as a result of insurgency which could deter researchers from conducting research [66].

According to data analyses for the isolate source, VRE prevalence was high in clinical, animal, and environmental sources and this is worrisome. These estimates indicate the depth of the spread of VRE in Nigeria and is one of the strengths of this study. Conducting these studies in different regions and isolates sources has provided a subtle picture of the prevalence in Nigeria. This does not give an in-depth explanation of the status of VRE in Nigeria, but it can be used as baseline information in its control.

In addition to obtaining isolates from different sources as strength of our study, our study also included a rigorous search with precise inclusion and exclusion criteria and we also observed frequently used specimens and methods of susceptibility testing. Several limitations also existed and these were our inability to report pooled estimates of VRE at the species level due to the limited number of included studies reporting enterococci at the species level, unavailability of studies from the Northeast region of Nigeria, which throws more question on the exact status of VRE in Nigeria, non-use of unpublished reports, and finally, the protocol of our study was not registered in PROSPERO.

4. Materials and Methods

4.1. Study Design and Protocol

The protocol of this study was designed according to the Preferred Reporting Items for Systematic Reviews and Meta-Analysis Protocol (PRISMA-P 2015) guidelines [67] (Supplementary file S1). The risk of bias across studies and the risk of bias graph are presented in Supplementary file S2.

4.2. Literature Review

A systematic review and meta-analysis were performed first by searching the PROSPERO database and database of abstracts of reviews of effects (DARE) (http://www.library.UCSF.edu) to check whether published or ongoing projects exist related to the topic. The literature search strategy, selection of studies, data extraction, and result reporting were done in accordance with the Preferred Reporting Items for Systematic Reviews and Meta-Analyses (PRISMA) guidelines. International databases MedLib, PubMed, ISI, Web of Science, Scopus, Google Scholar, and African journals online (AJOL) for published studies about the prevalence of VRE were also searched. PubMed was searched using the search strategy ("enterococcus"[MeSH Terms] OR "enterococcus"[All Fields]) AND ("nigeria"[MeSH Terms] OR "nigeria"[All Fields]), VRE [All Fields] AND ("nigeria"[MeSH Terms] OR "nigeria"[All Fields], ("epidemiology"[Subheading] OR "epidemiology"[All Fields] OR "prevalence"[All Fields] OR "prevalence"[MeSH Terms]) AND ("vancomycin-resistant enterococci"[MeSH Terms] OR ("vancomycin-resistant"[All Fields] AND "enterococci"[All Fields]) OR "vancomycin-resistant enterococci"[All Fields] OR ("vancomycin"[All Fields] AND "resistant"[All Fields] AND "enterococci"[All Fields]) OR "vancomycin resistant enterococci"[All Fields]) AND ("nigeria"[MeSH Terms] OR "nigeria"[All Fields]). Another search was also performed using keywords and their English equivalent (clinical infections, environmental

VRE, VRE in poultry and farm animals, Gram-positive bacteria, enterococci, antibiotic resistance, glycopeptide, vancomycin, and Nigeria) with all possible combinations. Also, the titles and references from selected articles were an additional search tool. To reduce bias, the search process was conducted independently by two authors.

4.3. Inclusion and Exclusion Criteria for Studies

We considered all cross-sectional or cohort studies that reported the prevalence of vancomycin resistance in *Enterococcus* isolates or numbers of VRE and total enterococci isolates in patients suspected of having clinical infection, in poultry, poultry/animal product, farmworkers, and the environment in Nigeria. We also included studies in which the standard method was used to detect VRE and were published or reported in English.

Exclusion criteria for the analysis were as follows: studies with insufficient information; studies on antimicrobial susceptibility tests other than vancomycin (studies that did not include VRE), studies having fewer than two isolates, studies not reporting enterococcal isolates separately (no population denominator), reviews, comments and duplications, case report studies, and studies that did not report the prevalence of VRE.

4.4. Data Extraction

After studies were identified based on their eligibility criteria, the first author's name, the publication year, the date of the study, the study location, the number of cases involved in the studies, the study method, the source of isolates, the sample size, and the prevalence of VRE infections were extracted from the manuscripts. Two independent reviewers extracted all data from the articles included, and the results were reviewed by the third reviewer. Inconsistencies between the reviewers were decided by a consensus. The published studies were examined in three steps: title, abstract, and full text.

4.5. Data Analysis

Prevalence of VRE was calculated and subgroup analyses were done according to the study region, isolate sources, and detection method. Considering the existence of heterogeneity in observational studies conducted in diverse settings, the random-effects model was used in determining the pooled prevalence of VRE which prompted the use of the DerSimonian and Laird method of meta-analysis [68,69].

4.6. Bias and Heterogeneity Analysis

The qualities of the study methods (study area, isolate source, and detection method) were used to assess the within-study biases. The across-study bias (small study effects) was examined by funnel plots. The heterogeneities of study-level estimates were assessed by Cochran's Q test. Non-significant heterogeneity was accepted if the ratio of Q and the degrees of freedom (Q/df) was less than one. The percentage of the variation in prevalence estimates attributable to heterogeneity was measured by the inverse variance index (I^2), and I^2 values of 25%, 50%, and 75% were considered low, moderate, and high heterogeneity, respectively [69]. In this meta-analysis, the I^2 value was high (96.26%) which is >75% an indication of significant heterogeneity. Due to this reason, the analysis was conducted using a random-effects model at 95% CI instead of the fixed-effects model. Funnel plot subgroup analyses were done if the heterogeneities were moderate to high. The sources of heterogeneity were analysed using the sensitivity analysis (leave-one-out meta-analysis), subgroup analysis, and meta-regression. Meta-analysis was performed using OpenMeta Analyst software version 10.10 [70].

5. Conclusions

We designed this study to obtain the pooled prevalence of VRE in Nigeria to provide baseline information to the National AMR Technical Working Group. The pooled prevalence of VRE in Nigeria was estimated at 25.3% (95% CI; 19.8–30.8%; $I^2 = 96.26\%$; $p < 0.001$) and *E. faecalis* is the most reported VRE. The prevalence of VRE is on the rise in Nigeria seeing the trend from the oldest to the earliest studies. High variability between studies may influence the estimate pooled prevalence at the national level. This can be overcome by using advanced diagnostic techniques in the detection of VRE and the implementation of a nationwide survey to estimate the true prevalence of VRE in Nigeria. This report indicates that a program directly targeting VRE nationally be in place and VRE be listed as a priority pathogen to reduce the burden of the infection. Adherence to proper and accurate antimicrobial usage, comprehensive testing and ongoing surveillance of VRE infections in the health care, community and environmental settings are required.

Availability of Data and Materials: The datasets used and/or analyzed during the current study are included in the manuscript.

Supplementary Materials: The following are available online at http://www.mdpi.com/2079-6382/9/9/565/s1, File S1: Preferred Reporting Items for Systematic Reviews and Meta-Analysis Protocol (PRISMA-P 2015) guidelines File S2: The risk of bias across studies and the risk of bias graph.

Author Contributions: Y.W. Conceived and designed the study; Y.W., C.Y.Y. select and assess quality of studies; extracted and analyzed data; Y.W., A.B.H. interpreted results; and drafted the manuscript. Y.W., A.R.Z. select and assess quality of studies; extracted data and interpret results. A.R.Z. interpret results and review the manuscript. All authors have read and agreed to the published version of the manuscript.

Funding: RUI Universiti Sains Malaysia (USM) grant with number 1001.PPSP.8012259 and the USM Fellowship.

Acknowledgments: This meta-analysis and systematic review are supported by the RUI Universiti Sains Malaysia (USM) grant with number 1001.PPSP.8012259 and the USM Fellowship.

Conflicts of Interest: The authors declare no conflict of interest.

References

1. Wada, Y.; Harun, A.B.; Yean, C.Y.; Zaidah, A.R.; Wada, Y. Vancomycin-Resistant Enterococcus: Issues in Human Health, Animal Health, Resistant Mechanisms and the Malaysian Paradox. *Adv. Anim. Veter-Sci.* **2019**, *7*, 1021–1034. [CrossRef]
2. Iseppi, R.; Di Cerbo, A.; Messi, P.; Sabia, C. Antibiotic Resistance and Virulence Traits in Vancomycin-Resistant Enterococci (VRE) and Extended-Spectrum β-Lactamase/AmpC-producing (ESBL/AmpC) Enterobacteriaceae from Humans and Pets. *Antibiotics* **2020**, *9*, 152. [CrossRef] [PubMed]
3. Adapa, S.; Naramala, S.; Boken, D.; Moreno, A.; Konala, V.M. Peritonitis from Anaerobic Gram-positive Cocci Likely Due to Translocation of Bacteria from Gut in a Patient Undergoing Peritoneal Dialysis. *Cureus* **2019**, *11*. [CrossRef] [PubMed]
4. Argudín, M. Ángeles; Deplano, A.; Meghraoui, A.; Dodémont, M.; Heinrichs, A.; Denis, O.; Nonhoff, C.; Roisin, S. Bacteria from Animals as a Pool of Antimicrobial Resistance Genes. *Antibiotics* **2017**, *6*, 12. [CrossRef]
5. Rostkowska, O.M.; Kuthan, R.; Burban, A.; Salińska, J.; Ciebiera, M.; Mlynarczyk, G.; Durlik, M. Analysis of Susceptibility to Selected Antibiotics in Klebsiella pneumoniae, Escherichia coli, Enterococcus faecalis and Enterococcus faecium Causing Urinary Tract Infections in Kidney Transplant Recipients over 8 Years: Single-Center Study. *Antibiotics* **2020**, *9*, 284. [CrossRef]
6. Folliero, V.; Caputo, P.; Della Rocca, M.T.; Chianese, A.; Galdiero, M.; Iovene, M.R.; Hay, C.; Franci, G.; Galdiero, M. Prevalence and Antimicrobial Susceptibility Patterns of Bacterial Pathogens in Urinary Tract Infections in University Hospital of Campania "Luigi Vanvitelli" between 2017 and 2018. *Antibiotics* **2020**, *9*, 215. [CrossRef]
7. Banik, A.; Halder, S.K.; Ghosh, C.; Mondal, K.C. *Enterococcal Infections, Drug Resistance, and Application of Nanotechnology*; Springer Science and Business Media LLC: New York, NY, USA, 2020; pp. 417–445.
8. Bhardwaj, S.B. Enterococci: An Important Nosocomial Pathogen. In *Pathogenic Bacteria [Working Title]*; IntechOpen: Rijeka, Croatia, 2019.

9. Bender, J.K.; Cattoir, V.; Hegstad, K.; Sadowy, E.; Coque, T.M.; Westh, H.; Hammerum, A.M.; Schaffer, K.; Burns, K.; Murchan, S.; et al. Update on prevalence and mechanisms of resistance to linezolid, tigecycline and daptomycin in enterococci in Europe: Towards a common nomenclature. *Drug Resist. Updat.* **2018**, *40*, 25–39. [CrossRef]
10. Wada, Y.H.; Harun, A.; Yean, C.; Nasir, N.M.; Zaidah, A.R.; Wada, Y. Vancomycin-resistant enterococcus, obesity and antibiotics: Is there a possible link? *Obes. Med.* **2020**, *18*, 100226. [CrossRef]
11. Freitas, A.R.; Tedim, A.P.; Coque, T.M.; Jensen, L.; Novais, C.; Peixe, L.; Sánchez-Valenzuela, A.; Sundsfjord, A.; Hegstad, K.; Werner, G.; et al. Multilevel population genetic analysis ofvanAandvanB Enterococcus faeciumcausing nosocomial outbreaks in 27 countries (1986–2012). *J. Antimicrob. Chemother.* **2016**, *71*, 3351–3366. [CrossRef]
12. Hammerum, T.M.; Pedersen, M.G.; Nielsen, L.C.; Ma, C.M.C.; Saee, L.M.; Worning, P.; Østergaard, C.; Westh, H.; Pinholt, M.; Schoenning, K. Emergence of a vancomycin-variable Enterococcus faecium ST1421 strain containing a deletion in vanX. *J. Antimicrob. Chemother.* **2018**, *73*, 2936–2940. [CrossRef]
13. Lee, T.; Pang, S.; Abraham, S.; Coombs, G.W. Molecular characterization and evolution of the first outbreak of vancomycin-resistant Enterococcus faecium in Western Australia. *Int. J. Antimicrob. Agents* **2019**, *53*, 814–819. [CrossRef] [PubMed]
14. Lee, B.J.; Vu, B.N.; Seddon, A.N.; Hodgson, H.A.; Wang, S.K. Treatment Considerations for CNS Infections Caused by Vancomycin-Resistant Enterococcus faecium: A Focused Review of Linezolid and Daptomycin. *Ann. Pharmacother.* **2020**, 106002802093251. [CrossRef]
15. Ross, J.L.; Rankin, S.; Marshik, P.; Mercier, R.-C.; Brett, M.; Walraven, C.J. Antimicrobial Stewardship Intervention and Feedback to Infectious Disease Specialists: A Case Study in High-Dose Daptomycin. *Antibiotics* **2015**, *4*, 309–320. [CrossRef] [PubMed]
16. Dagnaw, A.M.; Genet, C.; Andualem, T. Prevalence of Vancomycin resistant enterococci (VRE) in Ethiopia: A systematic review and meta-analysis. *BMC Infect. Dis.* **2020**, *20*, 1–12. [CrossRef]
17. Olawale, K.; Fadiora, S.; Taiwo, S. Prevalence of hospital acquired enterococci infections in two primary-care hospitals in Osogbo, Southwestern Nigeria. *Afr. J. Infect. Dis.* **2011**, *5*, 40–46. [CrossRef]
18. Oyedeji, O.; Olutiola, P.O.; Owolabi, K.D.; Adeojo, K.A. Multiresistant faecal indicator bacteria in stream and well waters of Ile-ife city, southwestern Nigeria: Public health implications. *J. Public Health Epidemiol.* **2011**. Available online: https://academicjournals.org/journal/JPHE/article-abstract/5C2D8F51666 (accessed on 22 March 2020).
19. Olawale, A.K.; Akinro, E.B.; Olawale, A.O.; Olakunle, T.P. Transmission of Antibiotic-Resistant Enterococcus faecalis through Currency Notes. *Am. J. Biol. Life Sci.* **2014**, *2*, 162–165. Available online: http://www.opensciencenonline.com/journal/archive2?journalId704&paperId1078 (accessed on 22 March 2020).
20. Olawale, A.; Salako, R.; Famurewa, O. Antibiotic-Resistant Enterococcus faecalis Isolated from Food Canteens in Osun States, Nigeria. *Br. Microbiol. Res. J.* **2015**, *6*, 196–206. [CrossRef]
21. Ayeni, F.A.; Odumosu, B.T.; Oluseyi, A.E.; Ruppitsch, W. Identification and prevalence of tetracycline resistance in enterococci isolated from poultry in Ilishan, Ogun State, Nigeria. *J. Pharm. Bioallied Sci.* **2016**, *8*, 69. [CrossRef]
22. Ekuma, A.E.; Oduyebo, O.O.; Efunshile, A.M.; Konig, B. Surveillance for Vancomycin Resistant Enterococci in a Tertiary Institution in South Western Nigeria. *Afr. J. Infect. Dis.* **2016**, *10*, 121–126. [CrossRef]
23. Adesida, S.A.; Ezenta, C.C.; Adagbada, A.O.; Aladesokan, A.A.; Coker, A.O. Carriage of Multidrug Resistant Enterococcus Faecium and Enterococcus Faecalis among Apparently Healthy Humans. *Afr. J. Infect. Dis.* **2017**, *11*, 83–89. [CrossRef] [PubMed]
24. David, O.M.; Imonitie, K.; Osuntoyinbo, R.T.; Olawale, A.K. Virulence Factors and Beta-Lactamase Production among Vancomycin-Resistant Enterococcus Faecalis Isolated from Clinical Samples and Hospital Environment. *Int. J. Biol. Res.* **2017**, *5*, 1–5. [CrossRef]
25. Oguntoyinbo, F.A.; Okueso, O. Prevalence, distribution and antibiotic resistance pattern among enterococci species in two traditional fermented dairy foods. *Ann. Microbiol.* **2012**, *63*, 755–761. [CrossRef]
26. Ndubuisi, J.C.; Olonitola, O.S.; Olayinka, A.T.; Jatau, E.D.; Iregbu, K.C. Prevalence and antibiotics susceptibility profile of Enterococcus spp. Isolated from some hospitals in Abuja, Nigeria. *Afr. J. Clin. Exp. Microbiol.* **2017**, *18*, 154. [CrossRef]
27. Shettima, S.A.; Iregbu, K.C. Antimicrobial Resistance Pattern of Enterococci Isolated from Stool Samples in a Tertiary Hospital in Nigeria. *Ann. Trop. Pathol.* **2019**, *10*, 126. [CrossRef]

28. Anyanwu, M.U.; Obetta, T.U. Prevalence and Antibiogram of Generic Enterococci in Ready-to-Slaughter Beef Cattle. *Not. Sci. Boil.* **2015**, *7*, 390–399. [CrossRef]
29. Nsofor, C.A. High Antibiotic Resistance Pattern Observed in Bacterial Isolates from a Tertiary Hospital in South East Nigeria. *Int. J. Res. Pharm. Biosci.* **2016**, *3*, 1–6.
30. Anyanwu, M.U.; Okorie-Kanu, O.J.; Ogugua, A.J.; Ezenduka, E.V.; Anidebe, C.O. Occurrence, Antibiogram and Vancomycin Resistance of Generic Enterococci in Horses in Nigeria. *Revue Méd. Vét.* **2019**, *170*, 46–52.
31. Foka, F.E.T.; Yah, C.S.; Bissong, M.E.A. Physico-Chemical Properties and Microbiological Quality of Borehole Water in Four Crowded Areas of Benin City, Nigeria, During Rainfalls. *Shiraz E-Med. J.* **2018**, *19*. [CrossRef]
32. Abasiubong, V.N.; Ikon, G.M.; Amadi, C.P. Enterococcus Isolates in Clinical Samples from In-Patients in Uyo, Nigeria. *Int. J. Life Sci. Res.* **2019**, *7*, 353–358.
33. Igbinosa, E.O.; Beshiru, A. Antimicrobial Resistance, Virulence Determinants, and Biofilm Formation of Enterococcus Species from Ready-to-Eat Seafood. *Front. Microbiol.* **2019**, *10*, 728. [CrossRef] [PubMed]
34. Igbinosa, I.H.; Raje, O.C. Characterization of Enterococcus species isolated from abattoir environment in Benin city, Nigeria. *Ife J. Sci.* **2020**, *21*, 81. [CrossRef]
35. Enenya, R.P.; Yakubu, S.E.; Ado, S.A.; Ella, E.E.; Igwe, J.C. Antibiotic Resistance Profile of Enterococcus species Isolated from Drinking Water Sources in Zaria, Kaduna State, Nigeria. *J. Trop. Biosci.* **2017**, *12*, 20–25. Available online: https://www.researchgate.net/profile/Rufus_Enenya/publication/325688794_Antibiotic_Resistance_Profile_of_Enterococcus_species_Isolated_from_Drinking_Water_Sources_in_Zaria_Kaduna_State_Nigeria/links/5b1e5cf745851587f29feef1/Antibiotic-Resistance-Profile-of-Enterococcus-species-Isolated-from-Drinking-Water-Sources-in-Zaria-Kaduna-State-Nigeria.pdf (accessed on 23 March 2020).
36. Federal Ministries of Agriculture, Environment and Health. In *National Action Plan for Antimicrobial Resistance 2017–2022*; 2017. Available online: https://ncdc.gov.ng/themes/common/docs/protocols/77_1511368219.pdf (accessed on 8 August 2020).
37. Wada, Y.; Harun, A.B.; Chan, Y.Y.; Mohamad Nasir, N.S.; Zaidah, A.R. Prevalence of Vancomycin resistant enterococcus in Malaysia: A meta-analysis and systematic review. *Int. J. Infect. Dis.* **2020**, Accepted Manuscript.
38. Ali, S.; Alemayehu, M.A.; Dagnew, M.; Gebrecherkos, T. Vancomycin-Resistant Enterococci and Its Associated Risk Factors among HIV-Positive and -Negative Clients Attending Dessie Referral Hospital, Northeast Ethiopia. *Int. J. Microbiol.* **2018**, *2018*, 1–9. [CrossRef]
39. Moghimbeigi, A.; Moghimbeygi, M.; Dousti, M.; Kiani, F.; Sayehmiri, F.; Sadeghifard, N.; Nazari, A. Prevalence of vancomycin resistance among isolates of enterococci in Iran: A systematic review and meta-analysis. *Adolesc. Health Med. Ther.* **2018**, *9*, 177–188. [CrossRef]
40. Alevizakos, M.; Gaitanidis, A.; Nasioudis, D.; Tori, K.; Flokas, M.E.; Mylonakis, E. Colonization with Vancomycin-Resistant Enterococci and Risk for Bloodstream Infection Among Patients With Malignancy: A Systematic Review and Meta-Analysis. *Open Forum Infect. Dis.* **2016**, *4*. [CrossRef]
41. Kramer, T.; Remschmidt, C.; Werner, S.; Behnke, M.; Schwab, F.; Werner, G.; Gastmeier, P.; Leistner, R. The importance of adjusting for enterococcus species when assessing the burden of vancomycin resistance: A cohort study including over 1000 cases of enterococcal bloodstream infections. *Antimicrob. Resist. Infect. Control* **2018**, *7*, 133. [CrossRef]
42. Emaneini, M.; Hosseinkhani, F.; Jabalameli, F.; Nasiri, M.J.; Dadashi, M.; Pouriran, R.; Beigverdi, R. Prevalence of vancomycin-resistant Enterococcus in Iran: A systematic review and meta-analysis. *Eur. J. Clin. Microbiol. Infect. Dis.* **2016**, *35*, 1387–1392. [CrossRef]
43. Toner, L.; Papa, N.; Aliyu, S.H.; Dev, H.; Lawrentschuk, N.; Al-Hayek, S. Vancomycin resistant enterococci in urine cultures: Antibiotic susceptibility trends over a decade at a tertiary hospital in the United Kingdom. *Investig. Clin. Urol.* **2016**, *57*, 129–134. [CrossRef]
44. Yang, K.-S.; Fong, Y.-T.; Lee, H.-Y.; Kurup, A.; Koh, T.-H.; Koh, D.; Lim, M.-K. Predictors of vancomycin-resistant enterococcus (VRE) carriage in the first major VRE outbreak in Singapore. *Ann. Acad. Med. Singap.* **2007**, *36*, 379–383.
45. Barger, M.; Blodget, E.; Pena, S.; Mack, W.J.; Fong, T.-L. VRE in cirrhotic patients. *BMC Infect. Dis.* **2019**, *19*, 1–8. [CrossRef]
46. Camins, B.C.; Farley, M.M.; Jernigan, J.J.; Ray, S.M.; Steinberg, J.P.; Blumberg, H.M. A Population-Based Investigation of Invasive Vancomycin-ResistantEnterococcusInfection in Metropolitan Atlanta, Georgia, and Predictors of Mortality. *Infect. Control Hosp. Epidemiol.* **2007**, *28*, 983–991. [CrossRef]

47. Jakovljevic, M.; Al Ahdab, S.; Jurisevic, M.; Mouselli, S. Antibiotic Resistance in Syria: A Local Problem Turns Into a Global Threat. *Front. Public Health* **2018**, *6*, 212. [CrossRef]
48. Zhussupova, G.; Skvirskaya, G.; Reshetnikov, V.A.; Dragojević-Simić, V.; Rančić, N.; Utepova, D.; Jakovljevic, M. The Evaluation of Antibiotic Consumption at the Inpatient Level in Kazakhstan from 2011 to 2018. *Antibiotics* **2020**, *9*, 57. [CrossRef]
49. Robertson, J.; Iwamoto, K.; Hoxha, I.; Ghazaryan, L.; Abilova, V.; Cvijanovic, A.; Pyshnik, H.; Darakhvelidze, M.; Makalkina, L.; Jakupi, A.; et al. Antimicrobial Medicines Consumption in Eastern Europeand Central Asia–An Updated Cross-National Study and Assessment of QuantitativeMetrics for Policy Action. *Front. Pharmacol.* **2019**, *9*. [CrossRef]
50. Jakovljevic, M.; Timofeyev, Y.; Ranabhat, C.L.; Fernandes, P.O.; Teixeira, J.P.; Rancic, N.; Reshetnikov, V. Real GDP growth rates and healthcare spending — comparison between the G7 and the EM7 countries. *Glob. Health* **2020**, *16*, 1–13. [CrossRef]
51. Shokoohizadeh, L.; Mobarez, A.M.; Zali, M.R.; Ranjbar, R.; Alebouyeh, M.; Sakinc, T.; Ali, L. High frequency distribution of heterogeneous vancomycin resistant Enterococcous faecium (VREfm) in Iranian hospitals. *Diagn. Pathol.* **2013**, *8*, 163. [CrossRef]
52. Adams, D.J.; Eberly, M.D.; Goudie, A.; Nylund, C.M. Rising Vancomycin-Resistant Enterococcus Infections in Hospitalized Children in the United States. *Hosp. Pediatr.* **2016**, *6*, 404–411. [CrossRef]
53. Leclercq, R.; Derlot, E.; Duval, J.; Courvalin, P. Plasmid-Mediated Resistance to Vancomycin and Teicoplanin in Enterococcus Faecium. *N. Engl. J. Med.* **1988**, *319*, 157–161. [CrossRef]
54. Uttley, A.; Collins, C.; Naidoo, J.; George, R. vancomycin-resistant enterococci. *Lancet* **1988**, *331*, 57–58. [CrossRef]
55. Werner, G.; Coque, T.M.; Hammerum, A.M.; Hope, R.; Hryniewicz, W.; Johnson, A.; Klare, I.; Kristinsson, K.G.; Leclercq, R.; Lester, C.H.; et al. Emergence and spread of vancomycin resistance among enterococci in Europe. *Eurosurveillance* **2008**, *13*, 19046.
56. Levitus, M.; Rewane, A.; Perera, T.B. Vancomycin-Resistant Enterococci (VRE). In *StatPearls 2020 Treasure Island (FL)*; StatPearls Publishing: Florida, FL, USA, 2020.
57. Arias, C.A.; Murray, B.E. The rise of the Enterococcus: Beyond vancomycin resistance. *Nat. Rev. Genet.* **2012**, *10*, 266–278. [CrossRef] [PubMed]
58. Davis, E.; Hicks, L.; Ali, I.; Salzman, E.; Wang, J.; Snitkin, E.; Gibson, K.; Cassone, M.; Mody, L.; Foxman, B. Epidemiology of Vancomycin-Resistant Enterococcus faecium and Enterococcus faecalis Colonization in Nursing Facilities. *Open Forum Infect. Dis.* **2020**, *7*, ofz553. [CrossRef]
59. Treitman, A.N.; Yarnold, P.R.; Warren, J.; Noskin, G.A. Emerging Incidence of Enterococcus faecium among Hospital Isolates (1993 to 2002). *J. Clin. Microbiol.* **2005**, *43*, 462–463. [CrossRef]
60. Deshpande, L.M.; Fritsche, T.R.; Moet, G.J.; Biedenbach, D.J.; Jones, R.N. Antimicrobial resistance and molecular epidemiology of vancomycin-resistant enterococci from North America and Europe: A report from the SENTRY antimicrobial surveillance program. *Diagn. Microbiol. Infect. Dis.* **2007**, *58*, 163–170. [CrossRef]
61. Hidron, A.I.; Edwards, J.R.; Patel, J.; Horan, T.C.; Sievert, D.M.; Pollock, D.A.; Fridkin, S.K.; Participating National Healthcare Safety Network Facilities. NHSN annual update: Antimicrobial-resistant pathogens associated with healthcare-associated infections: Annual summary of data reported to the National Healthcare Safety Network at the Centers for Disease Control and Prevention, 2006–2007. *Infect. Control Hosp. Epidemiol.* **2008**, *29*, 996–1011. [CrossRef]
62. Jakovljevic, M.; Gerdtham, U.-G.; McDaid, D.; Ogura, S.; Varavikova, E.; Merrick, J.; Adany, R.; Okunade, A.; Getzen, T.E. Comparative financing analysis and political economy of noncommunicable diseases. *J. Med. Econ.* **2019**, *22*, 722–727. [CrossRef]
63. Cattoir, V.; Giard, J.-C. Antibiotic resistance inEnterococcus faeciumclinical isolates. *Expert Rev. Anti-Infect. Ther.* **2014**, *12*, 239–248. [CrossRef]
64. Hollenbeck, B.L.; Rice, L.B. Intrinsic and acquired resistance mechanisms in enterococcus. *Virulence* **2012**, *3*, 421–569. [CrossRef]
65. Top, J.; Willems, R.J.; Bonten, M. Emergence of CC17Enterococcus faecium: From commensal to hospital-adapted pathogen. *FEMS Immunol. Med. Microbiol.* **2008**, *52*, 297–308. [CrossRef] [PubMed]
66. Madu Tella, C. Insecurity in Northern Nigeria: Causes, Consequences and Resolutions. *Int. J. Peace Confl. Stud.* **2015**, *2*, 23–36.

67. Shamseer, L.; Moher, D.; Clarke, M.; Ghersi, D.; Liberati, A.; Petticrew, M.; Shekelle, P.; Stewart, L.; the PRISMA-P Group. Preferred reporting items for systematic review and meta-analysis protocols (PRISMA-P) 2015: Elaboration and explanation. *BMJ* **2015**, *349*, g7647. [CrossRef]
68. George, B.J.; Aban, I.B. An application of meta-analysis based on DerSimonian and Laird method. *J. Nucl. Cardiol.* **2015**, *23*, 690–692. [CrossRef] [PubMed]
69. Higgins, J.P.T.; Thompson, S.G. Quantifying heterogeneity in a meta-analysis. *Stat. Med.* **2002**, *21*, 1539–1558. [CrossRef]
70. Wallace, B.C.; Dahabreh, I.J.; Trikalinos, T.A.; Lau, J.; Trow, P.; Schmid, C.H. Closing the Gap between Methodologists and End-Users:Ras a Computational Back-End. *J. Stat. Softw.* **2012**, *49*, 1–15. [CrossRef]

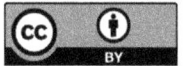

© 2020 by the authors. Licensee MDPI, Basel, Switzerland. This article is an open access article distributed under the terms and conditions of the Creative Commons Attribution (CC BY) license (http://creativecommons.org/licenses/by/4.0/).

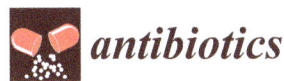

Article

Analysis of the Antibiotic Resistance Profiles in Methicillin-Sensitive *S. aureus* Pathotypes Isolated on a Commercial Rabbit Farm in Italy

Anna-Rita Attili [1,*,†], Alessandro Bellato [2,†], Patrizia Robino [2,†], Livio Galosi [1], Cristiano Papeschi [3], Giacomo Rossi [1], Eleonora Fileni [1], Martina Linardi [1], Vincenzo Cuteri [1], Francesco Chiesa [2] and Patrizia Nebbia [2]

1 School of Biosciences and Veterinary Medicine, University of Camerino, Via Circonvallazione 93/95, 62024 Matelica (MC), Italy; livio.galosi@unicam.it (L.G.); giacomo.rossi@unicam.it (G.R.); eleonora.fileni@studenti.unicam.it (E.F.); marti.linardi@gmail.com (M.L.); vincenzo.cuteri@unicam.it (V.C.)
2 Department of Veterinary Sciences, University of Torino, Largo P. Braccini 2, 10095 Grugliasco (TO), Italy; alessandro.bellato@unito.it (A.B.); patrizia.robino@unito.it (P.R.); francesco.chiesa@unito.it (F.C.); patrizia.nebbia@unito.it (P.N.)
3 Interdepartmental Animal Facility, University of Tuscia, Largo dell'Università snc, 01100 Viterbo (VT), Italy; papeschivet@gmail.com
* Correspondence: annarita.attili@unicam.it; Tel.: +39-(0)737-404002
† These authors contributed equally to this work.

Received: 31 July 2020; Accepted: 3 October 2020; Published: 5 October 2020

Abstract: The breeding of meat rabbits is an important sector in the livestock industry in Italy. The focus of this study was to describe the antibiotic resistance profile distribution among the Methicillin-sensitive *Staphylococcus aureus* isolated in a rabbit farm. From 400 animals of different ages and three farm workers, 96 randomly selected strains isolated from various anatomical sites and lesions were analysed. According to spa typing and the resistance profiles towards veterinary and human antibiotics, 26 pathotypes were identified. The highest resistance was observed against Tetracyclines (92.3%) and Macrolides (80.8%), while almost all were susceptible to Penicillins, according to the limited use of β-lactams on the farm. In total, 92.3% of pathotypes were multidrug resistant (MDRs). Two MDR pathotypes belonging to the t2802 spa type were isolated from both farmers and rabbits. Age categories harboured significantly different pathotypes ($p = 0.019$), while no association was found between pathotypes and lesions ($p = 0.128$) or sampling sites ($p = 0.491$). The antibiotic resistance was observed to increase with the time spent in the farm environment (age category). The selective pressure exerted by antibiotic use acted by giving advantage to more resistant strains rather than by lowering susceptibility to various drug categories within strains.

Keywords: *Staphylococcus aureus*; rabbits; pathotype; antibiotic resistance profiles; spa type; Italy

1. Introduction

The Italian rabbit industry annually produces about 24.5 million animals slaughtered for meat production and, in the European Union, takes third place after Spain and France. However, in recent years, rabbit breeding has seen a significant reduction in the number of commercial farms involved [1].

Rabbits are sensitive to many bacterial infections, such as respiratory and intestinal diseases, as well as skin infections. In general, farmers use various tools, such as biosecurity measures, good breeding conditions, alimentation, and behaviour. These protocols, when correctly implemented, give good results. Consequently, the use of antimicrobials has shown a steady decrease. Antibiotics are used as a therapy and include Fluoroquinolones, Trimethoprim-Sulfamethoxazole, Zinc Bacitracin, and Pleuromutilins, while other drug classes, such as Penicillins, Cephalosporins, and Lincosamides, need to be used with caution and should not be orally administered [2]. However, the use of antibiotics in livestock farming can increase antibiotic resistance prevalence, so it is also important to counteract this phenomenon under a One Health approach. Indeed, a low prevalence of antibiotic resistance in an intensive farm can be a sign of quality breeding [3,4].

Staphylococcus aureus is a zoonotic bacterium that occurs as both a commensal and opportunistic pathogen in many animals, including rabbits. It is associated with a wide variety of diseases, such as skin lesions, wound infections, mastitis, toxic shock syndromes, arthritis, endocarditis, osteomyelitis, and episodes of food poisoning [5–7]. In rabbits, this bacterium is an inhabitant of the skin, but it is also one on the main pathogens related to suppurative lesions [8]. For this reason, *S. aureus* could be used as indicator for the level of antimicrobial use in farms. Methicillin-resistant clones (MRSAs) are particularly monitored within the European community. In recent years, the presence of MRSAs in Italian rabbit breeding and the relationship between antibiotic use in farms and resistance have been evaluated [9,10]. High virulent strains (HV) were detected in Belgium, France, Greece, Italy, Portugal, Spain, and Hungary [8,11,12]. On the other hand, a recent study by Nemet et al. [12] provided evidence that low virulent (LV) strains can act as pathogens in rabbits.

Recently, a study showed various Methicillin-sensitive clones (MSSAs) in a rabbit farm, highlighting that some clonal strains (spa types) circulated in both animals and farm workers [13].

Although rabbit breeding is certainly a niche farm business, it has the potential risk for the spread of MDR, making it advisable to implement surveillance plans to control antibiotic resistance. In this research, following our previous study [13], the antibiotic resistance profile distribution among clones (spa types) isolated in an Italian rabbit farm was investigated. Moreover, to explore the evolution of antimicrobial resistance (AMR) in an intensively raised rabbit population, analyses and comparisons between the different pathotypes were carried out.

2. Results

2.1. Genetic Characterization

As previously reported by Attili et al. [13], in 96 randomly selected strains with low virulence and Methicillin-sensitive *S. aureus* (LV-MSSA), five different spa types were identified: t094, t491, t2036, t2802, and t605. The spa types most frequently found were t2802 (n = 51; 53.13%) and t491 (n = 37; 38.54%). Altogether, t094, t605, and t2036 accounted for 8.4%. Spa types were arranged into three spa-CCs: spa-CC267 (t2802), spa-CC084 (t094 and t491), and spa-CC012 (t2036). Due to its shortness, t605 could not be related to any clonal complex.

2.2. Antibiotic Susceptibility Testing

Antibiotic resistance was evaluated for each strain against 16 antibiotics belonging to 12 classes of antimicrobials. Table 1 reports the resistance prevalence for each of them.

All tested strains (n = 96) were susceptible to β-lactamase stable Penicillins (Cefoxitin), Lincosamides (Linezolid), Ansamycines (Rifampin), and Streptogramins (Quinupristin-Dalfopristin). The highest level of resistance was observed against Tetracyclines (n = 92, 95.8%). Out of the 96 strains, 90 (93.8%) were resistant to both of the Macrolides evaluated. Only three (3.1%) strains, obtained only from replacement rabbits, showed resistance to Penicillins. Susceptibility to Gentamicin and Tobramycin was highly correlated (r_{tet} = 99.0 ± 0.0), with 91 (94.8%) strains showing concordant responses. Therefore, these variables were shown to be dependent ($p < 0.001$). Moreover, resistance against Erythromycin and Clindamycin were dependent variables ($p < 0.001$), as they showed perfect concordance (r_{tet} = 1.0 ± 0.0). Among Glycopeptides, resistance against Teicoplanin and Vancomycin showed a weak negative correlation (r_{tet} = −0.2 ± 0.2), with only 27 (28.1%) strains showing concordant responses. Thus, the responses to the two antibiotics were shown to be independent from each other ($p = 0.425$). The overall resistance prevalence is shown in Figure 1.

Table 1. Frequency and resistance prevalence against the 12 antimicrobial classes and 16 antibiotics.

Antimicrobial Class	Freq.	% Prevalence (Mean ± s.e.)	Antibiotic	Freq.	% Prevalence (Mean ± s.e.)
Aminoglycosides	49	51.0 ± 0.5	Gentamicin	45	46.9 ± 0.5
			Tobramycin	48	50.0 ± 0.5
Ansamycins	0	0.0 ± 0.0	Rifampin	0	0.0 ± 0.0
β-lactamase labile Penicillins	3	3.1 ± 0.2	Penicillin G	3	3.1 ± 0.2
β-lactamase stable Penicillins	0	0.0 ± 0.0	Cefoxitin	0	0.0 ± 0.0
			Amoxicillin-Clavulanate	0	0.0 ± 0.0
Folate Pathway Inhibitors	9	9.4 ± 0.3	Sulfamethoxazole-Trimethoprim	9	9.4 ± 0.3
Fluoroquinolones	61	63.5 ± 0.5	Norfloxacin	61	63.5 ± 0.5
Glycopeptides	74	77.1 ± 0.4	Teicoplanin	71	74.0 ± 0.5
			Vancomycin	8	8.3 ± 0.3
Macrolides	90	93.8 ± 0.3	Clindamycin	90	93.8 ± 0.3
			Erythromycin	90	93.8 ± 0.3
Nitrofuranics	15	15.6 ± 0.4	Nitrofurantoin	15	15.6 ± 0.4
Lincosamides	0	0.0 ± 0.0	Linezolid	0	0.0 ± 0.0
Streptogramins	0	0.0 ± 0.0	Quinpristin-Dalfopristin	0	0.0 ± 0.0
Tetracyclines	92	95.8 ± 0.2	Tetracycline	92	95.8 ± 0.2

Legend: s.e. = standard error.

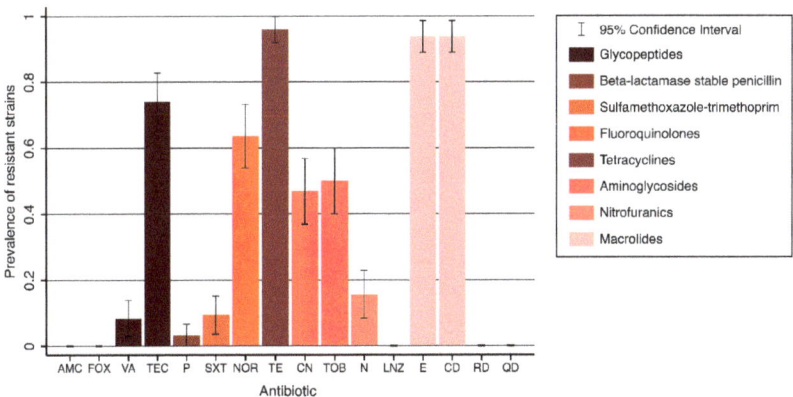

Figure 1. Prevalence of resistance against each antibiotic, with error bars showing 95% confidence intervals (AMC: Amoxicillin-Clavulanate; FOX: Cefoxitin; VA: Vancomycin; TEC: Teicoplanin; P: Penicillin G; SXT: Sulfamethoxazole-Trimethoprim; NOR: Norfloxacin; TE: Tetracycline; CN: Gentamicin; TOB: Tobramycin; N: Nitrofurantoin; LNZ: Linezolid; E: Erythromycin; CD: Clindamycin; RD: Rifampin; QD: Quinupristin-Dalfopristin).

Although an association between animal categories and resistance to antibiotics was observed only for Erythromycin and Clindamycin (Fisher's exact $p < 0.001$), the resistance percentages varied among different spa types and age categories. Out of 96 strains, 92 (97.9%) were MDRs and were not associated with spa types (Fisher's exact $p = 0.161$) but instead with age categories and adult and breeding rabbits (Fisher's exact $p = 0.010$). Not-MDR strains were observed only in young and replacement rabbits, with an MDR prevalence of 66.7 ± 33.3% and 75.0 ± 25.0%.

2.3. Analysis of Resistance Profiles

Among the 96 strains, 23 unique different resistance profiles were found based on the susceptibility to each antibiotic (*a* to *w*) (Table 2). Out of the 23, 9 were associated with only one strain each, while the other 14 together accounted for 90.6% of the strains. The most frequent resistance profiles were *p* (n = 23, 24.0%) and *j* (n = 20, 20.8%). The six resistance profiles (*b*, *f*, *j*, *p*, *r*, and *s*) that were observed in five or more strains were not associated with the age category ($\chi^2 = 12.447$, $p = 0.645$).

Table 2. Spa types associated to resistance profiles and pathotypes and their relative frequencies. All strains were susceptible to Amoxicillin-Clavulanate, Cefoxitin, Linezolid, Rifampin, and Quinupristin-Dalfopristin, so these antibiotics are not shown.

Spa Type	Freq. (%)	Resistance Profile	Pathotype	Freq. (%)	VA	TEC	P	SXT	NOR	TE	CN	TOB	N	E	CD
t094	4 (4.2)	e	A	1 (1.0)	S	S	S	S	R	R	S	S	S	S	S
		t	B	2 (2.1)	S	R	R	S	R	R	S	S	S	S	S
		w	C	1 (1.0)	R	R	R	S	R	R	S	S	S	S	S
t491	37 (38.5)	b	D	5 (5.2)	S	S	S	S	S	R	S	S	S	R	R
		f	E	5 (5.2)	S	S	S	S	R	R	S	S	S	R	R
		j	F	18 (18.8)	S	R	S	S	S	R	S	S	S	R	R
		m	G	1 (1.0)	S	R	S	S	R	R	S	S	S	R	R
		s	H	1 (1.0)	S	R	S	R	R	R	R	R	S	R	R
		u	I	3 (3.1)	R	S	S	S	S	R	S	S	S	R	R
		v	J	4 (4.2)	R	R	S	S	S	R	S	S	S	R	R
t605	2 (2.1)	c	K	1 (1.0)	S	S	S	S	S	R	R	R	R	R	R
		p	L	1 (1.0)	S	R	S	S	R	R	R	S	R	R	R
t2036	2 (2.1)	j	M	2 (2.1)	S	R	S	S	S	R	S	S	S	R	R
t2802	51 (53.1)	a	N	1 (1.0)	S	S	S	S	S	R	S	S	S	S	S
		d	O	2 (2.1)	S	S	S	S	R	S	S	S	S	R	R
		g	P	1 (1.0)	S	S	S	S	R	R	R	S	R	R	R
		h	Q	4 (4.2)	S	S	S	S	R	R	R	R	R	R	R
		i	R	2 (2.1)	S	S	S	R	R	R	R	R	S	R	R
		k	S	1 (1.0)	S	R	S	S	S	R	S	R	S	R	R
		l	T	2 (2.1)	S	R	S	S	R	S	S	S	S	R	R
		n	U	3 (3.1)	S	R	S	S	R	S	R	R	R	R	R
		o	V	1 (1.0)	S	R	S	S	R	R	S	R	R	R	R
		p	W	22 (22.9)	S	R	S	S	R	R	R	S	R	R	R
		q	X	1 (1.0)	S	R	S	S	R	R	R	R	S	R	S
		r	Y	5 (5.2)	S	R	S	S	R	R	R	R	R	R	R
		s	Z	6 (6.3)	S	R	S	S	R	R	R	R	S	R	R

VA: Vancomycin; TEC: Teicoplanin; P: Penicillin G; SXT: Sulfamethoxazole-Trimethoprim; NOR: Norfloxacin; TE: Tetracycline; CN: Gentamicin; TOB: Tobramycin; N: Nitrofurantoin; E: Erythromycin; CD: Clindamycin.

Farmer strains shared the same resistance profiles with the rabbits: Profile p was isolated from 17 adult rabbits, three breeding rabbits, one young rabbit, and two farmers; r was drawn from two adult rabbits, two breeding rabbits, and one farmer. Most of the profiles had resistance to Tetracyclines (n = 21, 91.3%) and Macrolides (Erythromycin and Clindamycin: n = 18, 78.3%). Only two (8.7%) profiles (t and w) showed resistance to Penicillin G.

Out of the 23 profiles, 15 (65.2%) were resistant to Glycopeptides: One was susceptible to Teicoplanin but resistant to Vancomycin; 11 were resistant to Teicoplanin but susceptible to Vancomycin; and two were resistant to both antimicrobials. Only two (8.7%) resistance profiles (i and s) were not susceptible to Sulfamethoxazole-Trimethoprim, and 16 (69.6%) were resistant to Norfloxacin. About half of the profiles (n = 11, 47.8%) showed resistance to Aminoglycosides: One was resistant only to Gentamicin; two were resistant to Tobramycin but susceptible to Gentamicin; and eight were resistant to both.

Only six (26.1%) were resistant to Nitrofurantoin, and two (8.7%) profiles (a and e) showed resistance to less than three classes of antimicrobial agents, while 14 (60.9%) were resistant to 3–5 antimicrobial classes, and 7 (30.4%) were resistant to 6–8 classes. Therefore, all but a and e were MDRs, with an average of 5.1 ± 1.9 resistance against single antibiotics and slightly fewer (5.0 ± 1.4) resistance against classes of antimicrobials. Out of the 11 rabbits from which multiple strains were obtained, all were MDRs. Among them, eight showed discordant resistance profiles, while three showed concordant profiles. Out of the seven rabbits whose isolates were obtained from different sampling sites, five (71.4%) profiles were discordant. Out of the four rabbits whose isolates were drawn twice from the same sampling site, three (75.0%) had discordant profiles. No evidence was found showing that different sampling sites hosted different resistance profiles (Fisher's exact $p = 0.721$).

2.4. Analysis of Pathotypes

By associating the 23 resistance profiles to spa types, 26 pathotypes were identified (A to Z) (Table 2). Out of these 26, 10 were associated to only one strain each, while the other 16 together were found in 88.3% of the strains. The most represented pathotypes were F and W, which were isolated from 18 (18.8%) and 22 (22.9%) strains, respectively, with an estimated prevalence among rabbits of 18.1% (95CI: 10.3–25.9%) and 23.4% (95CI: 14.8–32.0%). Pathotypes observed more than once were associated with age categories (Fisher's exact $p = 0.019$), but those that occurred at least five times (D, E, F, W, Y, and Z) were not ($\chi^2 = 12.115$, $p = 0.670$).

The two pathotypes isolated from farmers (W and Y) were also found in rabbits: W was isolated from 16 adult rabbits, three breeding rabbits, and one young rabbit; Y was drawn from two adult and two breeding rabbits. They were both spa type t2802 and resistant to six and seven classes of antimicrobials, respectively. Only two (7.7%) pathotypes (B and C), both drawn from replacement rabbits, showed resistance to Penicillin G.

Out of the 26 pathotypes, 17 (65.4%) were resistant to Glycopeptides; among them, one was susceptible to Teicoplanin but resistant to Vancomycin, 14 were resistant to Teicoplanin but susceptible to Vancomycin; and two were resistant to both antimicrobials. Only three (11.5%) pathotypes (H, R, and Z), drawn from fattening rabbits and breeders, were resistant to the Sulfamethoxazole-Trimethoprim combination, while 18 (69.2%) and 24 (92.3%), isolated from all four categories and farmers, showed resistance to Norfloxacin and Tetracycline, respectively. Half of the pathotypes (n = 13) obtained from all categories (except replacements) showed resistance to Aminoglycosides: One was resistant only to Gentamicin; two were resistant to Tobramycin but susceptible to Gentamicin; and 10 were resistant to both antibiotics. Only six (23.1%) pathotypes were resistant to Nitrofurantoin, while 21 (80.8%) drawn from all categories (except replacements) were found to be resistant to Macrolides (Erythromycin and Clindamycin). Only two (7.7%) pathotypes (A and N) were resistant to less than three classes of antimicrobial agents, while 15 (57.7%) were resistant to three to five antimicrobial classes, and nine (34.6%) to six to eight classes, with an overall 92.3% (n = 24) prevalence of MDRs.

Out of the 11 rabbits from which multiple strains were obtained, all reported MDRs. Among them, nine showed discordant pathotypes, while two showed concordant ones. Out of the seven rabbits whose isolates were obtained from different sampling sites, five (71.4%) pathotypes were discordant. All four rabbits whose isolates were drawn twice from the same site had discordant pathotypes. Consistently, no evidence showed that different sampling sites harboured different pathotypes (Fisher's exact $p = 0.491$).

The complexity of data, due to the high number of different pathotypes, and the scarcity of many of them in the population did not allow us to obtain further information on the distribution of the lineages among age categories in the rabbit population.

2.5. Clusterization and Factor Analysis

Since some pathotypes showed similar resistance profiles, factor analysis (FA) was used to reduce the complexity of the database and group strains based on the similarity of their phenotypic and genotypic features. As Erythromycin and Clindamycin were completely correlated, they were aggregated in FA to avoid a singularity of the correlation matrix. The sample was adequate to perform the factor analysis (Kaiser–Meyer–Olkin measure = 0.686). FA produced 11 factors, of which three were retained because they could explain 98.7% of the data variability. The variables that contributed the most to variability were Aminoglycosides (Gentamicin 90.4%, Tobramycin 94.7%), spa type (89.0%), Norfloxacin (72.1%) for the first factor; Penicillin G (79.4%) and Erythromycin (72.8%) for the second one; and Tetracycline (74.0%) for the third factor (Figure 2).

Other variables were less relevant to defining data variability. Since the first three factors were sufficiently informative to cover the variability of the whole dataset, they were used to produce the similarity matrix. Based on the matrix and a cut-off value of 0.0, five different clusters of strains were generated. Spa types were partly grouped together, but they were not completely separated from each other, with t491 showing high variability. Pathotypes were grouped together in a three-dimensional space as follows: Cluster 1: D, F, J, I, M; Cluster 2: A, B, C, E, G, N, X; cluster 3: O, T, U, V; cluster 4: H, K, L, S; and cluster 5: P, Q, R, W, Y, Z. The score-plot in Figure 3 shows the spatial distribution of the clusters and pathotypes in a two-dimensional space.

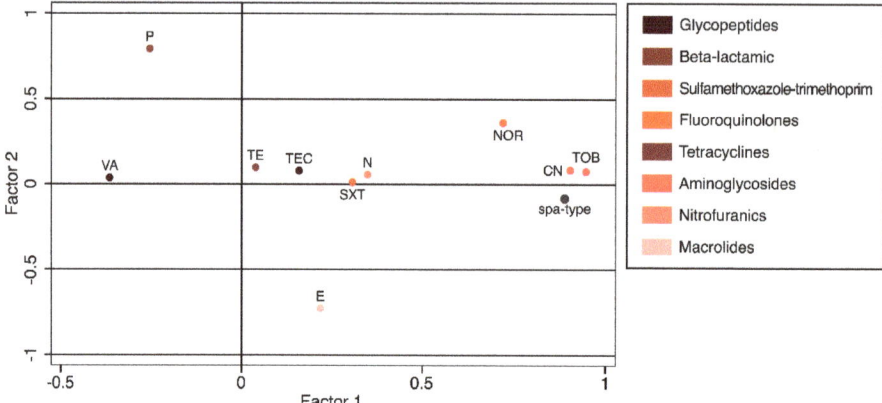

Figure 2. Loading plot showing the impact of each variable on the first two factors of the factor analysis. Legend: VA = Vancomycin; P = Penicillin G; TE = Tetracycline; TEC = Teicoplanin; E = Erythromycin; SXT = Sulfamethoxazole-Trimethoprim; N = Neomycin; NOR = Norfloxacin; CN = Gentamicin; TOB = Tobramycin.

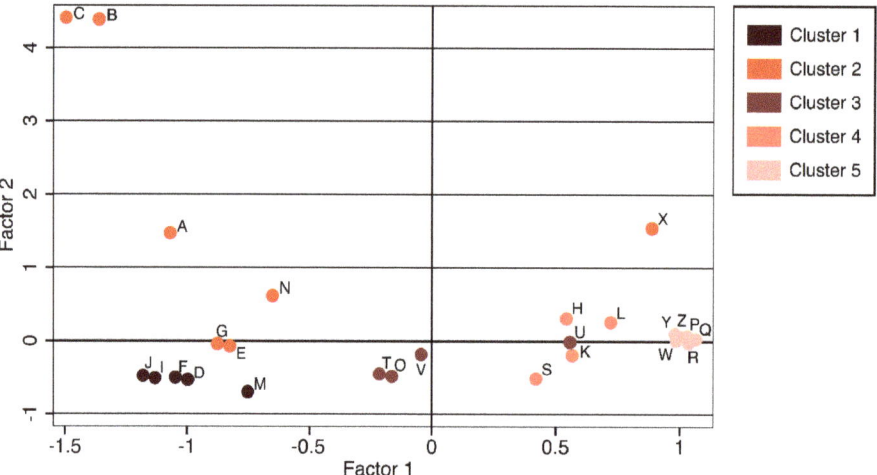

Figure 3. Scores of the pathotypes and their positions relative to the first two factors. Clusters are identified by different colours.

2.6. Analysis of Resistance Number

The resistance varied significantly among spa types (Friedman's test $p = 0.002$), ranging from 3.5 ± 1.0 in t094 to 5.9 ± 1.2 in t2802, but did not differ among age categories (Friedman's test $p = 0.815$), ranging from 3.5 ± 0.5 in replacement rabbits to 5.5 ± 0.3 in breeding rabbits. However, an increasing resistance trend was appreciable among the age categories of rabbits and the strains obtained from farmers, which showed the highest average resistance value (6.3 ± 0.6) (Figure 4).

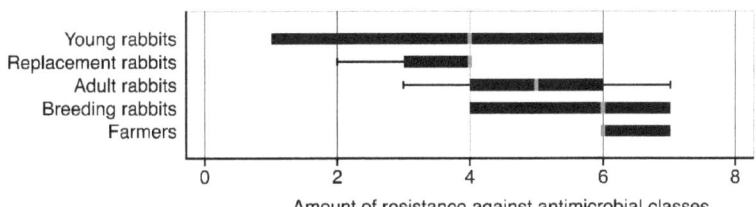

Figure 4. Resistance against antimicrobial classes for rabbits (age categories) and farmers. Legend: Error bars = Inter-quartile range.

According to the age categories, the resistance increased significantly with the time spent in the farm environment (Table 3).

Table 3. Observed and estimated number of class resistance by age category and in-farm time recorded groups. Risk ratios for the increase of youngest one.

Age Category	Resistance (Mean ± s.e.)	Time on Farm (Days)	Freq. (%)	Estimated Resistance (No.)	Estimated 95% C.I.	RR	p-Value
Replacement rabbits	3.5 ± 0.5	<60	7 (7.29)	3.6	2.5–4.7	1 (ref.)	-
Young rabbits	3.7 ± 1.5						
Adult rabbits	5.0 ± 0.2	60–80	71 (74.0)	5.0	4.7–5.3	1.4	0.035
Breeding rabbits	5.5 ± 0.3	≥240	18 (18.8)	5.6	5.1–6.2	1.6	0.007
Farmers	6.3 ± 0.3						

Legend: s.e. = standard error; C.I. = Confidence Interval; RR = Relative Risk.

Since spa types were associated with both age categories and time on the farm (Fisher's exact $p < 0.001$), as well as resistance profiles the categories needed to be added to the regression model to evaluate the "time on farm" effect on the resistance count. Due to including the fewest resistance, t2036 was set as the reference group. t605 and t2802 proved to be significantly related to an increase in resistance types. After the inclusion of spa types in the model, the effect of the time on farm was no longer significant ($p > 0.2$). Results and estimates for spa types are reported in Table 4.

Table 4. Observed and estimated resistance types for each spa type. Relative risks of gaining one more type(s) of resistance in each group compared to t2036.

Spa Type	Resistance (Mean ± s.e.)	Estimated Resistance (No.)	Estimated 95% C.I.	RR	p-Value
t094	3.5 ± 0.5	5.0	1.5–8.5	1.3	0.464
t491	4.0 ± 0.1	3.9	3.7–4.2	1.0	0.372
t605	5.5 ± 0.5	5.4	4.7–6.1	1.4	<0.001
t2036	4.0 ± 0.0	3.8	3.5–4.1	1 (ref.)	-
t2802	5.9 ± 0.2	5.9	5.5–6.2	1.5	<0.001

Legend: s.e. = standard error; C.I. = Confidential Interval; RR = Relative Risk.

Figure 5 shows that the significantly more resistant spa types (t605 and t2802, n = 53) increased with the time spent on the farm, while the other spa types (n = 43) reduced (Figure 5).

Although the time-on-farm effect vanished when spa types were considered, this effect could still affect the prevalence of different pathotypes. Therefore, to consider the full complexity of the data, an evaluation of the number of resistance types was performed in relation to pathotype clusters and the time-on-farm variable. The time spent in the farm environment proved not to be significant overall ($\chi^2 = 4.09$, $p = 0.129$), except between the first (<60 days) and the third (≥240 days) categories ($\chi^2 = 3.93$, $p = 0.047$).

Clusters had significantly different counts of resistance overall ($\chi^2 = 519.17$, $p < 0.0001$). Compared to cluster 1, cluster 2 did not have significantly more resistance ($\chi^2 = 0.68$, $p = 0.411$); cluster 3 had significantly more resistance than cluster 1 ($\chi^2 = 4.63$, $p < 0.032$) but not more than cluster 2 ($\chi^2 = 3.02$,

$p < 0.082$); clusters 4 and 5 had significantly more resistance than clusters 1 and 2 ($p < 0.001$) but not more than cluster 3 ($\chi^2 = 0.5, p < 0.480; \chi^2 = 2.58, p < 0.108$, respectively). The increasing trend acted on two different levels: Macroscopic variations were appreciable between clusters, while there were minor intra-cluster differences among the time-on-farm categories. Table 5 outlines the estimated counts of resistance by the clusters and time on farm of the categories.

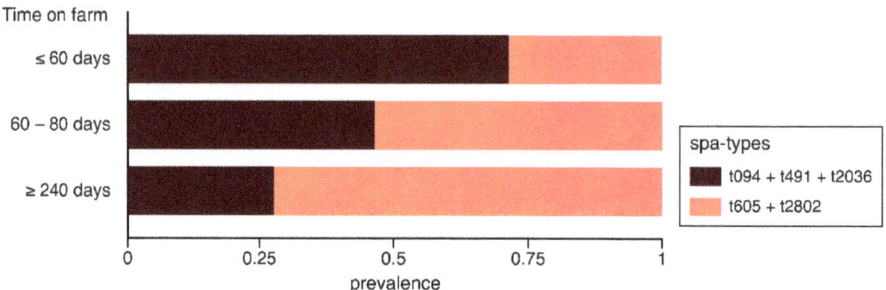

Figure 5. Prevalence of significantly more resistant spa types (t605 and t2802) against the less resistant ones for each in-farm time category.

Table 5. Predicted counts of resistance by the clusters and time on farm of the categories.

Cluster	Time on Farm (Days)	Estimated Resistance (No.)	Estimated 95% C.I.
1	<60	3.2	2.4–3.9
	60–80	3.9	3.7–4.0
	≥240	4.0	3.7–4.25
2	<60	3.3	2.5–4.2
	60–80	4.0	3.6–4.5
	≥240	4.2	3.6–4.7
3	<60	4.3	2.9–5.7
	60–80	5.2	4.0–6.5
	≥240	5.4	4.1–6.6
4	<60	4.8	3.4–6.1
	60–80	5.8	4.9–6.6
	≥240	5.9	5.0–6.8
5	<60	5.1	3.9–6.3
	60–80	6.2	6.0–6.4
	≥240	6.4	6.1–6.7

Figure 6 shows the predicted counts of resistance for each cluster, according to the on-farm time variable.

The chart shows that there is an effect of clusters that is also dependent from the time on farm, which had an additive effect between the first and the third category. There was also a break in the trend between the cluster 2 and 3 values.

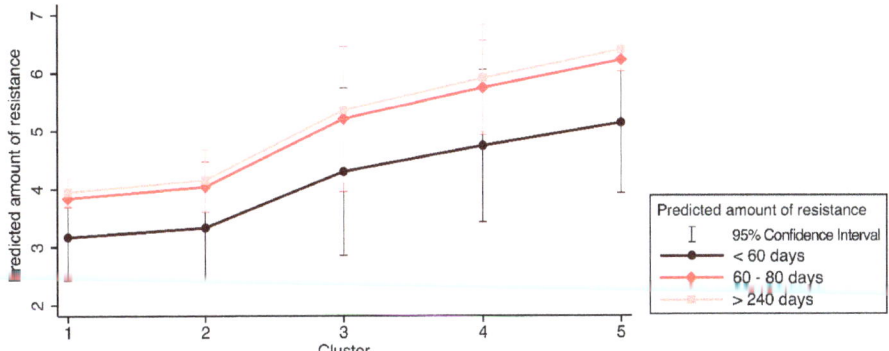

Figure 6. Predicted counts of resistance estimated considering the clusters and time on farm of the animal categories. Legend: error bars = 95% Confidence Interval of the predicted mean.

3. Discussion

The high prevalence of multidrug-resistant strains observed in this study (97.9%) agrees with what was previously described in intensively raised rabbits [14]. The highest resistance observed in this study, particularly against Tetracycline (95.8%), Macrolides (93.8%), and Quinolones (63.5%), is also similar to that observed against the same antibiotics in a recent study conducted in Spain and Portugal [14]. An unexpectedly high resistance was observed against Glycopeptides (77.1%), whose use is restricted to human medicine. This result suggests the possibility of human–animal transmission, although this study was not designed to test this factor. Moreno-Grua et al. [14] observed a 12.5% prevalence of Methicillin-resistant strains in the Iberian Peninsula, isolated from 22 out of 89 farms. We did not find any Methicillin-resistant strain, which is almost in agreement with the only MRSA case published on rabbits in Italy [9] that reported only one in 40 intensive rabbit farms having MRSA.

Due to its simplicity and affordability, spa typing has been described as a useful tool to survey the circulation of pathogenic strains in farm environments and among different farms and countries [15]. The clonal phylogenetic structure of *S. aureus* allows one to trace back the origin of the bacterial strains and map the lineages' evolution in a population, although it cannot fulfil all the needs of epidemiological surveillance of antimicrobial resistance. In this study, a representative sample of a relatively closed population of rabbits was chosen to investigate the prevalence of antibiotic-resistant Methicillin-sensitive *S. aureus* strains. Five spa types were found circulating among the animals, unevenly colonizing different body sites and age categories [15]. It was also observed that some spa types were more strongly related to some age categories, such as t094 in replacement rabbits. Since these animals were partly bought from outside the farm, it could be presumed that *S. aureus* strains were introduced along with the animals, while also bringing in new resistance genes. However, the overall group of newly introduced rabbits was very reduced (approximately 2.6%). Further, although these rabbits might host different spa types, those strains should have an evolutionary advantage in establishing themselves in a population already colonized by *S. aureus*. One of the main forces acting as selective pressure on bacteria in a farm environment is the usage of antibiotics, which act not only on pathogens but also on commensal flora that are being actively selected towards an increase in resistance [16,17]. To survey the evolution of resistant strains, spa typing showed its limit, as it was unable to differentiate strains at the level of detail needed. These details lay in the genomes of bacteria as resistance genes. However, for the purpose of this study, phenotypic manifestation was used to maintain a pragmatic approach since most laboratories do not have the resources to perform multiple types of molecular testing to identify resistance genes. Since phenotypic resistance patterns likely reflect underlying genotypic differences, susceptibility to each antibiotic could be considered a distinctive tract useful to define lineages circulating in the farm environment, along with spa types.

Out of the 8192 possible arrangements, only 23 different resistance profiles were found. Therefore, it is reasonable to expect that they are related to some other features of the strains or even to each other. The pathotype identification hinted at an association between spa types and resistance profiles, but such pathotypes were too dispersed to more deeply investigate. The implementation of factor analysis on the phenotypic data was intended to enhance the readability of the database, thereby improving our ability to understand how similar these pathotypes are. The results showed that spa typing does not describe all variability but remains a powerful tool to clarify clonal evolution mechanisms; further, the clusters of pathotypes generated by FA were associated with age categories.

Our objective was to explore how the selective pressure exerted by antimicrobial treatments affects the amount of resistance in S. aureus. Therefore, we assumed that the time spent in the farm environment would be a proxy for the quantity of exposure to antibiotics and that the farm environment would be a source of colonization for most resistant strains of S. aureus, which are considered to have the best survival chances. To test these assumptions, age categories were redefined while considering the physiology of rabbits and intensive-breeding times. By simply evaluating the frequencies of the most resistant spa types (t605 and t2802), it was observable that their prevalence increased with exposure to the farm environment and that the time on farm had a significant effect on the amount of resistance. A causal relationship was also supported by the dose–effect trend and prior knowledge of biological mechanisms. However, the time on farm was no longer able to statistically significantly explain this increase when the clusters of pathotypes were considered, although the trend remained evident. These findings confirm that the increase in resistance was due to antibiotic usage and the selective pressure exerted, while also suggesting another question: With an increase in time spent on the farm, do the resistant strains increase or does the resistance in strains increase? This sounds trivial, but, based on our findings, the former option seems more probable than the latter since the relationship between strains and resistance can completely hide the relationship between age and resistance. On the other hand, it is reasonable to assume that both mechanisms play a role in AMR, but they might proceed at different speeds.

More resistant strains are considered to have the best survival chances; therefore, their prevalence increased as they filled the space left empty by those that did not survive the antibiotic treatment. This finding indicates that rabbits who live for a long time in the environment play a key role in maintaining resistant strains and spreading them to newly introduced and new-born individuals. Furthermore, the role of farmers should not be underestimated, as farmers survive more often than animals and continue to spread resistant strains to newly introduced rabbits. The usefulness of the sanitary vacuum remains debated because it only applies to animals and the environment, but farmers could also act as a source of resistant strains.

4. Materials and Methods

4.1. Sampling and S. aureus Characterization

Sampling and bacteriological analysis (identification and molecular characterization of S. aureus isolates) were described in detail in our previous article [13] and are briefly summarized below.

Out of a total of 2066 samples taken from 400 rabbits of different ages reared in a commercial medium-sized intensive breeding farm in central Italy, and from farmworkers, 592 Methicillin-sensitive S. aureus strains (n = 552 from healthy skin and n = 40 from lesions) were isolated. A sample of 96 S. aureus was randomly selected to perform antimicrobial susceptibility tests (ASTs) and molecular analyses. The sample was so distributed: 72 strains representing the four breeding categories (n = 2, 2.8% of S. aureus infection in youngsters; n = 52, 72.2% in adults; n = 14, 19.4% in breeding rabbits; n = 4, 5.5% in replacement rabbits) were taken from healthy skin, 21 strains were isolated from lesions, and three from the healthy skin of the nose and hands of the farm workers, who gave their informed consent. Animals treated with antibiotics within 30 days were excluded from the study; the farm's veterinarian reported data about the antibiotic treatment in the previous three years: Enrofloxacin,

Sulfamethoxazole-Trimethoprim, Zinc Bacitracin, and Valnemulin were used to treat bacterial infections as need.

4.2. Antibiotic Susceptibility Testing

To determine the antibiotic profiles, 96 randomly selected *S. aureus*, *mecA*, and *mecC* negative (MSSA strains) were screened, and antibiotic susceptibility testing for 16 antimicrobial agents was performed according to the Clinical and Laboratory Standards Institute guidelines [18,19].

S. aureus subsp. *aureus* ATTC® 43300TM was used as a quality control strain for the zone diameter determinations and MIC evaluation. The standard disk diffusion method (Kirby-Bauer test) was used to test Penicillin G (P, 1 IU), Cefoxitin (FOX, 30 µg), Sulfamethoxazole-Trimethoprim (SXT, 25 µg), Norfloxacin (NOR, 10 µg), Tetracycline (TE, 30 µg), Gentamicin (GM, 10 µg), Tobramycin (TOB, 10 µg), Erythromycin (E, 15 µg), Clindamycin (CD, 2 µg), Rifampin (RIF, 5 µg), Nitrofurantoin (NT, 100 µg), Linezolid (LIN, 10 µg), and Quinupristin-Dalfopristin (Q-D, 15 µg). As recommended by CLSI (2018), Penicillin 1 IU was used to test the isolates against Penicillins and as a marker for penicillinase-labile beta-lactams, while Cefoxitin was used to test the strains against the penicillinase-stable ones (phenotypic resistance to methicillin). The E-test method was used to determine the MICs against Amoxicillin-Clavulanate, Vancomycin, and Teicoplanin, as described by the manufacturer (MIC Test Strip, Liofilchem, Roseto degli Abruzzi, Italy). Isolates that exhibited intermediate sensitivity were considered resistant to the antibiotic.

Some drugs were chosen for their importance in treating *S. aureus* infections in animals and others due to their ability to provide diversity in the representation of different antimicrobial agent classes. As Linezolid, Quinupristin-Dalfopristin, Vancomycin, and Teicoplanin are among the antibiotics that have become life-saving treatments for human patients suffering from different kinds of infections caused by multidrug-resistant bacteria, it was in our interest to assess sensitivity to these antimicrobials. Profiles of antibiotic resistance were investigated singularly and in association with clones (spa types) to define the unique combinations of phenotypical and genotypical characteristics as pathotypes. Alphabetical codes were used to identify resistance profiles (lowercase) and pathotypes (uppercase).

Finally, the pathotypes were grouped together in clusters based on spa types and resistance patterns.

4.3. Statistical Analysis

Many categorical variables were used to perform the statistical analyses, some related to the animals (rabbit's identification code, age category, site of sampling) and others to the bacteria (spa type). Resistance to antibiotics was coded as 1 if the strain was intermediate or resistant and 0 otherwise. From the previous variables, the other variables were derived: MDR strains were defined as those having resistance against at least three different antimicrobial classes [20]; the count of resistance was obtained by adding together all resistance types against single antibiotics.

According to a farmer's statement, on average, 30% of replacement rabbits were introduced from outside the farm at an adult age to replace the breeding rabbits (personal communication). For this reason, these rabbits could be conveniently associated with the young rabbits due to their short average time spent in the farm environment. On the other hand, breeding rabbits and farmers have spent a long time in the farm environment, hinting at a possible reunion of these two categories. Therefore, the age category variable was recorded as the time on farm as follows: <60 days, grouping together young rabbits that were 40–45 days of age with replacement rabbits; 60–80 days, for the age of adult rabbits that had lived on the farm since birth; and ≥240 days for grouping breeding rabbits whose reproductive activity started at least at 8 months of age with farmers. The time on farm analysis was performed as an exploratory survey since it was not defined from the beginning, but the need for it arose over the course of the analyses.

Data analysis proceeded as follows: (1) analysis of individual strains and the overall prevalence of resistant ones; (2) analysis of the resistance profiles and associations with age category and spa type and the prevalence of MDRs; (3) analysis of the pathotypes and their association with age categories;

(4) factor analysis and hierarchical clustering of pathotypes; and (5) analysis of the count of resistance and its association with other variables.

To investigate the prevalence of resistant strains *versus* antibiotics, as well as antimicrobial classes, an exploratory analysis was performed to calculate the mean, standard deviation, and standard error of the mean. Contingency tables were produced to investigate the relationships between resistance and spa types, age categories, and sampling sites using chi-square and Fisher's exact tests to assess the associations. The correlation between resistance to antibiotics belonging to the same class was evaluated with the tetrachoric correlation coefficient, r_{tet} [21]. Resistance profiles were obtained by collapsing the database to unique combinations of resistance to antibiotics and identified by lowercase letters from "*a*" to "*w*". The resistance profiles' prevalence and association with the age categories and spa types were estimated via the same methods described for individual strains. Pathotypes were defined as unique combinations of resistance profiles and spa types assigned uppercase letters from "*A*" to "*Z*". The prevalence of pathotypes resistant to every antibiotic and the association of this resistance with age categories were also investigated.

To improve data readability, enhance information quality, and avoid tautologies, a factor analysis (FA [22]) was performed on a set of 11 variables (spa types and resistance to antibiotics). FA produced some factors (vectors of eigenvalues) able to cover the variability of the related variables. The Kaiser–Meyer–Olkin measure was calculated to assess the usefulness of FA. The relationship among the former variables and the main factors was evaluated graphically by a loading plot and quantitatively by the explained cumulative variance. Using a graphical evaluation of the scree plot, some factors were chosen and then used for hierarchical clustering by applying Ward's criterion to the similarity matrix [23]. The obtained clusters resembled the groups of pathotypes circulating on the farm environment.

An analysis of variance to assess the resistance among age categories and spa types was performed using Friedman's test. The trend of the amount of resistance was evaluated using Poisson's regression models considering either the age category and spa types or the time on farm and clusters. The robust standard error was calculated.

Data were recorded on a Microsoft Excel spreadsheet, which was also used to build a database. Every subsequent analysis was performed using STATA 15.0 (Stata Corp. LLC, College Station, TX, USA).

5. Conclusions

This study showed that 92.3% of pathotypes were MDRs and associated with age categories and adult and breeding rabbits. The highest resistance was observed against the classes of Tetracyclines, Macrolides, and Glycopeptides in both animal and human *S. aureus* strains. According to the analysis of resistance, 23 unique different profiles were obtained, with farmer strains that shared the same resistance profiles with rabbits. In particular, when the 23 resistance profiles were associated with the spa types, 26 pathotypes were identified. Two pathotypes isolated from farmers were also found in rabbits, which were both spa type t2802 and resistant to six and seven class of antimicrobials, respectively, confirming the zoonotic risk that could occur in rabbit farms.

As Nemet et al. [14] observed, clonal types do not always correspond to spa types, through which only part of the bacterial genome is sequenced and evaluated. However, information on lineages circulating in the herd obtained by cluster analysis on antimicrobial resistance profiles could help us understand how the selective pressure exerted by antimicrobial treatment acts on *S. aureus* strains and thus provide useful management indications for antibiotic use.

Author Contributions: Conceptualization, A.-R.A., A.B., P.N., and P.R.; data curation, A.-R.A., and A.B.; formal analysis, A.-R.A., A.B., and F.C.; funding acquisition, P.R. and G.R.; investigation, A.B., E.F., and M.L.; methodology, A.-R.A., A.B., P.N., and P.R.; resources, L.G. and C.P.; supervision, A.-R.A., A.B., P.N., and P.R.; visualization, A.-R.A., A.B., and V.C.; writing—original draft preparation, A.-R.A, A.B., P.N., and P.R.; writing—review and editing, A.-R.A., A.B., P.N., and P.R. All authors have read and agreed to the published version of the manuscript.

Funding: This study was supported by NOVARTIS and by Ministero dell'Istruzione, dell'Università e della Ricerca (MIUR) under the programme "Dipartimenti di Eccellenza ex L.232/2016" to the Department of Veterinary Science, University of Turin.

Conflicts of Interest: The authors declare no conflict of interest. The funder had no role in the design of the study; in the collection, analyses, or interpretation of data; in the writing of the manuscript, or in the decision to publish the results.

References

1. EFSA ECDC. The European Union summary report on antimicrobial resistance in zoonotic and indicator bacteria from humans, animals and food in 2016. *EFSA J.* **2018**, *16*, 5182. [CrossRef]
2. Tyrrell, K.L.; Citron, D.M.; Jenkins, J.R.; Goldstein, E.C. Periodontal Bacteria in Rabbit Mandibular and Maxillary Abscesses. *J. Clin. Microbiol.* **2002**, *40*, 1044–1047. [CrossRef] [PubMed]
3. Van den Bogaard, A.E.; Stobbering, E.E. Time to ban all antibiotics as animal growth-promoting agents? *Lancet* **1996**, *348*, 1455–1456. [CrossRef]
4. Van den Bogaard, A.E. Antimicrobial resistance—Relation to human and animal exposure to antibiotics. *J. Antimicrob. Chemoth.* **1997**, *40*, 453–454. [CrossRef] [PubMed]
5. Von Eiff, C.; Becker, K.; Machka, K.; Stammer, H.; Peters, G. Nasal carriage as a source of *Staphylococcus aureus* bacteremia. *N. Engl. J. Med.* **2001**, *344*, 11–16. [CrossRef] [PubMed]
6. Gao, J.; Steward, G.C. Regulatory Elements of the *Staphylococcus aureus* Protein A (Spa) Promoter. *J. Bacteriol.* **2004**, *186*, 3738–3748. [CrossRef] [PubMed]
7. Penadés, M.; Viana, D.; García-Quirós, A.; Muñoz-Silvestre, A.; Moreno-Grua, E.; Pérez-Fuentes, S.; Pascual, J.J.; Corpa, J.M.; Selva, L. Differences in virulence between the two more prevalent Staphylococcus aureus clonal complexes in rabbitries (CC121 and CC96) using an experimental model of mammary gland infection. *Vet. Res.* **2020**, *51*, 11. [CrossRef] [PubMed]
8. Silva, V.; Sousa, T.; Gómez, P.; Sabença, C.; Vieira-Pinto, M.; Capita, R.; Alonso-Calleja, C.; Torres, C.; Capelo, J.L.; Igrejas, G.; et al. Livestock-Associated Methicillin-Resistant *Staphylococcus aureus* (MRSA) in purulent subcutaneous lesions of farm rabbits. *Foods* **2020**, *9*, 439. [CrossRef] [PubMed]
9. Agnoletti, F.; Mazzolini, E.; Bacchin, C.; Bano, L.; Berto, G.; Rigoli, R.; Muffato, G.; Coato, P.; Tonon, E.; Drigo, I. First reporting of methicillin-resistant *Staphylococcus aureus* (MRSA) ST398 in an industrial rabbit holding and in farm-related people. *Vet. Microbiol.* **2014**, *170*, 172–177. [CrossRef] [PubMed]
10. Agnoletti, F.; Brunetta, R.; Bano, L.; Drigo, I.; Mazzolini, E. Longitudinal study on antimicrobial consumption and resistance in rabbit farming. *Int. J. Antimicrob. Agents* **2018**, *51*, 197–205. [CrossRef] [PubMed]
11. Vancraeynest, D.; Haesebrouck, F.; Deplano, A.; Denis, O.; Godard, C.; Wildemauwe, C.; Hermans, K. International Dissemination of a High Virulence Rabbit *Staphylococcus aureus* Clone. *J. Vet. Med.* **2006**, *B53*, 418–422. [CrossRef] [PubMed]
12. Német, Z.; Albert, E.; Dán, Á.; Balka, G.; Szenes, Á.; Sipos, R.; Bódizs, S.; Biksi, I. Genomic Analysis of *Staphylococcus aureus* Strains Originating from Hungarian Rabbit Farms Reinforce the Clonal Origin of Various Virulence Types. *Animals* **2020**, *10*, 1128. [CrossRef] [PubMed]
13. Attili, A.R.; Nebbia, P.; Bellato, A.; Galosi, L.; Papeschi, C.; Rossi, G.; Linardi, M.; Fileni, E.; Cuteri, V.; Chiesa, F.; et al. The effect of age and sampling site on the outcome of *Staphylococcus aureus* infection in a rabbit (*Oryctolagus cuniculus*) farm in Italy. *Animals* **2020**, *10*, 774. [CrossRef] [PubMed]
14. Moreno-Grúa, E.; Pérez-Fuentes, S.; Muñoz-Silvestre, A.; Viana, D.; Fernández-Ros, A.B.; Sanz-Tejero, C.; Corpa, J.M.; Selva, L. Characterization of Livestock-Associated Methicillin-Resistant Staphylococcus aureus Isolates Obtained From Commercial Rabbitries Located in the Iberian Peninsula. *Front. Microbiol.* **2018**, *9*, 1812. [CrossRef] [PubMed]
15. Koreen, L.; Ramaswamy, S.V.; Graviss, E.A.; Naidich, S.; Musser, J.M.; Kreiswirth, B.N. *spa* Typing Method for Discriminating among *Staphylococcus aureus* Isolates: Implications for Use of a Single Marker To Detect Genetic Micro- and Macrovariation. *J. Clin. Microbiol.* **2004**, *42*, 792–799. [CrossRef] [PubMed]
16. Aminov, R.I.; Mackie, R.I. Evolution and ecology of antibiotic resistance genes. *FEMS Microbiol. Lett.* **2007**, *271*, 147–161. [CrossRef] [PubMed]
17. Summers, A.O. Generally overlooked fundamentals of bacterial genetics and ecology. *Clin. Infect. Dis.* **2002**, *1* (Suppl. 3), S85–S92. [CrossRef] [PubMed]

18. Clinical and Laboratory Standards Institute (CLSI). *M100 Performance Standards for Antimicrobial Susceptibility Testing*, 27th ed.; CLSI supplement M100S; Clinical and Laboratory Standards Institute: Wayne, PA, USA, 2017.
19. Clinical and Laboratory Standards Institute (CLSI). *VET08 Performance Standards for Antimicrobial Susceptibility Tests for Bacteria Isolated from Animals*, 4th ed.; Clinical and Laboratory Standards Institute: Wayne, PA, USA, 2018.
20. Magiorakos, A.P.; Srinivasan, A.; Carey, R.B.; Carmeli, Y.; Falagas, M.E.; Giske, C.G.; Harbarth, S.; Hindler, J.F.; Kahlmeter, G.; Olsson-Liljequist, B.; et al. Multidrug-resistant, extensively drug-resistant and pandrug-resistant bacteria: An international expert proposal for interim standard definitions for acquired resistance. *Clin. Microbiol. Infect.* **2012**, *18*, 268–281. [CrossRef] [PubMed]
21. Brown, M.B. Algorithm AS 116: The tetrachoric correlation and its asymptotic standard error. *Appl. Stat.* **1977**, *26*, 343–351. [CrossRef]
22. Afifi, A.A.; May, S.; Clark, V.A. *Practical Multivariate Analysis*, 5th ed.; CRC Press: Boca Raton, FL, USA, 2012; Chapters 14–16; pp. 369–432.
23. Ward, J.H., Jr. Hierarchical grouping to optimize an objective function. *J. Am. Stat. Assoc.* **1963**, *58*, 236–244. [CrossRef]

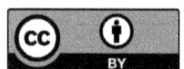

© 2020 by the authors. Licensee MDPI, Basel, Switzerland. This article is an open access article distributed under the terms and conditions of the Creative Commons Attribution (CC BY) license (http://creativecommons.org/licenses/by/4.0/).

MDPI
St. Alban-Anlage 66
4052 Basel
Switzerland
Tel. +41 61 683 77 34
Fax +41 61 302 89 18
www.mdpi.com

Antibiotics Editorial Office
E-mail: antibiotics@mdpi.com
www.mdpi.com/journal/antibiotics

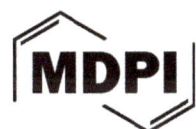

www.ingramcontent.com/pod-product-compliance
Lightning Source LLC
LaVergne TN
LVHW070634100526
838202LV00012B/801